Florence Kellogg
112 Allen
Lansing, Michigan

Urologic Nursing

Urologic Nursing

John G. Keuhnelian, M.D., F.A.C.S.

Clinical Assistant Professor of Surgery (Urology),
Cornell University Medical College;
Associate Attending Surgeon (Urology),
James Buchanan Brady Foundation of
The New York Hospital–Cornell Medical Center;
Associate Urologist, Lenox Hill Hospital

Virginia E. Sanders, M.N., M.A.

Assistant Professor of Nursing,
Cornell University–New York Hospital School of Nursing;
Formerly, Supervisor of Surgical Nursing (Urology),
The New York Hospital–Cornell Medical Center

The Macmillan Company

Collier-Macmillan Limited LONDON

This book is dedicated to

JACOB H. HEKIMIAN, M.D. (1889–1968),
whose example inspired more than one young man
to enter the medical profession

and

MARGARET SANDERS (1893–1963) and FRED SANDERS,
devoted parents

First Printing, 1970

Library of Congress catalog card number: 72-99024

THE MACMILLAN COMPANY
866 Third Avenue, New York, New York 10022

COLLIER-MACMILLAN CANADA, LTD., Toronto, Ontario

PRINTED IN THE UNITED STATES OF AMERICA

Preface

THIS textbook is designed as a primer of modern urologic nursing practice. It is divided into four sections. Unit I introduces the reader to the structure and function of the normal urinary tract and includes a discussion of the more common disorders and their treatment. The methods of urologic diagnosis are described in Unit II, with emphasis on the professional nurse's role in these studies. Unit III covers the more frequently performed urologic operations and stresses not only surgical techniques but also related preoperative and postoperative nursing care. The final section of the book, Unit IV, is concerned with the diagnosis and management of acute and chronic renal failure. The methods of dialysis are discussed, as are current problems in the area of renal transplantation. More detailed information on certain aspects of urologic nursing are included in the appendixes at the end of the text.

The techniques described are those employed in a large, active urology service, namely that of The New York Hospital–Cornell Medical Center. Although there are differences in technique and approach from hospital to hospital, the similarities are much greater than the disparities. Consequently, knowledge of the principles of, and rationale for, diagnosis and therapy, as outlined in this book, will permit the nurse to make the necessary adjustments quite easily.

This textbook can serve many purposes. By presenting principles in a concise, readable form, the nursing student should rapidly comprehend what the urologist is attempting to accomplish and how he does so. The more detailed application of these principles informs the professional nurse of diagnostic techniques and postoperative management, particularly in relation to catheter drainages. Considerable space is devoted to urinary collection systems, especially those for ileal conduit urinary diversion, a procedure that is being performed with increasing frequency. The management of these diversion patients is both an art and a science.

Therefore, detailed information is provided regarding the types of appliances available as well as their successful fitting, application, and care. Such information, which is very important for the complete rehabilitation of these patients, is useful to the nurse in the hospital setting as well as to the office nurse and the visiting nurse. The urologic office nurse will find the information in the diagnostic section especially useful, particularly in relation to the care and sterilization of instruments and catheters. Finally, the general surgical nurse should be able to adapt readily to urologic surgery with the information provided in Unit III. Suitable review questions are provided at the end of each chapter, and a list of references appears at the end of each unit.

The authors wish to express their gratitude to the many nurses on the staff of The New York Hospital–Cornell Medical Center, and most particularly Miss Virginia C. Dericks, clinical nursing specialist for ostomy care, who critically reviewed the manuscript and made constructive suggestions for the various units. The efforts of our illustrators—Helen Speiden, Caspar Henselmann, and William Thackeray—are appreciated. Dr. Victor F. Marshall, professor of surgery (urology), Cornell University Medical College, and attending surgeon-in-charge, James Buchanan Brady Foundation of The New York Hospital, was constantly available for advice and direction. Mr. Milton Zisowitz provided numerous useful editorial comments. The writers also appreciate the patient encouragement of Miss Joan C. Zulch, medical editor of The Macmillan Company. Last, but not least, they thank Mrs. Lynda Blount Nickelsen for the many hours spent in carefully typing and retyping the manuscript.

J. G. K.
V. E. S.

Contents

UNIT I
Pathophysiologic Considerations

CHAPTER 1
Introduction

UROLOGY is the study of the urinary tract in men and women, as well as the closely associated male genital tract. The urologist is a surgical specialist who studies and treats genitourinary disorders.

Urinary tract problems are among the earliest recorded diseases in man. The Egyptian physician Imhotep wrote a discourse on urinary infection, cystitis, and stone nearly five thousand years ago. Several mummies of that era have been discovered with renal and vesical calculi. Twenty-five centuries later, Hippocrates, the father of medicine, wrote about urinary calculi.

Circumcision is one of the earliest operations known to man. Perineal lithotomy for removal of bladder calculi, a fairly common problem, was one of the most frequently performed operations in medieval times. The "lithotomists" were usually barber-surgeons, whose operations would be followed by a high morbidity and mortality rate. Consequently, the surgeons would frequently operate at night and disappear by the following morning.

Many famous people in history have had their share of urologic difficulties. A historic autopsy was that of Pope Innocent XI, who in 1689 died with bilateral staghorn calculi and severely damaged kidneys. The famous composer Mozart died of chronic pyelonephritis. Dr. Samuel Johnson, the English critic and poet immortalized by Boswell, had polycystic kidney disease. Napoleon Bonaparte and Napoleon the Third had symptomatic bladder stones; the latter had such severe disability during the Battle of Sedan in the Franco-Prussian War that he had to be catheterized frequently and died as a result of his urinary problem less than one year later. Sir Arthur Sullivan of Gilbert and Sullivan fame had such severe attacks of pain from his bladder stones that he had to be carried off the podium during a performance on several occasions. Benjamin Franklin and his brother were plagued by bladder calculi, probably secondary to prostate trouble. Mr. Franklin's ingenuity arose to the occasion and included among his many accomplishments was the development of a flexible urethral catheter. The urologic problems of many contemporary famous people have become common knowledge to the average layman and are frequently described in minute detail by the press.

The connotation of venery has largely left the layman's concept of urologic practice, particularly following the advent of sulfa drugs, penicillin, and other antibiotics. Although venereal disease is still distressingly common, urology is now recognized as an expandingly broadened surgical specialty. The modern urologist possesses an impressive and efficient armamentarium of instruments: endoscopic equipment, catheters, and sounds. Radiographic techniques to delineate the urinary tract often reveal the finest anatomic details in the living patient. Refined microscopic techniques can identify cancer cells in the urine before the cancer is clinically evident. Improved chemical techniques can critically evaluate renal function and decompensation.

The ultimate effect of these advances has been a vast improvement in not only the diagnosis but also the treatment of urologic disorders even while the intricacies and magnitude of methods have been greatly enlarged. This improvement reflects better pre- and postoperative evaluation of the patient, safer anesthesia, careful surgical technique, improved resident training, and the judicious use of antibiotics and blood transfusions. For example, the mortality after prostatectomy at The New York Hospital–Cornell Medical Center during the past decade has been less than 1 per cent. This is in sharp contrast to figures of 10 per cent and higher only thirty years ago. These are respectable statistics when one considers the advanced age of many of these patients and the frequent association of serious nonurologic ailments.

In the future, urologic problems will play an expanding role in the panorama of medical ills. With an aging population, surgical disorders of the prostate will assume greater significance. Despite impressive strides in the treatment of urinary tract cancer, particularly cancer of the prostate, there is still much to be learned and done. Increased awareness of the congenital anomalies of the urinary tract and their treatment has completely changed and broadened the scope of pediatric urology. Children doomed to an early death from renal failure are being actively treated and have prospects of living to a ripe old age The number of patients with idiopathic pyelonephritis is shrinking as correctable deformities are being recognized. During the past twenty years the advances in pediatric urology have been truly amazing, and there is much interest in this branch of urology throughout the world. Increasing information is being accumulated in the recognition and treatment of hypertension secondary to abnormalities of the renal vasculature and their correction. Finally, increasing success in renal transplantation has spurred further activity in this area. The field of urology has come a long way from the days of the lithotomists and the venereologists.*

* References for Chapters 1–7 are listed at the end of Unit I (pages 56–57).

CHAPTER 2

Correlative Anatomy of the Urinary Tract

THE urinary tract consists of the kidneys, which constantly manufacture urine, and a collecting system consisting of various tubes and reservoirs necessary to carry it outside the body. The renal pelves and the ureters transport urine to the bladder, which functions as a reservoir, gradually filling until its capacity is reached. The bladder then discharges its contents to the outside through the urethra. Unlike the kidneys, which are vital organs, the bladder and urethra are not necessary for life, but loss of their functions, as occurs in the various forms of incontinence, can make a patient quite miserable.

The male genital tract is intimately associated with the urinary tract and consists of a major manufacturing source, the testis, and a drainage and reservoir system consisting of the epididymis, vas deferens, seminal vesicle, and prostate. The male urethra serves as the final conduit for the seminal fluid as well as for the urine.

Kidneys

The kidneys are paired, bean-shaped, retroperitoneal structures located below the diaphragm on either side (Fig. 2-1). They are usually 12 cm long. Because the liver presses down on the right kidney, it is usually lower than the left. Besides being covered with a tough fibrous capsule, the kidneys are surrounded by an insulation of perirenal fat. They are further protected by the abdominal contents in front and by the ribs and the thick musculature alongside the spinal column in back. Consequently, injury to a normal kidney requires either forceful blunt trauma or direct penetration, as with a knife or bullet.

The gross structure of the kidney can be divided into the solid *parenchyma* (the urine-producing part) and the *pelvis*, which is the beginning of the urinary transporting system (Fig. 2-2). Although the kidneys represent less than 1 per cent of the total body weight, they perform a truly massive amount of work. Over 50 gallons of blood plasma are filtered daily through the kidneys; in other words, the entire circulating volume of blood plasma is filtered every 30 minutes.

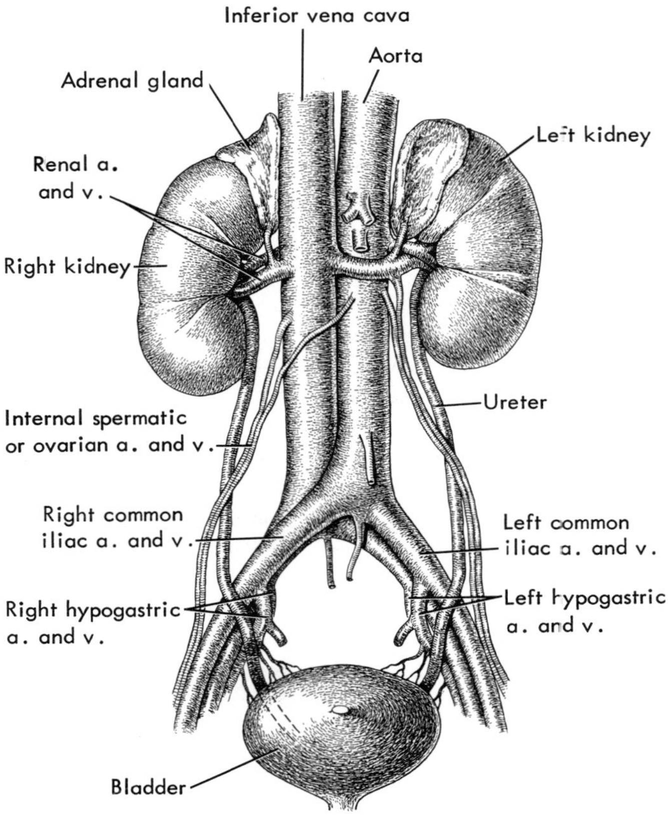

FIGURE 2-1. Gross anatomy of the kidneys, ureters, and bladder.

The kidneys have a threefold function. First, they excrete excess water and the nitrogenous waste products of protein metabolism, chiefly as urea, creatinine, and uric acid. Second, they regulate to a major degree the acid-base balance and the volume and electrolyte concentration of the plasma. Third, they have endocrine functions. Reductions in renal blood flow or arterial pressure may cause the release of an enzyme, renin. This enzyme, in turn, reacts with a circulating substrate of hepatic origin to produce angiotensin, a powerful compound that raises blood pressure. The kidneys also influence the adrenal glands in the production of aldosterone, a hormone that acts on the renal tubules in regulating sodium and water excretion. Another poorly understood renal substance is erythropoietin, which promotes red blood cell production. Indeed, all the functional aspects of the kidney are probably still unknown.

The functioning unit of the renal parenchyma is the *nephron*, and

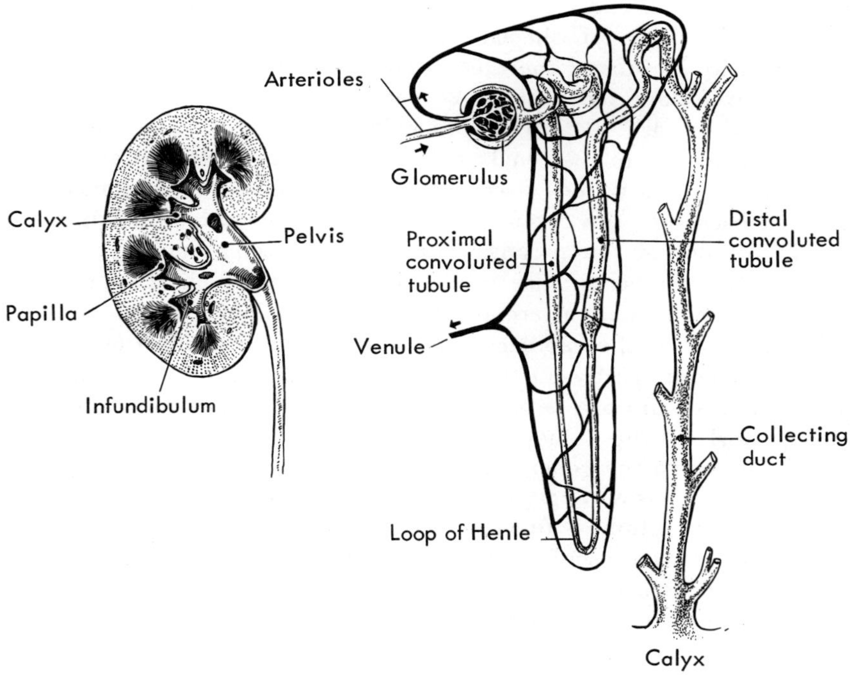

FIGURE 2-2. Gross structure of the kidney and a nephron unit.

each kidney contains one to one and a quarter million of these. The nephron is subdivided into the *glomerulus*, where plasma is filtered, and the *tubules*, where this filtrate is resorbed and actively concentrated. The majority of the glomeruli are located in the outer zone of parenchyma known as the *cortex*, and the tubules are mostly in the inner zone known as the *medulla*.

The glomerulus is essentially a tortuous capillary network which hangs in a space communicating with the inside (lumen) of the tubule. That portion of the renal arterial blood entering the *afferent arteriole* to the glomerulus is filtered of many constituents except for protein molecules and cells. This filtered blood leaves the glomerulus via the *efferent arteriole* to enter a second capillary network which surrounds the tubules in the medulla. The blood then enters the venous system. Approximately 120 to 130 ml of plasma are filtered every minute, and this is known as the normal glomerular filtration rate. The percentage of the plasma entering the kidney which is filtered is normally about 20 per cent and is known as the filtration fraction. The force for filtration is mainly provided by the incoming arterial pressure.

The tubular portion of the nephron leaving the glomerulus is known as the *proximal convoluted tubule*, which dips into the medulla. At the bottom of this dip is a U-shaped segment, the *loop of Henle*, which then connects with the *distal convoluted tubule*. Many such tubules join to form the *collecting ducts*. About 20 such ducts enter one renal *papilla*, of which there are 10 to 16 in each kidney. The papillae empty the completed urine into the renal pelvis. As the glomerular filtrate travels down the tubule, water, electrolytes, urea, and other substances are resorbed back into the circulation. As noted previously, the unfiltered protein content of the plasma, which exerts strong osmotic pressure, circulates in the peritubular capillaries, along with blood cells. Some substances, such as urea, are passively resorbed owing to this osmotic gradient between the capillary fluid and the fluid inside the tubules. Ionic shifts occur partly on this basis as well. Other substances such as glucose and sodium are resorbed by an active transport mechanism requiring work by the kidney. The degree of acidity or alkalinity of the blood returned to the general circulation is normally maintained within an amazingly narrow range. Importantly involved in this regulation and that of the fluid volume is an enzyme, carbonic anhydrase. Certain diuretics used clinically are carbonic anhydrase inhibitors. There is also a tubular excretory function. Compounds such as penicillin, para-aminohippurate, and phenolphthalein are excreted by the proximal tubule. Excretion of the last two substances is used to measure tubular function clinically. The kidney selectively filters, resorbs, and concentrates this 50 gallons of plasma daily to produce a quart or so of urine!

When a patient is in renal failure (uremia), poisonous wastes can be removed by various artificial methods—peritoneal dialysis or hemodialysis in particular. Electrolyte and fluid imbalances can be reduced by additions and subtractions, by infusions and ionic exchange resins, for example. If good renal function cannot return, a properly functioning transplanted kidney will usually improve the patient still more—for reasons not precisely defined.

The concentration or dilution of urine is a complicated process. Most of the filtered water is passively resorbed in the proximal tubule secondary to osmotic effects, but up to 20 per cent is resorbed in the distal tubule and collecting ducts under the action of a hormone of posterior pituitary origin, known as vasopressin (Pitressin) or the antidiuretic hormone. Hypertonic urine (urine more concentrated than the surrounding kidney tissue pulp and capillaries) is a result of the countercurrent multiplier mechanism; briefly stated, as the sodium concentration gradually rises in the medullary interstitium, farther along the tubule increasing amounts of water are resorbed until hypertonic urine is formed.

The urinary collecting system begins at the renal pelvis, a cup- or funnel-shaped structure with a normal capacity of 3 to 5 ml. The indentations of the peripheral pelvis by the papillae are known as the *calyces* (Greek for cups). Groups of calyces connect to the main pelvis itself by somewhat narrow common necks known as *infundibula*. The urine is transported by peristalsis out of the pelvis down another tubular structure, the ureter, to the bladder until voiding, or micturition, occurs. The normal *ureter*, which is about 25 cm long, is of uniform caliber throughout except for three relatively narrow places: its beginning (the ureteropelvic junction), its ending (the ureterovesical junction), and its crossing of the bifurcation of the common iliac arteries on either side. Ureteral peristalsis seems to be independent of an extrinsic nerve supply in that the determining stimulus to peristalsis is normally the distention from the accumulating urine.

Bladder

The urinary bladder is a marvelous contractile reservoir which empties abruptly at socially appropriate intervals. Under normal conditions it can readily hold up to 200 ml of fluid at essentially a constant pressure—so that it is distinctly different from a rubber balloon, for example. There is no significant resorption of water or electrolytes by the normal bladder. The wall of the bladder is constructed of three interwoven layers of smooth muscle known as the detrusor. These layers insert into the outlet, or neck, of the bladder. The concentration of fibers at the neck is known as the internal sphincter. Although urine under mild to moderate pressure is normally held at this level, a tightly closing bladder neck is not absolutely necessary for adequate urinary control. This neck is often divided or weakened by such procedures as prostatectomy or plastic surgery on the vesical neck without compromising continence. The lining, or mucous membrane, of the bladder is composed of transitional epithelium, a tissue that is unique to the urinary collecting system. For this reason it is also known as "urothelium." This lining has such great elasticity that it can vary from eight or ten cell layers in the contracted bladder to one of only two or three cells in thickness as the organ expands. Transitional epithelium lines the entire urinary collecting system from the renal pelves to at least the midprostatic urethra.

Lying on and attached to the floor of the bladder at its neck to the muscle layers previously mentioned is a thin triangle of muscle which is relatively immobile. This *trigone* normally measures an inch on either side. The apex is at the bladder outlet, and the ureteral orifices take up the remaining two angles. The side of the triangle between the orifices is known as the interureteric ridge.

The ureters enter the bladder not at right angles but obliquely through the muscle and the submucosa. This obliquity is an essential feature of the ureterovesical junction which prevents fluid from running back up the ureters. By means of the pressure built up by the ureteral peristaltic wave, urine descends into the bladder freely through this passive valve via the tunnel in the bladder wall. As the bladder contracts during the act of voiding, the walls of the tunnel collapse so that urine is expelled only through the vesical outlet. Regurgitation of urine back up the ureter is abnormal and is known as *vesicoureteral reflux.* Normally the ratio of the length of the intramural ureter to the diameter of the ureteral orifice must be at least 5:1 so that reflux will not occur.

In contrast to the function of the kidneys and ureters, retention in the bladder and micturition normally are under obvious nervous control and even influenced by the will. On the other hand, one cannot will or command the smooth muscle of the bladder to relax or contract without any other action elsewhere. Nor is any other mass of smooth muscle so controlled. The details of the sequence of events in voluntary micturition are surprisingly not well defined—yet this apparently simple act is performed millions of times each day! The effect of the will can be postulated as measured through the striated muscles of the pelvic outlet. The bladder is sensitive to distention, pain, and temperature; and these stimuli are transmitted via the pelvic parasympathetic nerves to the second, third, and fourth sacral roots in the spinal cord. It is generally believed that there are also stimuli transmitted out from the cord to the bladder via the parasympathetics. The sympathetic nerves have little to do with sensory function, being concerned mainly with sexual and vascular actions. Some at least low level of conscious recognition is part of urinary control. Otherwise the uninhibited voidings of the infant or the senile would result. Certainly there are important coordinating nervous connections within the cord, and these are influenced from still higher levels.

Certain facts seem established. As urine accumulates in the bladder, the smooth muscle accommodates, so that the intravesical pressure rises only slightly up to some general volume called the capacity, about 250 to 400 ml in the normal moderately hydrated adult. Then the previously faint rhythmic activity of the smooth muscle builds up toward a large massive contraction. If the striated perineal muscles, including the striated external sphincter, are contracted voluntarily, the vesical smooth muscle accommodates again to further increase in volume at a higher pressure and over a shorter range. Finally the perineal muscles relax, a little urine runs down into the posterior urethra, and this small but abrupt pressure drop sets off the already impending large vesical contraction and the person voids. At the conclusion of this incompletely understood phenomenon the perineal muscles tighten, the vesical muscle reaches its basic tone with the internal sphincter closed, and urine accumulation begins again.

Urethra

The sole function of the female urethra is to serve as the conduit for urine from the bladder to the outside (Fig. 2-3). This tube is only 3.5 cm long. It curves beneath the symphysis pubis to open below the clitoris just superior to the vagina. Proximally it is lined by transitional epithelium, but distally the lining changes to a squamous type. Many periurethral glands empty into its lumen, especially distally. These can be foci for

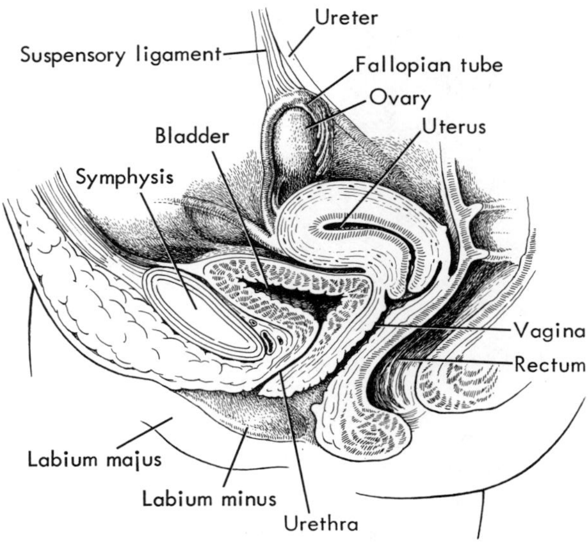

FIGURE 2-3. The female reproductive system and lower urinary tract.

chronic infection. Surrounding the urethra are smooth and striated muscle fibers which undoubtedly are important for urinary control, but there is no concentration of striated muscle comparable to the male external urinary sphincter.

The male urethra is much longer, mostly because of the length of the penis which it traverses (Fig. 2-4). It can be divided into an anterior and posterior portion, the point of division being the external urinary sphincter and urogenital diaphragm. The anterior urethra can be further subdivided into the *fossa navicularis* (the dilated area through the glans penis), the *pendulous urethra* (which traverses the remainder of the penis), and the *bulbous urethra* (another dilated portion which travels beneath the symphysis pubis to the urogenital diaphragm). The *posterior urethra* includes the *membranous urethra* (a 2-cm area that goes through the

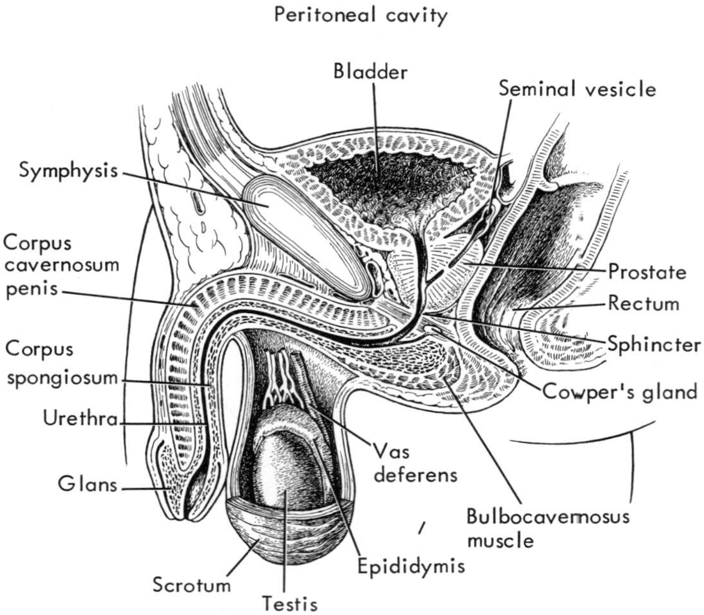

FIGURE 2-4. The male reproductive system and lower urinary tract.

diaphragm from the external sphincter to the apex of the prostate) and the *prostatic urethra* (that portion which traverses the length of the prostate). Two small glands, *Cowper's glands*, empty into the membranous urethra, and the anterior urethra is surrounded by numerous mucous secreting glands, the *glands of Littré*.

Male Reproductive System

The function of the male reproductive system is the manufacture of living spermatozoa and their discharge to the outside in such condition as to allow impregnation of the female ovum. Although only a single sperm cell is necessary for conception, at least 100 million are produced daily by the average adult male. This superabundance and inefficiency of nature is astounding!

Spermatozoa are produced by the seminiferous tubules of the *testes*, paired structures 4 cm in length which occupy a bilocular skin pouch, the *scrotum*. Thus the testes are in an exposed exterior position. The seminiferous tubules are very sensitive to changes in blood supply and temperature. If the testes are completely deprived of arterial blood for a period ranging from four to ten hours, there will be irreversible damage to spermatogenesis. Sperm production is markedly curtailed at normal body temperature, and the slightly cooler conditions afforded by the exterior position of the scrotum are necessary for maximum production. The testes also have an endocrine function. The interstitial cells, or Leydig cells, are exceedingly hardy, in contrast to the seminiferous tubules. They elaborate most of the androgenic hormones which are responsible for the secondary sexual characteristics of masculinity, such as the masculine body build, growth and distribution of facial, axillary and pubic hair, and development of the adult penis.

The spermatozoa travel through gradually enlarging channels in the comma-shaped *epididymis*, located behind the testis. These channels terminate in the *vas deferens*, a tubular structure only about 4 mm in diameter which begins at the bottom, or tail, of the epididymis. The vas deferens travels up the scrotum into the inguinal canal to the internal inguinal ring. Here it turns backward and downward to pass over the ureter and end in the ampulla behind the bladder. The *seminal vesicle* joins it to form the *ejaculatory duct*, which finally empties into the prostatic urethra. The seminal vesicles are paired, ear-shaped structures situated under and behind the bladder. They do not store spermatozoa, as was once thought, but do produce the protein and fructose necessary for nutrition of these cells. Their contents are discharged with the sperm and prostatic fluid at the time of ejaculation.

The *prostate gland* is located just distal to the bladder outlet. Through it courses the most proximal portion of the urethra. It daily produces 3 to 5 ml of a milky fluid, which is also nutritional to the sperm. It contains large quantities of an enzyme, acid phosphatase, the function of which is unknown. Finally it contains another enzyme, fibrinolysin, which is capable of dissolving clotted fibrin. Seminal fluid is a viscous material which, if allowed to stand in a test tube, liquefies. This liquefaction is presumedly from the fibrinolysin activity.

The *penis* is a skin appendage which can be transformed from a state of flaccidity to one of firm rigidity permitting introduction into the vagina. This characteristic (shared to a lesser degree by other erectile tissue, such as that of the clitoris or the nipples) is due to the capacity of erectile tissue, which consists of large vascular spaces. In some lower mammals, the penis contains a bony or cartilaginous strip, but the human organ does not. The two corpora cavernosa, which are bound by a tough fascial layer, contain most of this erectile tissue. Surrounding the urethra is some additional tissue of this type, the corpus spongiosum urethrae. Tight filling of these blood spaces produces the erection. The mechanism is complex in its details and is influenced by sympathetic nervous impulses as well as somatic ones. The impetus for this phenomenon is largely psychogenic. Aided and abetted by frictional stimuli, a complex of reflexes somewhat suddenly produces ejaculation and orgasm.

Ejaculation is the external discharge of the seminal fluid mixture derived from secretions of the testes, prostate, and seminal vesicles. Orgasm refers to the pleasurable erotic sensation emanating from the genital area, ordinarily accompanied by the rhythmical contractions of the perineal muscles which supply the force for ejaculation. Except that ejaculation does not occur in the female individual nor in the immature male, the process of orgasm is quite similar in both sexes.

REVIEW QUESTIONS

1. Describe the gross anatomy of the upper urinary tract.
2. Discuss three known functions of the kidneys.
3. Explain the specific functions of the glomerulus and the tubule in urine formation. Discuss the intrarenal circulation as it is related to these functions.
4. Describe the location and function of the trigone of the bladder.
5. Discuss the mechanism of micturition.
6. Define erection, ejaculation, and orgasm, and explain the mechanism of each.
7. Describe the route of a sperm cell from spermatogenesis to ejaculation and the function of the organs involved.

CHAPTER 3

Obstruction and Infection

OBSTRUCTIONS and infections are the most common causes of damage to the urinary tract. Although one can occur without the other, the combination is as natural as the chicken and the egg. Most naturally occurring obstructions are not complete. They may be congenital, such as various types of intrinsic narrowings and valve-like flaps, or they may be acquired. Common acquired obstructions are urinary tract calculi, neoplasia, and prostatic enlargement. With obstruction there is stagnation of urine. The combination of this stagnation with body warmth and the nutritious nitrogenous elements in urine establishes all the criteria for an excellent bacterial culture medium. An infection that gains a foothold in an obstructed urinary tract is usually difficult to eradicate permanently unless the obstruction is relieved.

Effects of Obstruction

The effects of obstruction on an infection have been demonstrated experimentally in numerous ways. Cox and Hinman used a urethral catheter to insert large numbers of pathogenic bacteria into the bladders of *normal* male volunteers. Within six to nine hours, the number of bacteria in the urine diminished markedly, and by 72 hours the bacteria had disappeared completely. Attempts to produce urinary tract infections with nonspecific bacteria in experimental animals have been unsuccessful unless other factors, usually obstructive in nature, have been introduced. These factors have included ureteral ligation, insertion of a foreign body into the bladder, and forceful massage of a kidney at the time of bacterial inoculation.

Let us review the mechanical effects of obstruction on the urinary tract. When there is obstruction to the outflow of a kidney, production of urine continues even when the obstruction is complete. Therefore, the blockage will cause an increase in the intrapelvic pressure. As a result of the continued production of urine with the increase in pelvic pressure, the renal pelvis and kidney will become dilated. The back pressure on the renal parenchyma gradually compresses the smaller intrarenal blood vessels. As more and more nephrons thus become ischemic, urine production will decrease, and as a result renal function will diminish. The amount of recovery after release of the obstruction will depend on the number of nephrons totally destroyed as compared to the number that are only partially disabled and have the ability to recover. The dilated obstructed kidney under these conditions is known as a *hydronephrotic* kidney.

Despite the continued production of urine by the hydronephrotic kidney, the accumulated volume rarely exceeds 3000 ml. In the presence of obstruction, there is a dynamic state of constant reabsorption of the urine produced by the obstructed kidney through the dilated tubules, venules, lymphatics, and directly from the interstitium of the kidney itself. Furthermore, the accumulated urine compresses the renal parenchyma and the internal vasculature so that the blood flow is diminished and less urine is produced. If an obstruction anywhere in the urinary tract below the level of the kidneys themselves is sufficiently prolonged and severe, it will gradually cause hydronephrosis. This may take place over a period of years with relatively mild obstructions or can occur within a matter of an hour or two, as with a calculus that suddenly occludes a ureter. Obstruction of the ureters will be manifested by dilatation proximal to the point of blockage. As the dilatation continues, the ureter will often become elongated and tortuous secondary to work hypertrophy of its musculature. These changes are known as *hydroureter*.

Obstruction to the bladder from its outlet distally produces profound changes in its appearance and function. Common obstructions are benign and cancerous enlargements of the prostate gland. Because of the increased effort necessary for micturition, the bladder musculature becomes hypertrophied and thickened. These changes are not unlike those seen in weightlifters with bulging muscles. If the bladder can empty itself despite the obstruction, it is compensated. As described in the previous chapter, the detrusor (the smooth muscle of the bladder wall) consists of an interlacing network of fibers. As these fibers hypertrophy, the intervening amuscular areas appear pitted owing to the prominence of the muscle bands. The resulting honeycombed appearance of the bladder wall is known as trabeculation. With further hypertrophy, however, the weak areas in the wall become more pitted and are known as cellules. Finally, the cellules can become actual bulges, or herniations, of the mucosa through the wall, not unlike the soft areas in an old rubber inner tube. These large bulges, or herniations, are known as diverticula. After micturition the normal bladder should have emptied itself, or at most contain a few milliliters. Under normal conditions, residual urine in the bladder of less than 15 to 20 ml is not considered too significant. However, when the leftover is 60 ml or greater, the bladder is said to be decompensating. In general, the likelihood of severe damage to the upper urinary tract increases with the volume of residual urine.

The back pressure established by prolonged bladder decompensation will gradually be transmitted to the upper urinary tract, and hydronephrosis will follow. If infection is superimposed on this situation, the damage can be truly severe. Bladder decompensation in its most complete form will be manifested by total urinary retention, so that the patient cannot void at all or at most can manage to release a few drops of urine at distressingly frequent intervals. This condition must be differentiated quickly from *anuria*, which is the cessation of urine production, not retention of that produced. Usually the differentiation is not difficult, but much needed information can be easily obtained in such a situation by simple urethral catheterization. Some of the commoner urinary obstructions are diagrammatically represented in Figure 3-1. The progressive damage from urinary obstructions is outlined in Figure 3-2.

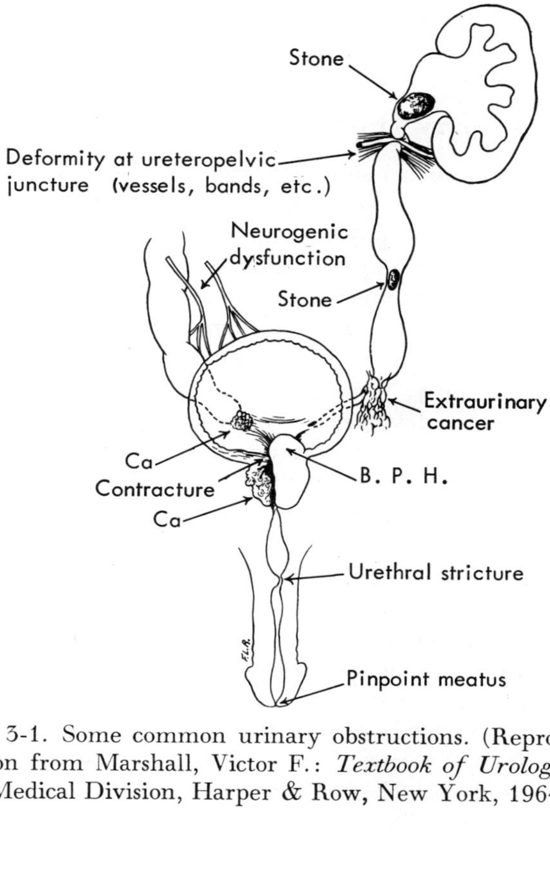

FIGURE 3-1. Some common urinary obstructions. (Reproduced by permission from Marshall, Victor F.: *Textbook of Urology*, 2nd ed. Hoeber Medical Division, Harper & Row, New York, 1964.)

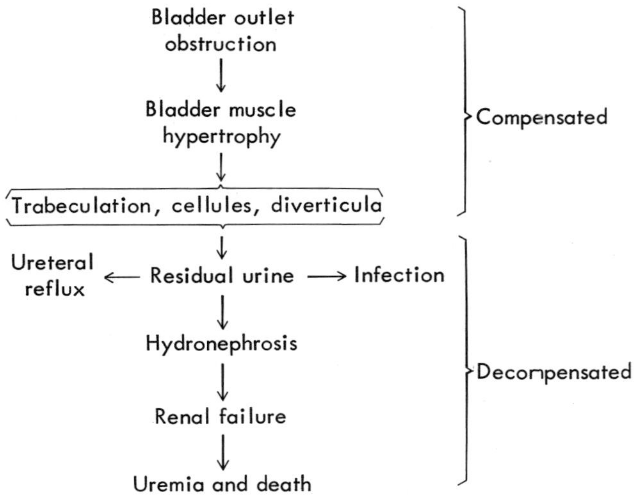

FIGURE 3-2. A diagrammatic representation of the consequences of urinary obstruction.

Nonspecific Urinary Tract Infections

Infections within the urinary tract can be caused by either specific or nonspecific organisms. Specific organisms can infect an anatomically normal urinary tract and produce specific diseases. Common invaders include virulent strains of *Staphylococcus aureus*, tubercle bacilli, and the various bacteria, viruses, and parasites that cause venereal diseases. Nonspecific organisms, on the other hand, nearly always require an anatomic abnormality of the urinary tract on which to obtain a foothold. As mentioned previously, it is difficult to produce an infection in an experimental animal unless there is an associated obstruction, or unless specific pathogens are used. Studies on autopsied patients confirm these laboratory findings. Pyelonephritis, or kidney infection, with nonspecific organisms is seldom found in a structurally and functionally normal urinary tract.

The usual nonspecific organisms are a group of gram-negative bacteria. The term *gram negative* refers to the staining characteristics with the gram stain, commonly used to identify bacteria. Organisms in this group are usually members of the *Proteus* species, the *Klebsiella* (*Aerobacter*) group, the *Pseudomonas* species, or *Escherichia coli*. They may appear as a pure culture of one group or often as a zoolike mixture with different bacteria predominating at various times. Other organisms not as commonly seen include the enterococci (*Streptococcus faecalis*).

The suffix *-itis* is usually added to the name of the organ involved in describing infections, but by definition, and despite common usage, this suffix usually describes inflammation rather than bacterial infection itself. An infection of the kidney is known as *pyelonephritis*, which implies inflammation of both the renal parenchyma and the collecting system. A *pyelitis*, or involvement of the renal pelvis *alone*, is extremely rare. Inflammation of the bladder is known as *cystitis* and that of the testis, *orchitis*. In the latter instance there in usually concomitant involvement of the epididymis, so that the term *epididymoorchitis* is more accurate. Involvements of the ureter and urethra are called *ureteritis* and *urethritis*, respectively, and that of the prostate, *prostatitis*. Involvement of the glans penis is known as *balanitis*.

Treatment of Infection

The first step in treating a urinary tract infection is to make an accurate diagnosis. The clinician is guided by the history, signs and symptoms, and the findings of pus cells and bacteria in the urine. It is pertinent to note that both cells and bacteria do not have to be present simultaneously with infection. Using the numerous diagnostic techniques available to him, the urologist must rule out obstructive uropathy and congenital malformations. Such a search is strongly indicated, since obstructions are so frequently encountered. An unrecognized obstruction may be the stumbling block to successful therapy.

It is usually necessary to launch a specific attack on the invading organism in the form of adequate antibacterial therapy. Such therapy should be based on the bacteriologic identification of the organism and determination of its in vitro sensitivity to the available antibacterial agents. These sensitivity studies are not foolproof but act only as a guide, since what may be effective in the laboratory is not necessarily so in the patient and vice versa.

The antibacterial agents may be divided into chemotherapeutic agents and the antibiotics. Chemotherapeutic agents are inorganic chemical compounds that can either slow bacterial multiplication (bacteriostatic agents) so that the natural defense mechanisms of the body can destroy the invader, or can actually kill bacteria by themselves (bactericidal agents). Antibiotics have similar antibacterial effects but are organic substances produced by living organisms, usually various fungi.

Control of the urinary acidity may aid in the treatment of infections, particularly chronic ones. Many of the gram-negative bacteria grow luxuriantly under alkaline conditions but fare less well in an acid medium. Consequently a change in the pH of the urine toward the acid side might be expected to discourage the growth of some of these bacteria when they are the cause of infection. Efforts to acidify urine in the presence of bacteria such as *Proteus* are very difficult and usually not too rewarding. These include the acid-ash diet, oral administration of ammonium chloride, large volumes of cranberry juice, and so forth. Besides being relatively ineffectual, these measures must be used with care if the patient has poor renal function and is already in a state of mild acidosis which may become worse with this treatment.

METHENAMINE AND MANDELIC ACID. Prior to the discovery of the present antibacterial drugs, the main available compounds were methenamine and mandelic acid, which are marketed in a combined form as methenamine mandelate (Mandelamine). Methenamine is a urinary antiseptic in use since 1894. Its action is to release formaldehyde and ammonia in acidic solutions. The formaldehyde further dissociates to formic acid, which is bactericidal to many gram-negative organisms, particularly *E. coli*. Its clinical usefulness is limited, but it does have the advantage of excretion by the kidneys, relatively few side reactions, and a minimal degree of development of bacterial resistance. Since one disadvantage is the rapid excretion of the drug, it has recently been marketed as methenamine hippurate, a form that slowly dissociates to hippuric acid and methenamine in the urine, the latter further breaking down as previously described.

Mandelic acid also has a mild bactericidal effect and is relatively nontoxic. It is most active in acid urine and, since it is an acid, does tend to lower the urinary pH. Thus in combination with methenamine the likelihood of dissociation of the latter drug is greater. Regardless, for practical application, this combination is best used for long-term therapy and has been in large part supplanted by newer medications in acute and severe urinary tract infections.

SULFONAMIDES. Sulfonamides are a group of drugs that act bacteriostatically by blocking an enzyme system necessary for bacterial growth. They are more effective in alkaline urine. The various sulfa drugs vary considerably in their absorbability from the intestinal tract and their solubility in the urine. The earlier sulfonamides were frequently very toxic owing both to drug idiosyncrasy and to precipitation within the renal tubules, the latter occasionally causing anuria. Consequently it was accepted practice in the past to prescribe alkalinizing agents with these drugs to increase their solubility. The sulfa drugs used presently for urinary infections are quite soluble and safe compared to their predecessors. Commonly employed examples are sulfisoxazole (Gantrisin), sulfamethoxazole (Gantanol), and sulfamethizole (Thiosulfil). There will be occasional instances of drug eruption or agranulocytosis with the modern sulfas but far less frequently than in the past. These drugs are usually administered orally, although some are available for intravenous use.

NITROFURANTOIN (FURADANTIN). This bactericidal chemotherapeutic agent acts locally within the urinary tract. It is rapidly absorbed from the intestinal tract. It does not attain significant tissue levels but is excreted promptly by both the renal glomeruli and tubules, resulting in a high urinary concentration. It is effective against many gram-positive and -negative organisms. Like the sulfonamides, it is particularly useful in long-term therapy. Gastrointestinal upsets with this drug are common, and toxic effects of various types are known but are not seen too frequently. The drug is usually given as an oral medication, although an intravenous form is available. Because of the high percentage of gastric irritability, it is best to take the medication with meals and with some food at bedtime. A newly marketed macrocrystal (Macrodantin) form is better tolerated.

NALIDIXIC ACID (NEGGRAM). This oral bacteriostatic agent, like nitrofurantoin, is primarily excreted in the urine. As its trade name implies, it is effective against many gram-negative organisms except for the *Pseudomonas* group. It is particularly effective against *Proteus* but often no more than other antibacterials. It has the disadvantage that bacteria, if not very sensitive to the drug, will rapidly become resistant to it. It appears to be fairly safe but there are occasional instances of nausea and vomiting and a peculiar ocular reaction consisting of sensitivity to light, blurring of vision, and the appearance of colored halos around objects.

ANTIBIOTICS. The advent of the antibiotics has made a substantial difference in the treatment of urinary tract infections, particularly in the acute and severe ones. *Penicillin*, the earliest available antibiotic, is still very effective. It remains the drug of choice for the treatment of syphilis and gonorrhea. With severe *Proteus* infection, especially when accompanied by bacteremia, it is probably the best available drug. To be effective it should be given in large dosages intravenously in the range of 10,000,000 to 20,000,000 units daily. Although sensitivity may appear with any of these drugs, a history of a reaction particularly to penicillin cannot be regarded too lightly. Before any of these drugs are administered, the patient is asked if he has ever received them and particularly if there were any untoward reactions. It is good practice for the nurse in her initial interview with the patient routinely to ask him if he knows of an allergy to *any* medication. In a desperate situation, where no other antibiotic will be satisfactory, penicillin can be given to a hypersensitive patient by a careful, rapid desensitization technique. This is risky, however, and must be supervised by a physician with considerable experience with this method. Penicillin is effective against staphylococci, but in recent years resistant strains have appeared. This resistance has developed from the organism's ability to produce penicillinase, an enzyme that deactivates penicillin. Recently developed synthetic penicillins—methicillin, oxacillin, and nafcillin—are effective against most such strains, but their overall effectiveness is less than that of penicillin itself. A newly introduced oral penicillin, *ampicillin*, has a wider spectrum for gram-negative bacteria. It can also be administered intravenously and intramuscularly. Penicillin is bacteriostatic and is available in oral, aqueous, and long-acting parenteral forms.

Streptomycin is a bactericidal drug effective against many gram-negative organisms. It must be administered by intramuscular injection and is excreted largely in the urine. Toxic effects include damage to the eighth cranial nerve with hearing loss and, in large dosages, renal toxicity. Therefore it must be administered with care. *Dihydrostreptomycin*, a similar compound, is now rarely used because of occasional damage to the vestibular apparatus causing permanent dizziness. *Kanamycin* (Kantrex) is similar to streptomycin in its administration and action but is even more toxic. Although a very effective and powerful drug, it should be given under careful surveillance, particularly to elderly patients and those with impaired renal function. *Colistin* (Colimycin) is also only available for intramuscular use and is particularly effective in severe *Pseudomonas* and *E. coli* infections. Again, with our present knowledge, it must be given under careful surveillance, particularly when renal function is impaired. Finally, *polymyxin B*, a compound very similar to colistin, can be used. This is available in an intravenous form for the desperately ill patient but must be given with extreme care because of its nephrotoxicity.

The *cycline* group of drugs is bacteriostatic. They can be administered orally, intramuscularly, and intravenously. Commonly used are *tetracycline*, *chlortetracycline* (Aureomycin), and *oxytetracycline* (Terramycin). Another recently introduced member of this family, *dimethylchlortetracycline* (Declomycin), can be used orally only. The drug in this group presently most useful for the urologist is tetracycline. Its spectrum is fairly broad.

Chloramphenicol (Chloromycetin) is particularly effective, but its use must be accompanied by frequent observations of the blood count, since it occasionally causes serious bone marrow depression. With adequate precaution, this drug is very effective and quite safe but is best used on an inpatient hospital basis. Chloramphenicol is a drug of choice against *E. coli* and *Klebsiella*.

Gentamycin (Garamycin) is a newly available bactericidal antibiotic similar to kanamycin for use by intravenous or intramuscular injection. The drug offers great promise against gram-negative infections, particularly those caused by *Pseudomonas* and *Proteus*. There is some danger of ototoxicity and nephrotoxicity from its use.

Cephalothin (Keflin) is a broad-spectrum, bactericidal antibiotic that must be used parenterally. It is especially effective against certain gram-negative organisms, particularly *Proteus mirabilis* and *E. coli* infections. When given intramuscularly, the injection must be deep in the muscle since the medication may be locally irritating. It is relatively nontoxic

and does not depress renal function. A few cross-reactions have been reported in patients known to be hypersensitive to penicillin.

A side effect from the use of antibiotics, particularly the broad-spectrum ones, is the suppression of bacteria to a degree that may promote fungal overgrowth, manifested chiefly by diarrhea and oral and vaginal lesions. Another type of disabling diarrhea with severe body fluid loss can occur when the majority of bacteria have been suppressed with a resultant overgrowth of staphylococci in the intestinal tract. Such an overgrowth can be recognized readily if a prompt gram stain of a stool specimen demonstrates large numbers of staphylococci.

The usual effectiveness of the commonly used urinary antibacterial agents against bacteria is summarized in Table 3-1.

TABLE 3-1

AVERAGE USEFULNESS OF ANTIBACTERIAL AGENTS IN URINARY TRACT INFECTIONS

ANTIBACTERIAL AGENTS	ORGANISM							
	Escherichia coli	*Proteus mirabilis*	*Proteus* (others)	*Klebsiella-Aerobacter*	*Pseudomonas aeruginosa*	*Streptococcus faecalis*	*Staphylococcus aureus*	*Neisseria gonorrhoeae*
Penicillin G	—	△*	—	—	—	●	△†	△
Ampicillin	△	+	●	—	—	△	—	△
Tetracyclines	+	—	—	△	—	—	+	+
Chloramphenicol	△	+	△	△	●	—	+	+
Erythromycin	—	—	—	—	—	+	+	+
Colistin	+	—	—	△	△	—	—	—
Kanamycin	+	●	●	+	●	—	+	+
Streptomycin	+	+	+	+	●	+	—	+
Cephalothin	+	△	—	—	—	●	+	—
Sulfonamides	+	●	●	●	—	●	—	●
Nitrofurantoin	+	—	+	●	—	—	—	—
Nalidixic acid	+	+	+	●	—	—	—	—

△ Drug of choice.
+ Usually effective.
● Inconstant.
— Usually resistant.
* In massive dosage intravenously.
† Sensitivity dependent on penicillinase production.

Specific Infections

Specific infections are those that can infect an anatomically normal urinary tract. As mentioned previously, nonspecific infections frequently require preparation of the soil before they can take hold.

STAPHYLOCOCCAL INFECTIONS. Infections caused by virulent staphylococci are usually blood-borne (hematogenous), arising from a focus of infection anywhere in the body but commonly in the skin. These bacteria settle in the renal parenchyma, initially in the cortex, where they create a pyelonephritis. Because these organisms produce enzymes that can cause local tissue necrosis, abscess formation is common. This may be manifested by multiple, small, discrete abscesses or a cluster of confluent ones which, when especially large, is known as a renal carbuncle. Adequate control of such an abscess, like one elsewhere, will require surgical drainage along with antibiotic therapy. These abscesses can rupture into the fat surrounding the kidney, where they are known as perinephric abscesses. They may be acute and fulminating but are often indolent without causing many symptoms for a long time.

TUBERCULOSIS. Tuberculosis of the urinary tract is usually secondary to a primary focus elsewhere, most often in the lungs. In this country the usual infecting organism is now the human tubercle bacillus and not the bovine or avian form. Since tuberculosis usually progresses very slowly, the primary focus may be difficult to uncover and may be ostensibly healed. The tubercle bacilli arrive in the kidney by hematogenous spread. Here they form small cortical abscesses accompanied by caseation necrosis. The difficulty of diagnosis may pose a serious problem, a significant part of which is the degree of suspicion on the part of the clinician. One clue is the demonstration of pus cells in an acid urine wherein bacterial cultures are repeatedly sterile—the so-called sterile acid pyuria of tuberculosis. However, secondary nonspecific bacterial invaders are frequently found, and their presence does not rule out the diagnosis. The x-ray picture shows the characteristic changes of the kidneys, the earliest of which is the moth-eaten appearance in the calyces, particularly those of the upper pole. The pyelographic appearance of the kidneys is usually much more benign than the actual degree of tissue involvement, which may occasionally be quite extensive despite normal-appearing x-rays. The most important factor in making the diagnosis is the actual demonstration of tubercle bacilli in the urine by acid-fast smears and subsequent culture and identification of the organism. Few bacilli other than tubercle bacilli will pick up the acid-fast stain, but the best way to differentiate these organisms is by culture. However, tubercle bacilli grow slowly and it may be four to eight weeks before there is significant growth on the culture plates. Furthermore, since tubercle bacilli are often present in small quantities in the urine in the presence of urinary tract tuberculosis, it is good practice to obtain at least three separate, negative, smears and cultures before ruling out the disease. Usually the first voided specimen of the morning offers the best chance of making the diagnosis. The disease probably progresses within the urinary tract by lymphatic spread down the ureters to the bladder, prostate, seminal vesicles, testes, and epididymides. With bladder involvement severe frequency and urgency may develop owing to irritation and a gradual decrease in the bladder capacity secondary to fibrosis within the bladder wall.

The treatment of urinary tract tuberculosis has been revolutionized with the use of antituberculous agents such as streptomycin, isoniazid, para-aminosalicylic acid, and cycloserine. These drugs must be given for long periods of time, and most programs call for a course of treatment lasting one or two years or longer, using at least two or three of these drugs in combination. Surgery, however, still plays an important role. There are instances indicating partial or complete nephrectomy, particularly with severe unilateral involvement, abscess formation, or hydronephrosis. Other indications for surgery include the hopelessly contracted bladder or scrotal abscess formation. The term *autonephrectomy* is often heard in conjunction with renal tuberculosis. The word implies that somehow the kidney has removed itself from the patient. Actually autonephrectomy is used to describe the situation in which a kidney has been totally destroyed by the tuberculous process and remains in the patient as a nonfunctioning mass of tissue. Usually such kidneys are also obstructed by fibrotic stenosis of the ureter and are potentially a site of further enhancing infection elsewhere or becoming secondarily infected. Usually no extraordinary care is necessary in handling the urine of these patients.

VENEREAL DISEASE. Venereal diseases are usually transmitted by sexual intercourse. The portal of entry is therefore the penis or vagina. Other portals are available, of course, but necessarily involve alternate sexual practices.

Syphilis is caused by the spirochete *Treponema pallidum*. About three weeks after contact a hard, ulcerating, nontender lesion, the chancre, will appear, usually on the glans penis or foreskin (primary syphilis). At this point, the lesion is highly contagious; the treatment consists in courses of therapy with penicillin. If unchecked, the spirochetes will travel through the bloodstream resulting in an indolent chronic disorder particularly affecting large arteries and the nerve cells of the spinal cord and brain. At four to six weeks after infection, the diagnosis can be made by various complement-fixation tests and demonstration of the spirochetes in the chancre by dark-field microscopic examination. Except for its portal of entry, the disease is really not a urologic disorder.

Gonorrhea is caused by the gram-negative diplococcus *Neisseria gonorrhoeae.* It is manifested by a purulent urethritis seen within two or three days, sometimes as long as ten days, after intercourse. The diagnosis can be made readily by the history of contact and demonstration of gram-negative intracellular diplococci on a smear of the urethral discharge. If not treated, the acute symptoms may well subside spontaneously. However, the persistence of viable organisms in the periurethral glands can cause an indolent periurethritis with gradual scarring as healing occurs. The constricting effect of the healing periurethritis can cause a narrowing, or stricture, of the urethral lumen. Such a stricture will become symptomatic, resulting in a thin urinary stream and difficulty in voiding. The treatment of these strictures includes gradual dilatation of the urethra. The infection may progress to acute involvement of the prostate, testes, and epididymides with abscess formation. Unchecked, the infection may spread via the bloodstream and occasionally involve joints or the valves of the heart.

Penicillin is highly effective against the majority of strains of *Neisseria*, and often a single injection of 600,000 units will eradicate the infection in its acute stage. Presently, because of attenuated strains, the recommended dosage is 4,800,000 units as an initial injection. In the presence of resistance or hypersensitivity to penicillin, tetracycline seems to be a good second choice. It is interesting that although syphilis and gonorrhea can be very serious infections to human beings, the causative organisms are very delicate and will survive for only short periods outside the body. They are very sensitive to drying, heat, and the effect of soap and water. Yet these devils thrive luxuriantly on human mucous membranes. Culture techniques are very difficult and unreliable.

There are several other venereal diseases worthy of mention. *Lymphogranuloma venereum* is a disease caused by a large virus which responds to treatment with either chloramphenicol or the tetracyclines. One to three weeks after sexual contact a small penile papule appears and heals spontaneously almost as quickly as it came. Shortly thereafter there will be painful enlargement of the inguinal lymph nodes which suppurate, form multiple sinuses accompanied by chills, fever, and generalized malaise. In untreated cases, the sinuses may persist or may close with resultant local chronic lymphatic obstruction. Late rectal stricture formation is a common complication of this disease.

Chancroid, or soft chancre, is an ulcerating lesion of the penis occurring several days after exposure, caused by the Ducrey bacillus. Inguinal node suppuration is common and occurs in two to three weeks. This disease responds promptly to the tetracyclines or sulfonamides. *Granuloma inguinale* is caused by the bacterium *Donovania granulomatis.* The disease progresses slowly as a swelling of the skin of the genitalia followed by ulceration and secondary infection. The response to chloramphenicol and the tetracyclines is prompt.

Trichomonas infestation of the male urethra and prostate is probably more prevalent than commonly recognized. Infection is by sexual contact with a woman harboring trichomonads in the vagina. This parasite seldom infects the female urinary tract. The diagnosis is usually made by demonstration in the male of organisms in the urine or prostatic fluid. Culture techniques are difficult. Treatment is usually quite successful after a ten-day course of oral metranidazole (Flagyl), particularly if the female partner is treated simultaneously.

REVIEW QUESTIONS

1. Explain the structural and functional changes in the hydronephrotic kidney.
2. Describe the changes in the bladder with progressive distal obstruction. How can these changes cause renal failure?
3. Differentiate between specific and nonspecific urinary infections; name the commoner invaders in each category.
4. Name four possible factors in the genesis of nonspecific infections.
5. List some of the commoner obstructive urologic disorders.
6. Discuss the etiology and treatment of the venereal diseases.
7. Describe the antibacterial agents commonly used in the treatment of urinary infection, their mode of action, and possible side effects.

CHAPTER 4

Congenital Malformations

VARIATIONS from the normal anatomy of the genitourinary tract can be demonstrated in 10 per cent of the population as determined by autopsy studies. These variations cover the gamut from minimal deformity to extreme abnormalities such as complete agenesis of the kidneys and exstrophy of the bladder. Since these changes frequently are associated with malfunction, a brief review of the embryology and study of the more common and severe disorders is warranted. A more complete description of anomalies of the urinary tract with an excellent list of references can be found in most of the standard textbooks of urology. Some of the more common and significant anomalies will be discussed here. The important point is to appreciate the frequency of these disorders.

Embryology of the Urinary Tract

Formation of the adult kidney begins at the hind end of the embryo and goes through three stages reflecting evolution of the kidney in lower forms of life. These are successively the pronephros, mesonephros, and metanephros. This last stage becomes the adult human kidney and supplies the adult nephrons. The ureter grows out as a bud from the wolffian duct, the remnant of the excretory duct of the second stage. One end of the wolffian duct opens into the cloaca, a common terminus for both the urinary and intestinal tracts. The ureteral bud grows toward the metanephros, subdividing to form the renal pelvis, infundibula, calyces, and collecting ducts. As this development is occurring, the kidneys ascend both relatively and actually as the tail end of the embryo grows, until the final normal position opposite the first three lumbar vertebrae is reached. This ascent is accompanied by a ladderlike acquisition and loss of blood supply; i.e., blood vessels from the lower aorta and its branches are lost, and newer ones higher up are acquired. As the kidneys ascend, they also rotate 90° inwardly so that the renal pelvis changes from a ventral to a dorsal position. A *malrotated* kidney is not uncommon.

By the end of the sixth week in utero, the cloaca is divided into anterior and posterior compartments by a transverse membrane, the urorectal septum. The closed external end of the cloaca, the cloacal membrane, then perforates both in front and behind this septum to form an anterior urogenital sinus and a posterior anal opening. The bladder is formed from the higher portion of this anterior segment, and the female urethra and male posterior urethra from the lower portion. An upper connection of the bladder to the umbilicus, the urachus, eventually closes but persists in the adult as a midline ligament from the bladder dome to the umbilicus. A rounded projection near the end of the urogenital sinus, the genital tubercle, elongates rapidly and, as it does, becomes grooved. The distal end becomes the phallus, and the sides of the groove grow together to form the anterior urethra in the male. The prostate is derived from multiple outpocketings of the posterior urethra.

Formation of the gonads (sperm- and ovum-producing organs) is intimately related to the development of the urinary tract. They begin as undifferentiated thickenings near the early wolffian ducts known as the "germinal ridge." These become ovaries or testes, which reside within the peritoneal cavity attached by a ligament known as the round ligament in the female and the gubernaculum in the male. The male organ, the testis, then travels through the inguinal canal to the scrotum, taking with it the epididymis and vas deferens, which are persistences of the wolffian duct. The relationship of testicular descent to formation of the kidney can be emphasized by the fact that 17 per cent of male patients with an undescended testicle have an associated congenital abnormality of the upper urinary tract on the same side.

Anomalies of Kidney and Ureter

More than two separate kidneys is almost unknown. The term *double kidney* means one kidney containing two pelves with varying degrees of ureteral duplication. The two ureters may be present down to the bladder or may join each other anywhere along the way. In the presence of duplication it is common to find a separate renal artery to each collecting system. The term *reduplication* is commonly used to describe this situation. The correct term would be *duplication*, since this means a doubling whereas reduplication implies a fourfold increase. Absence of one kidney is not rare and is usually associated with nondevelopment of the ureter and corresponding half of the trigone on that side. *Bilateral agenesis*, of course, is incompatible with life. Newborn infants with this defect can be recognized readily because of a peculiar facies, the most striking aspects of which are malformed and low-set ears, small lower jaw, epicanthal folds, and widely separated eyes. Kidneys may be unusually small (*congenital hypoplasia*), or unusually large (*congenital hypertrophy*). Hypoplastic kidneys are frequently *dysplastic* also; that is, their nephrons are inadequately developed as well as reduced in number. At times it becomes difficult to differentiate the shrunken kidney secondary to pyelonephritic atrophy from congenital hypoplasia, particularly since the latter is so prone to infection. Several varieties of *cystic* change may or may not be congenital. The most striking example is the *congenital multicystic kidney*, wherein the organ is replaced by a mass of grapelike cysts with little, if any, functioning parenchyma. This deformity is usually associated with atresia (narrowing or absence of the lumen) of the upper ureter. The cystic disorders will be discussed in more detail in Chapter 7.

Variations in the location and form of the kidney are common. Owing to persistence of an embryonic blood supply, the kidney may be located lower than usual, with its arterial supply arising from the lower aorta or its branches. Examples include the *ectopic* and *pelvic* kidney. Failure of rotation of the kidney during ascent is often accompanied by some degree of obstruction at the ureteropelvic junction. Nonrotation may be bilateral, and if the lower poles of the kidneys remain joined, the result is a *horseshoe kidney*.

Congenital ureteropelvic junction obstruction may result from malrotation of the kidney, as previously mentioned, but is more often caused by abnormal blood vessels or their fibrous remnants which compress or distort the ureteropelvic area. Again, the obstructive features of an anomalous blood supply are noted. The termination of completely duplicated ureters into the bladder is almost always reversed, so that the ureter draining the superior pole of the kidney enters the bladder at a point *lower* than that from the inferior pole. This is known as the *Weigert-Meyer rule* and exceptions are almost unknown. Many of the common abnormalities of the ureter involve its terminus in the bladder. An *ectopic* ureter is one that does not enter the bladder at the corner of the trigone; in fact, it might not enter the bladder at all but open into the urethra or vagina. If such an opening is distal to the sphincter mechanism, a history of normal micturition accompanied by continuous leakage from the urinary fistula thus created can often be obtained. A *ureterocele* is a cystic ballooning of the lower end of the ureter which, besides obstructing the ureteral orifice, can also act as an obstruction to the bladder neck if sufficiently large and properly located. Ureteroceles are frequently associated with duplication of the upper tract on the same side, and most of them involve the orifice of the ureter from the upper renal pole—thus, the orifice lowermost in the bladder, as per the Weigert-Meyer rule. Congenital strictures at the ureterovesical junction will act as obstructions and may require surgical correction. Vesicoureteral reflux, discussed in detail in Chapter 2, may be due to malformation of the ureterovesical junction, and its consequences to the upper urinary tract on that side are usually serious.

Anomalies of the Bladder

Anomalies of the bladder are apparently more common than was once thought. A *urachal fistula* is a direct connection from the dome of the bladder to the umbilicus due to lack of the normal atresia of the urachus. Incomplete closure with formation of cysts anywhere along this tract may occur. *Exstrophy* of the bladder is a distressing anomaly manifested by separation of the symphysis pubis with an accompanying defect in the lower abdominal wall through which the open bladder everts. Treatment of this defect presents a major challenge to the urologist. Fortunately it is quite rare. Recent experiments on chick embryos have shown that this

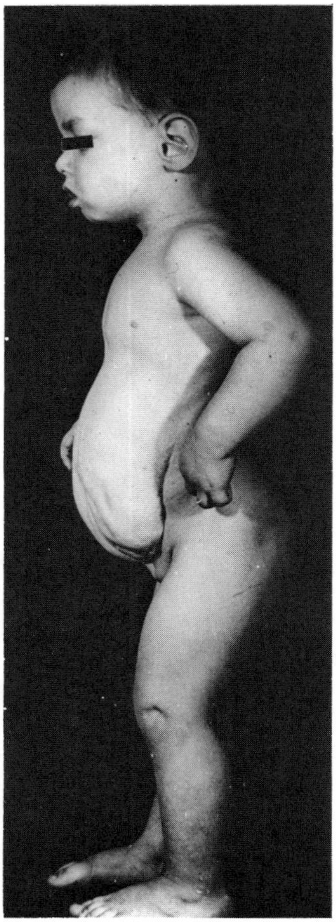

FIGURE 4-1. The appearance of the abdomen in the prune-belly syndrome.

defect is primarily due to prolonged presence of the cloacal membrane. By far the more common anomalies are subtle changes at the bladder base due to maldevelopment in and about the trigone. These less obvious deformities have been shown to be responsible for serious renal infection not only in children but also in adults. Some of these seemingly minor changes have gone unrecognized for years. Consequently, both the diagnosis and treatment of these disorders are presently subjects of great controversy among urologists.

A *bladder neck contracture* results from a fibrous ring at the bladder neck, which may vary from the obviously tight to the uncertainly snug. Whether or not a child can "outgrow" such a condition is a matter of debate, especially how the maturation can occur, whether apparent or real. Classically, the bladder behind such an obstruction shows the hypertrophic, trabeculatory changes similar to prostatic obstruction in the adult. The *megacystis syndrome*, on the other hand, usually is accompanied by a thin-walled, smooth, large-capacity bladder. The size of the trigone is larger than normal, and the intramural ureteral tunnels are short, so that vesicoureteral reflux can readily occur. Recurrent urinary tract infections usually play a prominent role in the clinical presentation of these conditions. These abnormalities in trigonal development are seen more commonly in girls.

A rare but interesting anomaly of unknown cause is the *prune-belly syndrome*. It is manifested by a flaccid wrinkled appearance of the abdominal wall due to hypoplasia of the muscle layers, which are unusually thin. The only serious element is the massive hydronephrosis with marked dilation and hypertrophy of the ureters, so that death often occurs early from uremia and sepsis. The appearance of these patients is worth remembering as the diagnosis can be made with a knowledgeable glance (Fig. 4-1).

Anomalies of the External Genitalia

Anomalous development of the penis proper is rare, but disorders of the urethra are common. Absence of the penis, duplications, and other malformations fall into the realm of curiosities. *Hypospadias*, a common congenital defect of the distal urethra, seems to be caused by incomplete closure of the embryonic urethral groove. The urethral opening is therefore located proximally along the ventral surface of the penis or in more severe cases in the scrotum or perineum. The scar tissue comprising the distal atretic urethra acts like the string of a bow, causing the penis to curve downward on itself in a condition known as *chordee*. A dorsal urethral defect is the relatively rare condition of *epispadias*. Nearly all cases of vesical exstrophy have an associated epispadias, in which there is separation of the corpora cavernosa, with an unclosed urethra above them.

If the defect also involves the sphincteric area, there can be urinary incontinence. Malformations of the prostatic urethra are rare. The most common are the presence of congenital *prostatic valves*, usually located at the apex, which can cause very serious trouble from obstruction.

The most common testicular abnormality is the *undescended testis* (cryptorchidism). The testis may be located anywhere in its normal path of descent from the pelvic brim down through the inguinal canal, where the majority are found. The usual defect seems to be a relative shortening of the spermatic vessels, which must be mobilized during surgical correction. The condition is almost always associated with a congenital indirect inguinal hernia. If such testes are not brought into the scrotum by age five or six years, they will be poor sperm producers because of their prolonged exposure to normal body temperature as compared to the relative coolness of the scrotum necessary for adequate spermatogenesis. Even if surgically corrected, undescended testes undergo malignant degeneration much more commonly than those normally situated, especially if they were originally located within the abdomen. Nevertheless, the incidence of cancer in cryptorchids is not high, since testicular neoplasms generally are quite infrequent.

REVIEW QUESTIONS

1. Discuss the embryologic development of the kidneys.
2. Define the following terms: ectopic kidney, malrotated kidney, horseshoe kidney, duplicated kidney, multicystic kidney.
3. Discuss the possible urologic significance of a newborn infant with (a) "low-set" ears and (b) "prune belly."
4. What is the significance of the undescended testis? Discuss its correlation with anomalies of the upper urinary tract.
5. Describe the following: megacystis syndrome, urachus, ureterocele, hypospadias, chordee, epispadias, and exstrophy.

CHAPTER 5
Urinary Calculi

STONE formation in the urinary tract is a common problem. The actual cause (and prevention) of the majority of calculi is unknown, despite continuing research. Some stones are formed secondary to disorders within the urinary tract; others are urinary manifestations of systemic metabolic disease. Yet in many of the latter instances, for some unknown reason, one kidney may be repeatedly involved with calculi whereas the other may remain normal.

Composition of Calculi

Urinary tract calculi are concretions precipitated on an organic matrix of mucoproteins and polysaccharides. This matrix may be derived from small amounts of these substances filtered through the glomeruli or may originate from desquamated cells from the renal papillae. The majority of stones contain calcium, which makes them visible radiographically. The calcium precipitates with oxalates, phosphates, or carbonates in either pure or mixed forms. Calculi containing mixtures of calcium carbonate and magnesium ammonium phosphate are usually associated with infection. Uric acid stones, on the other hand, are radiolucent in their pure form. They cannot be visualized by x-ray unless contrast material is introduced to outline the filling defects caused by them. The rare stone of cystine is faintly visible by x-ray because of its sulfur content.

The appearance and consistency of urinary calculi are often suggestive of their composition prior to an actual chemical analysis. Calcium oxalate stones are usually black to gray, quite hard, and tend to be spiculed or angular. Calcium phosphate and carbonate stones are often smoother and lighter in color, like plaster. Urate calculi have a greenish-tan hue, tend to be smooth, and are usually softer than those containing calcium. Cystine stones are yellowish and characteristically have a waxy or greasy surface.

Factors in the Urine

Urine is a complex solution of numerous substances, many of which are present in a supersaturated state. Consequently, precipitation is less likely to occur in a dilute urine. Therefore, a large fluid intake becomes an important basis for all stone-prevention regimens. It is a wonder that stones do not form more often! The acidity of the urine will affect the solubility of its various components. For example, uric acid is almost a hundred times more soluble in urine that is slightly alkaline as compared to a pH of 5.5, as seen in very acid urine. Conversely, calcium salts are much more soluble in acid urine.

Metabolic Disorders

Although recognized systemic metabolic disorders are not the most common causes for calculous formation, they should always be sought out since they may be in large part corrected or controlled.

Hyperparathyroidism, overactivity of the parathyroid glands, is usually caused by noncancerous neoplasia of these organs. The tumors are functionally active, producing increased amounts of parathormone which is released into the circulation. The neoplasia may be multiple. The disorder is characterized by an increased blood level of ionized calcium and a correspondingly high urinary calcium excretion. The serum phosphorus level is usually decreased, probably from diminished renal tubular resorption of phosphorus. Therefore, the high urinary output of both calcium and phosphorus promotes precipitation of phosphatic calculi—this is the urologic manifestation of the disorder. The diagnosis is not always made easily and may require repeated blood and urine studies of a more sophisticated nature to detect these findings, which may not be consistently present. Once the diagnosis is established, the cause is eliminated by surgical extirpation of the offending parathyroid adenomas. This curable disorder accounts for less than 5 per cent of all patients with urinary tract calculi. In neglected cases, there is extensive skeletal calcium resorption with bone cyst formation and pathologic fractures. Peptic ulcer is often an associated finding.

Abnormal amounts of calcium may be excreted in the urine under other circumstances. One is *idiopathic hypercalciuria*, which must be differentiated from hyperparathyroidism. This is most probably a renal tubular defect with a relative inability to resorb urinary calcium. The hypercalciuria is accompanied by normal or slightly depressed serum calcium levels, contrasted to the elevated values in hyperparathyroidism. The urinary calcium loss stimulates increased parathyroid activity, so that blood levels of phosphorus also decrease and the urinary excretion is elevated. Prolonged immobilization of a patient is likely to cause resorption of calcium from the skeleton and an increased likelihood of urinary calculous formation. A large ingestion of milk over a long period of time has a similar effect.

Hyperuricemia may or may not be associated with clinical gout. An increase in the production of uric acid is followed by an increase in the total body uric acid pool and an increase in the serum level of this substance. When uric acid precipitates in or around joints, the clinical manifestations of gout will appear. Particularly in the presence of acid urine (which is usually the case) excessive amounts of uric acid in the urine will precipitate to form calculi.

Cystinuria is a familial renal tubular defect wherein abnormal amounts of four amino acids appear in the urine. Three of these acids are highly soluble, but the fourth, cystine, is not and precipitates to form calculi. Numerous other disorders are associated in varying degrees with stone formation. These include oxalosis, xanthinuria, renal tubular acidosis, sarcoidosis, and certain blood dyscrasias.

Local Factors

The most important local factors are obstruction and infection. Infection with urea-splitting organisms such as *Proteus* is associated with alkaline urine and a high incidence of magnesium ammonium phosphate calculi. Often it is difficult to decide which came first—the stone or the infection. Acting as a foreign body in the urinary tract, the stone tends to perpetuate the infection. Local stasis is a common background for calculous formation, particularly in the lower urinary tract. In modern times, vesical calculi are almost always secondary to obstruction and infection from an enlarged prostate, urethral stricture, or neurogenic dysfunction.

Consequences of Calculi

Calculi in the urinary tract act as foreign bodies and are therefore irritating. More often than not, there is associated infection. Most important, however, are the obstructions they cause. Eighty to ninety per cent of calculi that enter the ureter will pass spontaneously. If there is no intrinsic obstruction in the urinary passages, calculi 1 cm or less in diameter will usually pass. Many of these patients can be followed on an outpatient basis. Unless the hydronephrosis above the stone is unusually severe or infection is marked, one can often wait several months before considering surgical or instrumental intervention. Instructions are given to the patient to strain the urine so that the stone can be recovered (thus clinching the diagnosis) and analyzed to determine its composition and plan a program to prevent recurrences.

Depending on the estimated size of the stone from x-ray, the urine may be strained in one of several ways. If the calculus is large enough to see easily (3 mm or greater), the patient can simply void into a clear water glass thus screening each specimen. For smaller calculi, the patient is advised to strain the urine through a fine gauze pad. If the urine is infected, an oral antibacterial medication is prescribed. Oral analgesics such as meperidine (Demerol) will be necessary to allay the pain of colic. The patient is instructed to keep up a large oral fluid intake and to notify the doctor immediately should there be chills, fever, severe pain not responding to the analgesic, or grossly bloody urine. Fever, particularly, is an indication for inpatient management of the stone patient.

Prevention of Stone Recurrence

A large fluid intake with a correspondingly large urinary output is a most important common denominator in all programs to prevent stone recurrence, regardless of the type of stone. Additional general measures to decrease the incidence of stone include correction of congenital or acquired obstructions in the urinary passageways and control of associated infections. Measures to dissolve calculi in the kidney or ureter by continuous irrigations with various solutions have yet to be consistently successful. Furthermore, they may be traumatic to the kidney tissue, with serious complications. Dissolution of calculi in the bladder, particularly in the presence of drainage tubes is possible but often not practical. The solutions used are described on pages 170–71.

Various regimens have been proposed for prevention of uric acid calculi. The best preventative seems to be the use of the drug allopurinol. This compound is a xanthine oxidase inhibitor, interrupting the metabolic sequence in the production of endogenous uric acid by the body. A low-purine diet (see Appendix I) is prescribed to decrease the oral intake of uric acid precursors. Attempts can be made to alkalinize the urine because of the marked increase in solubility of uric acid at a neutral or slightly alkaline pH. This is difficult to accomplish and may require large amounts of oral sodium bicarbonate. The amounts required may be a serious consideration in patients with hypertension and cardiovascular disease for whom the oral sodium intake must be kept to a minimum. The patient is given nitrazine or litmus paper and advised to adjust the intake of bicarbonate depending on the pH. This procedure requires laborious attention on the part of the patient, and most lose interest after a while. Uricosuric agents such as probenecid are occasionally used to decrease the uric acid pool. These must be monitored carefully since too much mobilization of uric acid into the urine may further increase precipitation of uric acid.

A successful program for the prevention of recurrent phosphatic calculi is the Shorr regimen. This consists of a low-calcium, low-phosphorus diet (see Appendix I), limiting the oral intake of phosphorus to

1300 mg per day. To be effective, the diet must be accompanied by the oral intake of aluminum carbonate gel, 30 to 40 ml, taken 30 minutes after meals and at bedtime. The gel combines with the oral phosphate to form an insoluble precipitate in the intestinal tract, thus reducing further the amount of phosphorus offered to the nephron. If, with a good urinary output, the 24-hour excretion of phosphorus is kept below 300 mg/day, the incidence of recurrent calculi is significantly diminished.

Although the regimen is very effective, patients need constant encouragement to continue with the program. The aluminum gels are relatively tasteless and tend to be constipating. They can be made more palatable by refrigeration and the addition of a few drops of peppermint or lemon oil as flavoring. The constipation can be treated by increasing the amounts of roughage in the diet or the use of milk of magnesia at bedtime. The efficacy of the diet is monitored by periodic x-rays of the urinary tract for recurrent stone and measurements of the 24-hour urinary excretion of calcium and phosphorus. Although the diet is aimed primarily at the prevention of recurrent phosphatic calculi, it is also effective against other types of calcium concretions, even in the face of alkalinizing infection. Studies have shown the incidence of recurrent stone following complete nephrolithotomy to be 75 to 85 per cent on a general diet, whereas it is less than 10 per cent if the Shorr program is followed. Consequently, it is our practice not to embark on such a major operation for stone removal unless the patient can demonstrate to us prior to operation his ability to cooperate with this regimen.

Acidification programs for prevention of calcium stones have been popular but relatively ineffectual. A long-time favorite has been the use of cranberry juice. To even begin to be effective, a minimum of 1 quart must be ingested daily. Low oxalate diets are also popular and are easily tolerated. The patient is advised to moderate his intake of dairy products and oxalate-containing foods such as rhubarb, spinach, nuts, and chocolate. The 24-hour excretion of oxalate under all circumstances is quite low and difficult to measure accurately. The dietary intake does not influence it much. Again, the most effective measure is a large oral fluid intake.

The dietary regimen for cystine consists primarily of a massive intake of water—up to 6 or 8 liters per day. The patients are advised to awaken by the clock during the middle of the night to ingest more water. Alkalinization of the urine, as with uric acid formers, is pursued. Experimentally, and of clinical value, is the use of oral *d*-penicillamine. This drug offers hope in that it competes metabolically in cystine synthesis, thus decreasing its output in the urine. However, toxic complications of the drug are common, and it has yet to be fully assessed. Fortunately, patients who are cystine stone formers are relatively rare.

REVIEW QUESTIONS

1. Describe the chemical composition of the commoner types of urinary calculi.
2. List some of the commoner metabolic disorders responsible for stone formation.
3. What local factors in the urinary tract predispose to stone formation?
4. Explain the relationship between urinary pH and calculous disease.
5. Discuss the general principles in the management of the recurrent stone-forming patient.

CHAPTER 6
Neoplasia of the Urinary Tract

Kidney and Adrenal Tumors

NEOPLASMS of the kidney can be grossly subdivided according to their origin in the parenchyma or in the collecting system. Since the collecting system is lined by urothelium common to the ureter, bladder, and proximal urethra, a more complete description of that pathology will be found in the discussion on bladder tumors.

Benign parenchymal tumors such as adenomas and fibromas are usually of little consequence except when the question of malignancy arises, particularly when they become large. The common parenchymal malignancy is an adenocarcinoma. Owing to its cellular appearance, it is known as a "clear-cell" carcinoma. These cells resemble those seen in the normal adrenal cortex, and it was once thought that these tumors arose from embryonic rests of adrenal tissue within the kidney. Recent electron microscopic techniques may revive this old theory. Since the adrenal gland sits on top of the kidney (or is "hyper" to it), the name *hypernephroma* was established and is still frequently but incorrectly used.

These growths, and in fact all renal parenchymal masses, can become quite large before they cause symptoms. As previously described, the kidneys are located in a very protected area with large muscle masses behind and the intestinal contents in front. The classical triad of pain, mass, and hematuria is not always seen. The pain is due to tension on the renal capsule by the gradually enlarging mass. Hematuria occurs when the tumor erodes into the collecting system. This may be painless or, if accompanied by the passage of clots, may give rise to the symptoms of renal colic. Other symptoms are malaise, weight loss, or intermittent fevers due to necrosis within the tumor. Hypernephroma tends to metastasize to the lungs and bone via the bloodstream.

The only adequate treatment for this neoplasm is its total physical removal. None of the presently available chemotherapeutic agents is significantly effective, and the response to radiation therapy is not impressive. The surgical removal can be accomplished through a transabdominal approach, the classical lumbar route, or transthoracically by division of the diaphragm. The goal is wide exposure and early ligation of the blood supply before the tumor is mobilized. Usually the fatty envelope surrounding the kidney is removed en bloc with the specimen, and lymph nodes along the aorta are excised. The five-year survival rate after excision of this tumor is approximately 35 per cent, but variations in the rapidity of growth are not unusual. Death from tumor recurrence after an apparent cure has been reported as long as forty years after nephrectomy!

Another parenchymal malignancy, which fortunately is less common, is the highly malignant *Wilms' tumor*, *nephroblastoma*, mostly seen in childhood. The diagnosis is usually begun by demonstration of a large abdominal mass, and surgery must be performed promptly. A rapid differential diagnosis must be made, most often between a large hydronephrosis or a neuroblastoma, a childhood sarcoma of neural origin, often arising in the adrenal area. Hydronephroses are the most common abdominal childhood masses of renal origin. The incidence of Wilms' tumor and neuroblastoma is about equal. The most successful results in the treatment of Wilms' tumor have come from immediate nephrectomy, generally through the transabdominal approach, accompanied by vigorous postoperative radiation therapy. The reported cure rates vary considerably from clinic to clinic, reflecting not only difference in techniques but especially the nature of the cases that present. The results with small encapsulated growths and those in patients under two years of age are vastly better than the opposite circumstances. Because of the highly malignant nature of this tumor, an apparent absence of disease two years after treatment makes recurrence thereafter infrequent. Recently, significant palliation and even apparent short-term cures, particularly of pulmonary metastases, have been accomplished by the addition of the systemic use of either actinomycin D or vincristine.

Neuroblastoma is a tumor arising from sympathoblasts in the adrenal medulla or from such cells in ganglia along the sympathetic chain. Like Wilms' tumors, they are usually seen in young children and are equally malignant, if not more so. The diagnosis is most often suspected by discovery of an abdominal mass or from the signs of metastases. The latter most often invade the liver or bones. A common presentation of metastases is a bulge of the skull or an anterior displacement of the eye where there is cranial spread. Involvement of the bone marrow can sometimes be demonstrated by simple biopsy, the same technique as employed in hematologic studies. The outlook with bone spread is virtually hopeless, but surprisingly metastases in the liver are not as hopeless as such are in other cancers. The treatment is total surgical removal (often impossible at the time of diagnosis), radiation therapy, and chemotherapy. In circumstances that are unfortunately rare, the tumor may spontaneously mature to a benign neuroma or disappear entirely. It has been suggested that partial removal of the tumor or administration of large amounts of vitamin B_{12} might aid this transformation, but this does not seem likely. The most useful chemotherapeutic agents to date have been the systemic administration of cyclophosphamide (Cytoxan) and vincristine.

Urothelial Tumors (Renal Pelvis, Ureter, and Bladder)

The treatment of urothelial tumors is a complex affair for several reasons. One is that these growths vary from relatively benign neoplasms to highly anaplastic, rapidly growing lesions. Perhaps nowhere in the body is the variation in malignancy so great. Consequently, an important factor in prognosis is the histologic appearance of the tumor. In comparison, although there are variations in the microscopic appearance of lung and stomach cancers, the overall degree of malignancy of the common tumors is rather similar. The usual location for a urothelial neoplasm is in the bladder, and 90 per cent of these growths are transitional-cell tumors. The remaining 10 per cent of these growths include skinlike epidermoid tumors, adenocarcinomas, sarcomas, and so forth.

The reported results of treatment of these malignancies varied considerably from clinic to clinic in past years because of the variations and differences in nomenclature. With eventual classification of these lesions as to grade and stage by Jewett, Marshall, and Whitmore, comparative order has been made of chaos. These tumors can be graded from 1, the lowest degree of malignancy, to 4, the highest. Grade 1 tumors are called papillomas; Grade 2, very low-grade carcinomas; Grade 3, well-differentiated but fully malignant cancers; and Grade 4, unusually anaplastic carcinomas. Papillomas are delicate, friable tumors formed on thin stalks covered by frondlike excrescences. They are often multiple and very rarely metastasize. By hemorrhage, infection, and occasionally obstructions they may produce a malignant course for the patient as a whole even though microscopically they are benign.

There is a direct correlation in the survival rate not only with the degree of malignancy but also with the stage of the tumor at the time of treatment. Usually the stage and grade of the tumor go hand in hand. Stage 0 tumors are confined to the mucosa only and are most commonly histologically benign papillomas. Stage A means a depth of penetration no deeper than the submucosa. Stage B_1 and B_2 describe invasion of the muscle, halfway and deeper, respectively. Involvement of the perivesical fat is Stage C, and distant metastases or involvement of adjacent organs, such as the prostate, Stage D. Figure 6-1 is a diagram of staging. The prognosis varies from a 70 per cent five-year survival for low-grade, low-stage neoplasia to 15 per cent in high-grade, high-stage lesions. This system, or the similarly based international classification, is presently

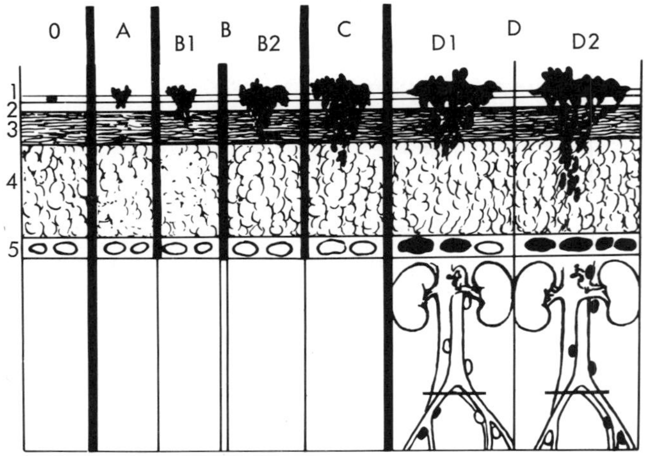

FIGURE 6-1. A method of staging bladder tumors.

O, limited to mucosa.
A, not beyond submucosa.
B_1, not more than halfway through muscle layer.
B_2, beyond the halfway level of the muscle layer, but not into fat.
C, beyond the muscle layer, but not metastatic, or invading the substance of adjacent organs.
D_1, metastatic to the pelvic lymph nodes and/or invading the substance of adjacent organs.
D_2, metastatic beyond the pelvis.

(Modified from Marshall, Victor F.: *Textbook of Urology*, 2nd ed. Hoeber Medical Division, Harper & Row, New York, 1964.)

used, although an even more detailed classification has recently been proposed by Whitmore.

Adenocarcinomas of the bladder are quite rare and most often are associated with a tumor arising from glandular tissue residual in the urachus or a preexisting cystitis glandularis. Leukoplakia, a form of chronic cystitis, is thought by some to be a precursor of squamous-cell carcinoma. Although this holds true for such lesions in the mouth and vulva, a transformation to carcinoma in the urinary bladder has been rare in our experience except in severe cases of this change. Sarcomas are generally very malignant, rare, and encountered mainly in children.

Although low-grade papillomas of the renal pelvis and ureter might be treated by local excision in exceptional instances, such as a uremic patient who needs all the renal function he can retain, the accepted therapy is complete removal of the kidney, entire ureter, and a cuff of bladder at the ureteral orifice. The reason for such extensive surgery is that tumor recurrence in the ureteral stump is very high.

The primary modality for bladder tumors is surgical. The method used will depend on the location of the tumor, grade of malignancy, the depth of bladder wall penetration, and the ability of the surgeon. Methods used are transurethral resection, wherein the tumor (or tumors) is removed piecemeal by use of an electrified wire cutting loop. This can also be accomplished by open surgery on the bladder. A portion of the bladder may be removed (segmental resection), or a total cystectomy can be done. A radical cystectomy is an en bloc removal of the entire bladder and the pelvic lymph nodes along with prostate and seminal vesicles in the male patient or en bloc removal with uterus, tubes, ovaries, and upper vagina in the female. The margins of resection in a radical cystectomy are limited only by the lateral walls of the bony pelvis, whereas in a simple cystectomy the margin is close to the bladder. If there are lymph node metastases, the prognosis for cure is bleak indeed unless these metastases are close to the bladder and few in number. After the bladder has been removed, the urinary stream must be diverted elsewhere. The problem of such urinary diversion will be discussed later in this text.

The present status of radiation therapy for bladder neoplasia is uncertain. Occasionally it has produced remarkable remissions—even cures—but it is not generally used by us as the only means of treatment. One of the present regimens includes preoperative radiation to the bladder of 2000 roentgens tumor dose followed by surgery a month later. The complications encountered after higher doses have been impressively frequent. Chemotherapy against vesical carcinomas has so far been disappointing. Systemic treatment for disseminated disease presently offers no significant benefit. A useful adjunct against superficial low-grade cancers or papillomas may be local instillations of triethylenethiophosphoramide (Thio-TEPA) about once a month for a year or more.

Benign Prostatic Hypertrophy

Noncancerous enlargement of the prostate gland is a common affliction of the elderly male. Its practical significance is not the enlargement itself but obstruction to free flow of urine consequent to narrowing of the prostatic urethra. The symptoms of this obstruction (prostatism) follow, and compensatory changes occur in the bladder musculature. As the obstruction progresses, the bladder eventually decompensates, and increasingly larger amounts of residual urine are left behind. Infection is frequently associated with the residual urine. Finally, the effects of back pressure and infection are transmitted to the upper urinary tracts with ensuing hydroureter, hydronephrosis, and progressive renal damage leading to uremia and death from renal failure in the neglected patient.

The changes that occur in the prostate are due to the hyperplasia of the periurethral prostatic glands, which, as they grow, form an adenoma that compresses the true capsule of the prostate.

Therefore, in the last analysis, the term *benign prostatic hypertrophy* is a misnomer. Although noncancerous, it can be malignant enough to kill the patient if the severity of obstruction is not appreciated. The condition is a newgrowth (hyperplasia) rather than a true hypertrophy of preexisting tissue. The treatment of benign prostatic hypertrophy is surgical removal of the adenoma. Once developed, the condition cannot be changed by hormonal therapy, although it can be prevented by castration in youth—a drastic form of prophylaxis. Recently some experimental improvement has been accomplished with testosterone enanthate but apparently not to a useful degree.

Carcinoma of the Prostate

Carcinoma of the prostate is a common cancer of the aging male. The majority of prostate cancers begin in the posterior lobe (true capsule), an area that is not removed in the usual enucleation procedures for benign enlargements. Since the posterior lobe is located farther away from the prostatic urethra than the remainder of the gland, the presence of urinary symptoms as a presenting complaint usually indicates advanced disease. Another common presenting complaint is low backache or hip pain due to metastases to the vertebrae, pelvis, and femur. Consequently, the best method to discover an early curable prostatic carcinoma is by careful routine rectal digital examinations of men over the age of 45 years.

Most prostatic cancers are adenocarcinomas. The tumor spreads locally to the seminal vesicles and the base of the bladder. The lymph nodes of the pelvis are involved early. Spread to the skeleton can occur through the lymphatics but does so primarily by venous channels which anastomose luxuriantly up and down the vertebral column. The upper urinary tract eventually becomes damaged from local enlargement with bladder outlet obstruction and gradual impingement on the lower ureters with hydronephrosis and superimposed infection.

The diagnosis is made by the histologic demonstration of the carcinoma. Rectal digital examination may reveal a small suspicious nodule in the prostate or a stony hard, fixed gland in the more advanced situation. In the early, potentially curable patient, a biopsy should be obtained by an open perineal exposure of the prostate, at which time a frozen section is obtained and ablative surgery is performed. If curative operation is indicated, provided the lesion is carcinomatous, open exploration will be needed whether or not a needle biopsy shows cancer, since the exclusive value of such a biopsy is rather low. With advanced disease, tissue can be obtained by the perineal needle biopsy or by transurethral resection. X-rays of the lower lumbar vertebrae, bony pelvis, and upper femora may show the characteristic osteoblastic metastases. These must first be differentiated from other disorders of bone, particularly Paget's disease. Several blood studies can be of value, particularly determination of acid phosphatase. This is an enzyme produced by prostatic tissue and is elevated in the blood in about 75 per cent of patients in whom the tumor has extended beyond the prostatic capsule. Only rarely will other disorders raise this value. However, a normal acid phosphatase determination is of little help in ruling out prostate cancer. Alkaline phosphatase is an enzyme that is usually elevated in the blood when bony metastases are present. This nonspecific elevation is seen in numerous conditions involving the production of bone and also with biliary osbtruction. Another enzyme that should be evaluated is fibrinolysin, particularly in patients for whom surgery is contemplated. A high level of this enzyme of prostatic origin in the blood may lead to uncontrollable hemorrhage from dissolution of blood clots.

A small carcinoma of the prostate with no demonstrable extension of the tumor beyond the prostatic capsule can be treated by a radical prostaticoseminal vesiculectomy. In contrast to the enucleation procedures for noncancerous conditions, a radical removal is defined as removal of the entire prostate, including the true capsule and the seminal vesicles en bloc. The divided bladder neck and membranous urethra are then approximated to fill in the gap. Such an operation can be performed via a retropubic or a perineal approach.

What of the patients who are not candidates for radical surgery? This group certainly represents the large majority of patients with prostatic cancer. Are they doomed to a rapid painful death?

Fortunately, although most patients with prostatic cancer are not curable when first seen, much can be done for the "incurable" patient. The majority of prostate cancers are hormonally dependent. They grow with androgens and regress with estrogens. Most of the male sex hormone is produced by the Leydig cells of the testis, although some is of adrenal origin. Therefore, orchiectomy will remove most of the androgens. Small doses of estrogens can be given orally to suppress growth. There is no good evidence that larger doses of estrogens give any additional benefit. With such treatment, 50 per cent of patients with incurable prostate cancer will be alive five years later. The five-year survival after radical prostatectomy is not much different. The difference lies, however, with the survival at ten years and later. At this time only 5 to 10 per cent of the conservatively treated patients and 30 per cent of those treated by radical prostatectomy will be alive. To complicate the problem further, patients who have undergone such surgery will certainly be impotent, and about 5 to 10 per cent will have deficient urinary control, varying from stress incontinence to complete incontinence. Consequently, factors other than local operability, such as the life expectancy of the patient if he did not have prostate cancer, must be weighed before advice is given. Removal of the adrenal glands or the pituitary gland has not generally prolonged life significantly, i.e., years, although such surgery can afford much relief of pain from bone metastases when the patient no longer responds to estrogens. Although hormonal therapy certainly provides great symptomatic relief—and one would think an increased longevity on that account alone—serious doubts are being raised as to when therapy should be begun. Some physicians feel that hormonal treatment (with transurethral resection) to relieve obstruction, if present, is the method of choice even in apparently "curable" cases.

Tumors of the External Genitalia

The usual neoplasm of the penis is an epidermoid carcinoma. This cancer is rare in a person who has been circumcised in infancy and is associated with a lack of personal cleanliness. Penile cancer is not common in this country, and one intrepid observer noted that if a surgeon performed a circumcision every ten minutes, eight hours a day, and five days a week, he would have to operate somewhere between six and twenty-nine years to prevent one cancer of the penis! This disease is treated by wide excision (usually partial penectomy) and dissection of the inguinal lymph nodes.

Papillomatous lesions of the penile urethra are treated by ablative surgery, although a tissue differentiation must be made between a neoplastic lesion and condylomata acuminata, a noncancerous papilloma of viral origin.

Scrotal tumors are usually epidermoid carcinomas and are uncommon. These are also treated by wide excision with or without inguinal node dissection. At one time in history, this was an occupational hazard of two kinds of laborers—chimney sweeps and mule spinners in cotton factories. Constant exposure of the scrotal skin to coal tars lining chimneys or oil in the cotton mill was the irritant.

Malignant neoplasms of the testis are not common. Statistically the inguinal undescended testes have a ten times greater chance of developing cancer than the normally descended ones, and the intraabdominal ones about forty to fifty times greater. However, cancers in normally descended testes are so rare that even this increased chance is so low that prophylactic removal seems at least no more than elective. Ninety five per cent of testis tumors arise from the germinal epithelium. They may be composed of a uniform cell type, or several cell types may appear concomitantly in a single tumor. The various types include seminoma, embryonal-cell carcinoma, teratocarcinoma, and choriocarcinoma. Such tumors are commoner in younger men and all have a high degree of malignancy. Metastases are lymphatic and blood borne. Spread is directly to the periaortic lymph nodes, following which the mediastinal and supraclavicular nodes are involved.

Treatment following the removal of the primary tumor is directed to the sites of metastases and is surgical, radiologic, and chemical, or combinations thereof, depending on the tumor type. The high sensitivity of seminomas to radiation results in an 80 to 90 per cent five-year survival rate following excision of the primary tumor and such therapy to the node-bearing areas when metastases are not discernible on presentation of the patient. Less desirable results are obtained with embryonal-cell carcinoma and teratocarcinoma, which are much less sensitive to radiation. Periaortic retroperitoneal node dissection and radiotherapy are used, frequently complemented by chemotherapeutic agents, of which actinomycin D seems most effective. Pure choriocarcinoma is extremely malignant, and, despite all means of treatment, the five-year survival rate in male patients is almost zero. This is in contradistinction to female patients with the histologically identical cancer, for whom methotrexate has wrought great improvement.

REVIEW QUESTIONS

1. Define the following tumors: hypernephroma, Wilms' tumor, neuroblastoma. Describe common presenting symptoms of each.
2. Discuss the staging and grading of bladder tumors and how they affect prognosis and treatment.
3. Why is the term *benign prostatic hypertrophy* a misnomer?
4. What blood tests are useful in the diagnosis of prostatic cancer? How accurate are they?
5. Discuss the hormonal treatment of prostatic cancer.
6. List the varieties of testicular cancer and the methods of treatment for each.

CHAPTER 7

Miscellaneous Disorders of the Urinary Tract

Injury of the Urinary Tract

SINCE the kidneys are well protected, a fair degree of force is necessary to injure them. The majority of renal injuries are *contusions*, wherein the capsule remains intact but there is intrarenal bleeding often accompanied by some degree of hematuria. A *laceration* implies more severe injury accompanied by tearing of the capsule progressing to a frank *rupture*. Severe damage to a kidney is more likely if a preexisting renal disorder, usually hydronephrosis, is present. The majority of renal injuries can be treated expectantly with frequent observation of the patient for signs of hemorrhagic shock, a progressively enlarging flank mass, or ecchymosis in the flank. Surgery for renal injury often ends with nephrectomy, since little safe reparative work may be possible. Consequently, a knowledge of the status of the opposite kidney early in the course of treatment is important. If necessary, an intravenous pyelogram can be performed directly in bed to assess the status of both kidneys.

Injuries to the ureters by external force or even direct penetrating injuries are relatively uncommon. More common by far are injuries sustained as a result of surgery on adjacent structures, such as the large bowel, uterus, ovaries, and lumbar sympathetic ganglia. These injuries include complete and incomplete tears and unrecognized ligation. Treatment depends on the severity of the injury and its location in the ureter. For example, injuries of the upper ureter are best treated by reanastomosis with drainage by a splinting catheter. Injuries close to the bladder are best treated by reimplantation of the ureter into the bladder.

Bladder injuries are more common when the organ is full of urine. The most common cause of such injury is a fracture of the bony pelvis wherein a spicule of bone pierces the full bladder. Proper treatment includes continuous drainage of the bladder, preferably by a cystostomy catheter, and closure of the injury site. Injuries of the external genitalia are usually avulsions of the loosely applied skin of this area. Trauma to the urethra is mostly blunt straddle injury wherein the urethra is forcefully compressed against the pubis. Treatment involves repair of the injury, adequate drainage of the area, and usually temporary diversion of the urinary stream.

Cystic Disorders of the Kidneys

The two commonest cystic disorders of the kidneys are *solitary* cysts and *polycystic* kidney disease. Solitary cysts are probably acquired lesions occurring most frequently in the fifth decade of life and later years. Their origin may be related to an interference of the blood supply to a localized area of kidney with associated tubular obstruction. Their greatest importance is that they must be differentiated from other mass lesions of the kidney, particularly cancer. Of secondary importance is local compression of the surrounding renal parenchyma by the cyst as the lesion expands. Rarely, cancer is present within a cyst cavity.

Once a mass lesion of the kidney is discovered by physical examination and intravenous or retrograde pyelograms, a differential diagnosis between cyst and tumor can be reached in the majority of patients by means of renal arteriography or nephrotomography. An absolute diagnosis for a specific patient can be settled only by surgical exploration. Removal of that portion of the cyst wall extending beyond the kidney (decapsulation) will cure a cyst nicely. An attempt to remove the entire cyst wall is not necessary for cure and converts a benign operation into a bloody and dangerous one. Rarely, in very poor-risk patients, a reasonably correct diagnosis can be made in large cysts by percutaneous aspiration and examination of the cyst fluid for malignant cells accompanied by x-ray after injection of contrast material into the cyst cavity. The discovery of bloody rather than the characteristically clear fluid within a solitary cyst greatly increases the likelihood of an occult malignancy.

Polycystic kidney disease is a condition wherein the majority of the kidney tissue is eventually replaced by thousands of cysts of varying sizes. The condition is often hereditary and may appear in several members of a family. It is usually bilateral and such kidneys may become so large as to entirely fill the abdomen. Often, such cystic changes may appear along with the kidney involvement in other organs, particularly the liver, pancreas, and lung. As time progresses, intracystic hemorrhages, infection, and loss of functioning kidney tissue by enlarging cysts result in uremia, anemia, and death. This process is slow and the average patient dies in the fourth or fifth decade. There is no adequate treatment except the supportive management of anemia, uremia, and infection. Operative decapsulation of the cysts has had little to offer.

There are many other kinds of renal cystic disorders, many of which are incompatible with life. *Multicystic kidney disease* is a congenital disorder, usually involving only one kidney, wherein the organ is completely replaced by several large cystic masses and often associated with an absent (or nondemonstrable) renal artery on that side and atresia of the ureter.

Hypertension

It has long been known that hypertensive patients frequently have changes within their kidneys consisting of arteriolar thickening. Assuming that the thus decreased intrarenal blood flow was the cause of hypertension, Goldblatt constricted the renal arteries of dogs and was able to produce sustained hypertension. Further investigation has shown that partial blockage of the main renal arteries or their branches in hypertensive patients is not rare and that such a situation frequently represents a curable form of hypertension. This is generally referred to as renovascular hypertension. The causative mechanism is not completely understood. A decrease in either pulse pressure or blood flow acts to release renin into the bloodstream. Renin acts on an inert circulating decapeptide, which is then converted to an octapeptide called angiotensin. Angiotensin has a powerful effect on maintaining vascular tone and blood pressure. Unfortunately, blood assays for circulating renin and angiotensin are not simple or readily available. The diagnosis must be made on clinical suspicion, changes in the intravenous pyelogram, renal arteriograms, and the findings of specific divided renal function studies. The treatment consists of either improving the defective blood supply by various angioplastic techniques or nephrectomy.

Another form of hypertension of interest to the urologist is that caused by neoplasia of the adrenal medulla known as pheochromocytoma. These tumors are usually noncancerous and most often arise in the adrenals, but they may arise anywhere along the sympathetic chain. By their production of norepinephrine, these tumors usually cause spasmodic episodes of marked hypertension. The demonstration of an increased 24-hour urinary excretion of catecholamines is the best way to make the diagnosis. Another form of hypertension of adrenal origin is hyperaldosteronism. This is caused by increased secretion of the mineralocorticoid aldosterone, which has a strong effect on sodium and water retention. The hormone may be produced either by hyperplasia of the adrenal or by a functioning tumor.

Disorders of the Bladder and Urethra

Infections and inflammations of the bladder and urethra of nonspecific causes are common in both sexes. Such diagnoses imply that specific factors have been ruled out. These specific factors include obstructions, foreign bodies, neoplasia, and specific infections such as tuberculosis.

Cystitis symptoms in the female patient include urgency, frequency, burning, nocturia, and suprapubic discomfort. These symptoms may come on acutely and be associated with severe frequency and burning, often with terminal or total gross hematuria. An associated fever is rare and, if present, implies kidney infection also. Cultures may show nonspecific bacteria and the symptoms will respond readily to hot sitz baths, increased fluid intake, and administration of relatively benign chemotherapeutic agents. The bladder, at this stage, is usually quite inflamed.

Chronic cystitis symptoms are common among women. Frequently there will be few findings on urinalyses, and cultures are often sterile. The symptoms frequently respond to local therapy such as gentle urethral dilation, insertion of agents such as 1:5000 silver nitrate solution, etc. Occasionally a source of irritation may be infected Skene's glands, which surround the urethral meatus. Fulguration of these glands occasionally prevents recurrent attacks. Local and oral estrogens in the elderly patient may toughen these tissues to increase the resistance to irritation. Treatment with appropriate antibacterial agents as determined by urine cultures may be indicated.

Other less common kinds of cystitides are those resulting from radiation therapy and interstitial cystitis. The latter is fortunately rare but an interesting, poorly understood disorder. It is manifested by ulceration of the bladder mucosa and a gradual decrease in bladder capacity due to fibrosis of the wall. Consequently, these patients must urinate at frequent intervals day and night with much associated pain. The bladder mucosa is pale and fragile. Distention of the bladder may result in a stellate crack with accompanying ulceration and bleeding. Treatment consists of bladder dilatations under anesthesia, fulguration of the ulcers, surgery to divide sacral nerve roots ad infinitum. The results are generally unsatisfactory.

Chronic nonspecific urethritis in the male patient is another common disorder of little consequence but of great concern to the patient. This is usually manifested by a mild urethral discharge, particularly in the morning, burning or "tingling" on urination, and vague aches and pains. After specific causes have been ruled out, treatment consists of eradication of any demonstrable infection, adequate sexual hygiene, occasionally prostatic massage, and much reassurance. Infection within the prostate may be assessed by examination of prostatic secretions after massage.

Incontinence

Incontinence, or lack of urinary control, can vary from the extremes of a slight leakage of urine on rare occasions to complete loss of urinary control. *Stress* incontinence by definition is the loss of urine under conditions such as coughing, laughing, and lifting of heavy packages. This condition is most commonly found in women after traumatic labor with damage to bladder supports. When the condition is severe, surgical correction is indicated. This may involve a vaginal repair of the bladder and urethral supports or a suprapubic vesicourethral suspension (Marshall-Marchetti operation). There are many other causes of incontinence, including traumatic damage to the urinary sphincters, urinary fistulas as a result of surgery, radiation, or cancer, and congenital fistulas such as ectopic ureteral orifices.

Disorders of the nerve supply to the bladder and perineum can also cause incontinence in a condition known as a *neurogenic bladder*. The defect may involve the sacral reflex arc (lower motor neuron), a level above this arc (upper motor neuron), or a combined lesion. Lower motor neuron lesions are usually manifested by a flaccid bladder with poor motor power. Upper motor neuron lesions manifest themselves by spasticity, a low capacity, and frequent uncontrollable contractions. In both situations, there is often damage to the upper urinary tracts by ineffectual bladder emptying. Hydronephrosis, vesicoureteral reflux, and infection follow. Frequently the only thing that can be done is to divert the urinary stream out of the bladder to preserve renal function. Recent attempts have been made to insert indwelling electronic stimulators to improve bladder function but, by and large, these have not been successful.

REVIEW QUESTIONS

1. Discuss the various degrees of renal injury.
2. What is the condition most commonly associated with traumatic rupture of the bladder?
3. Discuss the forms of cystic kidney disease and their significance.
4. Describe the present concept of renovascular hypertension.
5. What is cystitis? Discuss several forms of the disorder.
6. What is meant by urinary incontinence, and what are some common causes of this problem?

REFERENCES—UNIT I

Abbott Laboratories: *Fluid and Electrolytes.* Abbott Laboratories, North Chicago, Ill., 1960.

Albright, Fuller, and Esther Bloomberg: "Hyperthyroidism and Renal Diseases," *J Urol*, **34**: 1–7, 1935.

Albuquerque, Paulo F., Rodolpho Forster, and Roberto Zanandrea: "Etiological Factors in Urolithiasis: A Clinical Analysis of 275 Cases," *J Urol*, **89**: 325–28, 1963.

Barnes, Roger W.: "Prostatic Tumors—Surgical Treatment," Part I, *Amer J Nurs*, **56**: 982–85, 1956.

Campbell, Meredith F., ed.: *Urology*, 3 vols. W. B. Saunders Co., Philadelphia, 1963.

Cooper, H. G.: "Treatment of Genito-Urinary Tuberculosis: Report After 14 Years," *J Urol*, **86**: 719–27, 1961.

Cox, C. E., and F. Hinman, Jr.: "Experiments with Induced Bacteriuria, Vesical Emptying and Bacterial Growth on the Mechanism of Bladder Defense to Infection," *J Urol*, **86**: 739, 1961.

Davis, Joseph E.: "Drugs for Urologic Disorders," *Amer J Nurs*, **65**: 107–12, 1965.

Dick, Vernon S.: "Carcinoma of the Prostate Gland with Metastases," *Surg Clin N Amer*, **42**: 771–97, 1962.

Dixon, Frank J., and Robert A. Moore: "Testicular Tumors. A Clinicopathological Study," *Cancer*, **6**: 427–54, 1953.

Franks, L. M.: "Benign Nodular Hyperplasia of Prostate: Review," *Ann Roy Coll Surg Eng*, **14**: 92–106, 1954.

Friedman, Nathan B., and Robert A. Moore: "Tumors of the Testis," *Milit Surg*, **99**: 573–93, 1946.

Goldblatt, Harry: *The Renal Origin of Hypertension.* Charles C. Thomas, Springfield, Ill., 1948.

Grant, John Charles Boileau: *An Atlas of Anatomy*, 5th ed. Williams & Wilkins, Baltimore, 1962.

Grayhack, John T.: "Hormonal Treatment of Prostatic Cancer," *Surg Clin N Amer*, **39**: 13–27, 1959.

Guyton, Arthur C.: *Textbook of Medical Physiology*, 3rd ed. W. B. Saunders Co., Philadelphia, 1966.

Hand, John R.: "Infections of the Urinary Tract," *Amer J Nurs*, **57**: 1008–10, 1957.

Heckel, Norris J.: "Kidney Stones: Their Etiology and Treatment," *Amer J Nurs*, **55**: 194–97, 1955.

Higham, A. R. C.: "Stone in the Urinary Tract," *Nurs Mirror*, **122**: 8–10, 1966.

Huggins, Charles, R. E. Stevens, Jr., and Clarence V. Hodges: "Studies on Prostatic Cancer: The Effects of Castration on Advanced Carcinoma of the Prostate Gland," *Arch Surg*, **43**: 209–22, 1941.

Keuhnelian, John G., Francis Bartone, and Victor F. Marshall: "Practical

Considerations from Autopsies on Azotemic Patients," *J Urol*, **89**: 467–73, 1964.

Kimber, Diana C., Carolyn E. Gray, Caroline E. Stackpole, and Lutie C. Leavell: *Anatomy and Physiology*, 15th ed. The Macmillan Co., New York, 1966.

Lattimer, John K.: "The Treatment of Tuberculous Infections of the Genitourinary tract," *J Urol*, **74**: 291–300, 1955.

Littlepage, Sylvia: "Genitourinary Injuries—Nursing Care," *Amer J Nurs*, **55**: 973–74, 1955.

Marshall, Victor F.: *The Diagnosis of Genitourinary Neoplasms*. American Cancer Society, New York, 1949.

Marshall, Victor F.: *Textbook of Urology*, 2nd ed. Hoeber Medical Division, Harper & Row, New York, 1964.

Methany, Norma M., and William D. Snively, Jr.: *Nurses Handbook of Fluid Balance*. J. B. Lippincott Co., Philadelphia, 1967.

Morin, Lawrence J., and Charles H. Hemminger: "Bladder Tumors: A Ten-Year Review," *J Urol*, **87**: 368–72, 1962.

Musser, Ruth D., and Joseph G. Bird: *Modern Pharmacology and Therapeutics*, 2nd ed. The Macmillan Co., New York, 1962.

Osathanondh, Vitoon, and Edith L. Potter: "Pathogenesis of Polycystic Kidneys," *Arch Path*, **77**: 459–65, 1964.

Parkhurst, Edward, and Ernest K. Landsteiner: "Management of Renal Trauma," *Surg Gynec Obstet*, **105**: 393–400, 1957.

Rose, John F.: "Management of the Patient with Trauma of the Urinary Tract," *Med Clin N Amer*, **48**: 1633–54, 1964.

Smith, Donald R.: *General Urology*, 5th ed. Lange Medical Publications, Los Altos, Cal., 1966.

Smith, Homer W.: *Principles of Renal Physiology*. Oxford University Press, New York, 1956.

Spence, Harry M.: "Urinary Tract Infections in Infants and Children," *J Urol*, **91**: 623–38, 1964.

Statland, Harry: *Fluids and Electrolytes in Practice*, 3rd ed. J. B. Lippincott Co., Philadelphia, 1963.

Winter, Chester C., Marilyn M. Roehm, and Harriet Grant Watson: "Urinary Calculi, Medical and Surgical Management," *Amer J Nurs*, **63**: 72–74, 1963.

Zinsser, Hans H.: "Urinary Calculi." *JAMA*, **174**: 2062–65, 1960.

UNIT II

Diagnosis of Urologic Disorders: General Principles and Nursing Considerations

CHAPTER 8
History and Physical Examination

THE patient with a disorder of the genitourinary system undergoes a thorough diagnostic evaluation before treatment of his condition is undertaken. Basic essentials of the evaluation are a careful history and physical examination as well as appropriate laboratory studies of the blood and urine. Following these the urologist has at hand a wide variety of highly refined instruments and diagnostic techniques that permit visual and radiographic examination of the urinary tract. With a complete history, physical examination, and the available diagnostic procedures, it is rare that an accurate diagnosis cannot be made prior to any necessary surgery.

The nurse's responsibilities during the diagnostic phase of the patient's illness are many and varied. Because of her frequent and often intimate contacts with the patient, she may elicit facts or make observations that give the doctor data essential to fit together the pieces of the diagnostic puzzle. The nurse must understand the purpose of the various diagnostic procedures, how they are performed, and her specific responsibilities in relation to their successful completion. In her zeal to perform the technical functions related to the study, the nurse must not forget that the patient is vitally concerned with all the proceedings and needs understanding, reassurance, and explanation. It has been shown repeatedly that the patient who knows why and how a test is to be done is less fearful, is more cooperative, and has greater confidence in those responsible for his care. Diagnostic studies, when accurately performed, will lead to more prompt diagnosis and treatment. This is certainly the ultimate goal desired by the patient, doctor, and nurse.

History

An accurate history is the first and most important step in diagnosis, and this must include the general history as well as the genitourinary history.

In the general history, it is important to learn of abnormal conditions associated with other body systems. Since the urologist sees many patients in the older age group, he must be particularly familiar with those disorders related to the aging process. Commonly encountered disorders are those of the cardiovascular system such as coronary artery disease, cerebrovascular disease, and peripheral vascular insufficiency. Pulmonary problems such as chronic bronchitis, emphysema, and bronchiectasis are common. Metabolic disorders such as diabetes mellitus and gout are more frequent in the elderly. With the presence of any of these conditions, it may be necessary for the urologist to modify or revise the plan of treatment of the genitourinary disorder.

An accurate, precise genitourinary history is often difficult to obtain. Because of limited knowledge resulting from various cultural and social taboos, the patient may have a poor understanding of the anatomy and function of this system. Often, too, because of fear, embarrassment, or guilt, he may be vague in describing his symptoms. It is also true that symptoms of certain genitourinary disorders are subtle and insidious in onset or transient in occurrence, so that the patient may be unaware of any abnormality. Therefore, the urologist must be skillful in eliciting facts by an attitude of sincere interest and sympathetic understanding to allay the patient's fear and gain his confidence.

The first step in the history is to record the patient's presenting symptoms in his own words—the chief complaint. From this point, the doctor's questions will be directed toward a precise amplification of these symptoms. How long have these symptoms been present? Have they been getting worse, or are they about the same? Have they been persistent or intermittent? If there has been pain, what have been its character, location, and severity? Did the symptoms appear suddenly, or have they been developing gradually? Frequently, one can evaluate the severity of pain by comparison with other pain in the patient's past experience. For example, it is not uncommon for women to voluntarily state that the pain of renal colic is more severe than the discomfort of childbirth.

The examiner can then inquire about seemingly unrelated facts. Has there been an unexplained weight loss and lethargy suggestive of a slowly developing disorder such as neoplasm, tuberculosis, or chronic renal failure? Have there been any fevers suggestive of infection? Is there a recent history of a streptococcal pharyngitis leading toward a suspicion of glomerulonephritis? What disturbances have there been in urinary habits, and have there been any observable color changes in the urine?

The family history and occupational history may be significant. A history of numerous deaths of family members from a kidney disorder at age 40 to 50 might suggest polycystic kidney disease. Renal calculous disease frequently seems to run in families. The urinary tract is subject to certain occupational hazards. Of purely historic interest is the chimney sweep's disease. In nineteenth-century England, chimney sweeps climbed down chimneys brushing away accumulated soot. The coal tars in the soot chronically irritated the scrotum, and these workers commonly incurred carcinoma in this part of the body. Other known occupational hazards are the high incidence of bladder tumors in aniline dye workers and a significant incidence of renal brucellosis in packinghouse workers.

If the patient is a child, the doctor will want the mother to describe any unusual occurrences during pregnancy and delivery. A history of maternal medication during pregnancy may be significant. For example, progestational compounds during early gestation may result in female pseudohermaphroditism. The recently documented effects of thalidomide are only too well known. The developmental history is important. At what age was the child toilet-trained, and at what age did bed-wetting cease or is it still present? After five years of age, enuresis is usually considered abnormal and may be caused by a urinary tract disorder. Did the child sit, stand, and talk at the expected time? Has the mother noted the size and force of the child's voiding stream? Does the child void with ease, or is micturition accompanied by straining, grunting, or visible signs of pain? Does the child, on the other hand, void infrequently as compared with siblings? Is there any history of abdominal pain, recurrent unexplained fevers, or documented urinary tract infections? Have urinalyses or urine cultures been obtained in the past, and if so what were the findings?

Symptoms frequently associated with genitourinary disorders are abnormalities related to micturition and abnormalities in the appearance of the urine.

Symptoms Related to Micturition

There is a large vocabulary to describe the symptoms related to micturition. Many of these terms have precise meanings and are related to a specific physiologic process. Other terms, however, are more general and if used out of context are inaccurate and misleading. It is important, therefore, that the nurse know the definition of these terms and their correct usage, so that she will better understand her patient's condition and be able to communicate accurately and more effectively with the doctor and her co-workers.

Three terms—*micturition*, *voiding*, and *urination*—are commonly used to describe the act of discharging urine from the body. *Frequency* is a relative term which implies urination more often than usual for that specific patient. The volume at each voiding may be the usual amount or may be diminished. Frequent urination accompanied by small volumes usually indicates a urinary tract disorder, although psychogenic factors must be considered. Frequent urination with normal or larger volumes at each passage can better be termed *polyuria*. This may be due to a correspondingly high oral fluid intake or suggest disease such as diabetes mellitus or diabetes insipidus. Another cause can be the ingestion of diuretics such as are used for congestive heart failure. A well-known plebeian diuretic effect, usually manifested by frequent large voidings, follows the drinking of large amounts of beer.

A small total urinary output (*oliguria*) requires immediate investigation. Output in any 24-hour period less than 100 ml is referred to as anuria. Rarely will this be noted in extreme dehydration. The critical differential is to determine whether urine is being produced and retained or whether there is actual cessation of urine production. The first step the urologist would take would be to insert a catheter into the bladder. If urine still failed to appear, he would investigate more thoroughly to demonstrate the patency of at least one upper urinary tract. If the problem still remained unsolved, he could investigate the integrity of the renal circulation.

Frequent urination with small volumes suggest irritation and sensitivity of the lower urinary tract from various causes. These may include infections, foreign bodies, contracture of the bladder, or a relatively diminished capacity due to large amounts of residual urine. *Urgency*, another symptom of irritation is a sudden almost uncontrollable desire to urinate. If this is severe enough so that there is actual loss of urine, it is then called *urgency incontinence*. *Nocturia* means voiding during the night. Voiding once during the night is not necessarily abnormal, but when it is more frequent, an abnormality must be suspected. It is again important to determine whether the patient voids only a small amount, as seen in urinary tract disorders, as contrasted to a large amount from a large fluid intake or systemic disease such as diabetes mellitus. One must also differentiate as to whether he is awakened from a sound sleep by the necessity to urinate or whether he is a poor sleeper who eases the tedium of sleeplessness by relieving his bladder.

Severe, frequent, painful urination of the worst sort is called *strangury*, a most descriptive term. This is seen with marked irritation and with pronounced decrease in bladder capacity, such as in tuberculous or interstitial cystitis.

Hesitancy, *intermittency*, and *dribbling* are often associated with lower tract obstruction, most commonly prostatic enlargement. *Hesitancy* implies difficulty in starting to urinate. *Intermittency* refers to temporary cessation of the stream during micturition; one of its causes may be an intermittent corklike obstruction by a bladder calculus. The word *dribbling* is self-explanatory.

The combination of symptoms such as frequency, urgency, nocturia, hesitancy, and poor stream results so often from obstruction by an enlarged prostate that the clinical syndrome is called prostatism. This does not mean that prostatic enlargement is the sole cause for such a history, but it is the usual offender. *Burning*, as its name implies, is an uncomfortable warm sensation on voiding and usually signifies inflammation in the passages, particularly in the urethra. The term *dysuria* is quite nonspecific and merely implies painful or difficult urination.

One of the most distressing symptoms is *incontinence* or the loss of voluntary urinary control. *Total incontinence*, the continuous leakage of urine, may result from trauma to the urinary sphincter, from damage to the nerves supplying the lower urinary tract, or from a urinary fistula. An ectopic ureter is in effect a congenital fistula which may cause incontinence if it opens distal to the external sphincter or into the vagina. If the other ureter enters the bladder normally, these patients give a history of apparently normal micturition with persistent dribbling in between. The patient who has a large residual urine because of bladder outlet obstruction or neurogenic dysfunction may have *overflow incontinence*. Small amounts of urine will be expelled when the volume of retained urine raises the intravesical pressure enough to partially overcome the obstruction. A frequent complaint of women who have had injuries or weakening of bladder supports, most often after a difficult childbirth, is that of *stress incontinence*. It occurs at a time of physical strain. Sneezing, coughing, or lifting a heavy object may cause a sudden jet of urine to be expelled from the urethra.

Abnormalities in the Appearance of the Urine

Hematuria means blood in the urine. Not all red urine is due to blood. It can be caused by certain medications, such as phenolphthalein and pyridium. Metabolic disorders such as porphyria or simply the over-ingestion of beets can make the urine red. In the female patient, it is important to determine if the blood that is seen is coming from the urinary tract or the genital tract. Even though hematuria may be accompanied by no other significant symptoms, its appearance demands a thorough urologic evaluation, since this bleeding may be the first sign of serious disease. A clinical survey of 1000 patients with gross hematuria showed that 20 per cent of them had cancer of the urinary tract. Hematuria is a symptom in 80 per cent of cases in which a urinary neoplasm is eventually diagnosed.

The urologist will want to know when the bleeding first occurred, how long it was present, and if it was associated with other symptoms such as pain. The pain of renal colic would imply upper urinary tract bleeding. Were actual clots seen? A shoestring clot, for example, suggests ureteral bleeding. Was the bleeding *initial* (at the beginning of voiding), or *terminal* (at the end of voiding), or *total* (throughout the voiding). Initial and terminal hematuria usually imply a lower urinary tract origin. Total hematuria may arise anywhere from within the urinary tract. If there are no immediate contraindications to the procedure, a cystoscopic examination should be done at the time of bleeding if at all possible—this opportunity may never present itself again. Under such circumstances, the origin of the bleeding may be determined, resulting in earlier diagnosis and treatment.

Cloudy urine may or may not represent an abnormal condition. Cloudiness caused by the precipitation of phosphates in an alkaline urine is of little clinical significance and can be cleared by the addition of acetic acid to the specimen. Significant, however, is the cloudiness caused by pus cells. These cells can be readily identified by microscopic examination of the urine, and in this case the urine does not clear by the addition of acid. Lymph in the urine (*chyluria*) gives it a distinctly milky appearance. This, however, is a rare condition which can be proven by the demonstration of fat, rather than pus or phosphates, in the urine. The urine of patients with biliary tract disease, especially if jaundice is present, may contain bile pigments and appear yellow-brown. To check for these pigments, shake a small sample of urine. A yellow foam suggests the presence of bile, which can then be proven by more specific chemical determinations. Gas in the urine is called *pneumaturia*. The most common cause is from the introduction of air into the bladder during instrumentation, such as catheterization or cystoscopy. When disease is the underlying cause, it is usually due to a fistulous connection to the bladder from an air-containing organ, usually the large intestine. Such fistulas can be caused by pelvic neoplasms, infections, or trauma. A simple demonstration for pneumaturia is to have the patient urinate in a bathtub under water and observe the bubbles during micturition. Another rare cause of such a phenomenon is a gangrenous cystitis caused by gas-forming bacilli—a condition most often associated with diabetes.

Pain as Related to the Urinary Tract

Pain may be local or referred. Local pain occurs in the area of the involved organ. Referred pain originates in the involved organ but is felt at a distance owing to transmission along a common nerve supply. Thus, a stone obstructing a ureter can cause nausea, vomiting, ileus, and severe abdominal pain, symptoms also associated with an acute process of the gastrointestinal tract related to renovisceral reflexes.

Pain in the upper urinary tract is usually caused by an acute infectious or obstructive process. Kidney pain is felt at the level of the costovertebral angle, around the flank, and may radiate toward the umbilicus at the level of the twelfth rib on the affected side. This pain occurs when there is sudden overdistention of the capsule of the kidney, such as that produced by the edema of acute pyelonephritis or back pressure from a calculus obstructing the ureter. The absence of pain does not necessarily mean the absence of disease. If the disease process is gradual in onset, the compensatory ability of the kidney is such that a disorder may be present for a long time before giving rise to symptoms. This compensatory ability is true of other structures in the genitourinary tract and all too frequently accounts for the presence of far-advanced disease at the time of diagnosis. Ureteral pain occurs when the lumen of the ureter is suddenly obstructed. The cause of obstruction may be a blood clot or stone. This pain is usually severe, intermittent, and radiates from the costovertebral angle along the course of the ureter anteriorly to the lower abdominal quadrant and inner thigh. In men, the pain may be felt in the scrotum or testicle. In women, it may be felt in the vulva. The pain results from the overdistention of tissue, hyperperistalsis, and smooth muscle spasm as the ureter attempts to overcome the obstruction. Because the pain is paroxysmal in character, it is commonly referred to as renal colic. Figure 8-1 illustrates the usual pain radiation.

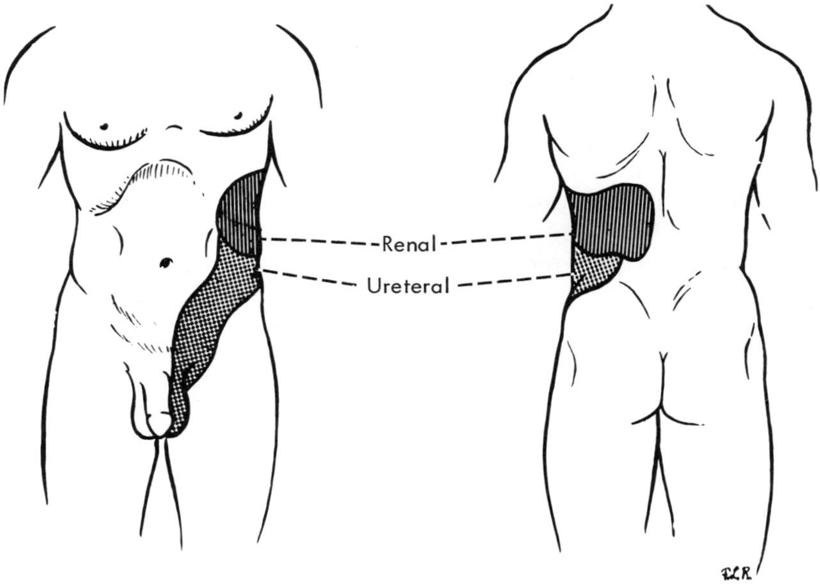

FIGURE 8-1. Location of renal and ureteral pain. (Reproduced by permission from Marshall, Victor F.: *Textbook of Urology*, 2nd ed. Hoeber Medical Division, Harper & Row, New York, 1964.)

Pain in the lower urinary tract is usually the result of infection and irritation such as might be caused by stones, tumors, obstructions, or specific infections. The various subjective symptoms associated with urination have been previously described in this chapter. Often with lower tract disturbances there is referral of pain, as an accompanying dull ache, to the rectum, perineum, and low back.

The Physical Examination

Following the history, the doctor performs a complete physical examination. This includes an examination of all systems, but particularly of the genitourinary system. The doctor will palpate the abdomen for tenderness and unusual masses. In normal individuals, except for those who are unusually thin, the kidneys are not palpable. If the kidney is enlarged or has an abnormal contour, as in hydronephrosis or tumor, these abnormalities can often be identified. In extremely thin patients or young children transillumination of a suspected renal mass may differentiate between a solid tumor or a hydronephrosis. Transillumination must be performed in a darkened room. A light source is placed behind the mass and the doctor notes whether the mass will or will not transmit light. If the light is transmitted, the likelihood is that the mass contains fluid and is not a neoplasm. A strong light source is the fiberoptic light (see Chap. 13). Tenderness in the lumbar region at the level of the costovertebral angle may indicate an acute infection or obstruction of the kidney. Since normal kidneys are a little tender to deep palpation, this sign may not be clinically significant. A bladder containing less than 150 ml of urine is usually not palpable. However, many an abdominal mass has been known to disappear when the patient has voided or a catheter has been introduced into the bladder! Lymph nodes in the groin may be palpable normally in thin people but may indicate an infection or tumor in the pelvic or genital organs.

The external genitalia should be carefully examined for the presence of masses, rashes, or unusual discharge. No urologic physical examination is complete without a pelvic and rectal examination. In the female patient, besides evaluation of the genital organs, information can be obtained regarding the bladder supports and palpatory findings along the urethra. A bimanual pelvic examination can be performed on the male patient with one finger placed in the rectum and a palpating hand on the abdomen. Useful information for the urologist would include a more complete examination of the prostate gland, palpation for solid vesical neoplasia, and the presence of palpable lower ureteral calculi. On rectal examination, the normal prostate gland will be approximately the size of a quarter, smooth, symmetrical, of even consistency, and slightly movable. Asymmetry of the gland or a firm fixed position may indicate neoplasm or chronic infection. Examination of the male genitalia includes transillumination of scrotal masses. A cystic mass will be translucent whereas a solid tumor will not. The penis should be palpated and examined with the foreskin retracted.

The patient who is to have a history taken and a physical examination may be nervous or anxious. The patient with genitourinary symptoms may feel guilty or embarrassed. The male patient may fear loss of sexual potency. The female patient may be uneasy about the impending pelvic examination. Many patients fear that their disease may be incurable. A calm, systematic approach by the nurse is reassuring. Sincere interest and thoughtful explanation can greatly allay a patient's anxiety. The nurse can explain that the doctor will want to know not only all of the details related to the patient's present difficulty but also the details of other illnesses, even those going back to childhood. It is also important to emphasize that all information given to the doctor will be held strictly confidential. During the history and physical examination, the nurse should make certain that the doctor and his patient have the utmost privacy and are not unnecessarily interrupted.

When the doctor is ready to examine the patient, the nurse should see that all the equipment he will need is available and in good working order. When a complete physical examination is to be done, the patient should remove all his clothes and be given a gown to wear. If clothes are not removed, inspection, palpation, percussion, and auscultation cannot be performed properly. While the patient is undressing, the nurse should allow him privacy by leaving the room. It may be necessary, however, for the nurse to assist the patient with physical limitations or the mother with a crying, squirming child. It is important that the patient be as relaxed as possible during the examination. The male patient will be less embarrassed if the female nurse is not in the room. During the examination of the female patient, however, a nurse should be present. The adult patient's family or friends should not ordinarily be present during the examination unless there are unusual problems such as language difficulties.

When the doctor is ready to do the pelvic examination on the female patient, he will indicate which position he wishes and may leave the room while the nurse makes preparations. One of three positions is commonly used: the Sims (or lateral) position, the knee-chest position, or the lithotomy position, this last being the most common (Fig. 8-2). The patient should be draped so that only the area to be examined is exposed. The pelvic examination will include careful inspection of the external genitalia, speculum examination of the vagina and cervix, and bimanual palpation of the cervix, uterus, and uterine adnexa. Samples of the secretions of the cervix and vagina can be taken for Papanicolaou studies. During this procedure, the nurse should encourage the patient to breathe deeply and easily, set the light for adequate visualization, and see that sufficient quantities of lubricating jelly are available. Following the procedure, the nurse should quickly remove excess jelly from the external genitalia and assist the patient into a supine position. If the patient, because of some physical limitation, cannot assume the position requested

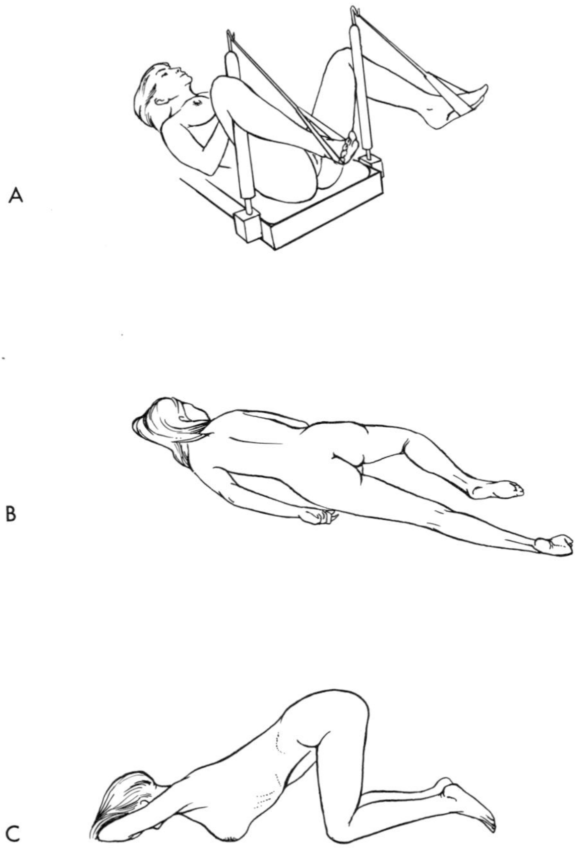

FIGURE 8-2. Common positions for examination of the female patient. *A*, lithotomy; *B*, Sims or lateral; *C*, knee-chest.

by the doctor, the nurse should bring this to his attention. Gentleness, dignity, and care cannot be overemphasized in the performance of a pelvic examination on female patients. Undue jocularity and unrelated conversation tend to be unsettling and divert needed attention. A pelvic examination is at least uncomfortable, but the inconveniences, physical and psychic, can be kept to a minimum to the benefit of both patient and physician.*

* References for Chapters 8–14 are listed at the end of Unit II (pages 157–58).

REVIEW QUESTIONS

1. Explain the nurse's responsibilities during the history and physical examination.
2. Define the following terms: frequency, urgency, hesitancy, intermittency, dribbling, nocturia.
3. What condition is most frequently associated with the symptoms listed in Question 2, and what is the physiologic explanation for their occurrences?
4. Define oliguria and anuria. What steps would be used to determine which condition existed?
5. Differentiate between the frequency of polyuria and that associated with urinary tract obstructions.
6. Why is it vitally important that blood in the urine be investigated? What kinds of information will the doctor want to know about the bleeding?
7. What considerations are important for the nurse assisting both the patient and physician with the pelvic examination?
8. By what simple technique can pneumaturia be demonstrated?
9. Describe the pain of ureteral obstruction in men and women.

CHAPTER 9

Examination of the Urine

THE most important single laboratory test for the urologist is the urinalysis. A carefully performed urinalysis must be considered an essential step in urologic diagnosis. Many urologic disorders will be reflected by abnormalities in the urine. The reliability of the examination largely depends on proper preparation of the patient and accurate collection and handling of specimens—matters for which the nurse is usually responsible. Many errors occur because the nurse either did not understand the procedure or failed to communicate pertinent information to the patient or other nursing personnel. Most health agencies have laboratory manuals which specifically outline the procedure for and purpose of each test. Where such a manual is not available, necessary instructions can be obtained from the physician or the laboratory technician. Instructions to the patient should be phrased in concise, understandable terms. Written instructions are helpful, particularly if the patient is to collect the specimen at home.

Collection of Specimens

A routine or plain voided specimen requires no special preparation of the patient and is collected by simply voiding into a clean, dry container. Plain voided specimens are usually satisfactory for most 12- and 24-hour studies and for the initial urinalysis. Abnormalities in the urine such as red or white blood cells and bacteria require examination of a specimen obtained by the "clean-catch" technique or by catheterization, since contaminants may be causing the abnormal findings. This is particularly true in the female patient where vaginal secretions may be mixed with the urine.

The "clean-catch" method consists of a midstream voided specimen collected after the area of the urethral meatus has been thoroughly cleansed. In the female, the labia are separated and the urethral and vaginal orifices are cleansed. Using a clean cotton ball for each front to back stroke, the area is first washed with soap and water. This is followed by a wash with an appropriate antiseptic solution such as 1:1000 benzalkonium chloride. Once cleansing has begun, separation of the labia must be maintained until after the specimen has been collected in a clean, dry container. This container must naturally be sterile if a culture is to be obtained. Usually the patient needs the continued assistance of the nurse. In the male patient, the urethral meatus is similarly cleansed and after voiding and discarding an aliquot of urine, a "midstream" specimen is obtained. Given proper instruction and the necessary equipment, the male patient can usually perform this procedure unassisted. Since innocuous bacteria often exist as normal occupants in the distal urethra, it is best not to include the very first part of the voiding, particularly if the specimen is collected for bacterial colony count. If, on the other hand, the patient clinically has a urethral infection, the first part of the voiding will be sent for culture in order to identify the infecting organism.

Fractionated Urine Specimens

Fractionated urine specimens are useful, particularly in male patients, in an attempt to localize the source of red or white cells and bacteria in the urine. Commonly used are the "two-glass" and "three-glass" tests. One common type of three-glass test is as follows: The patient is in-

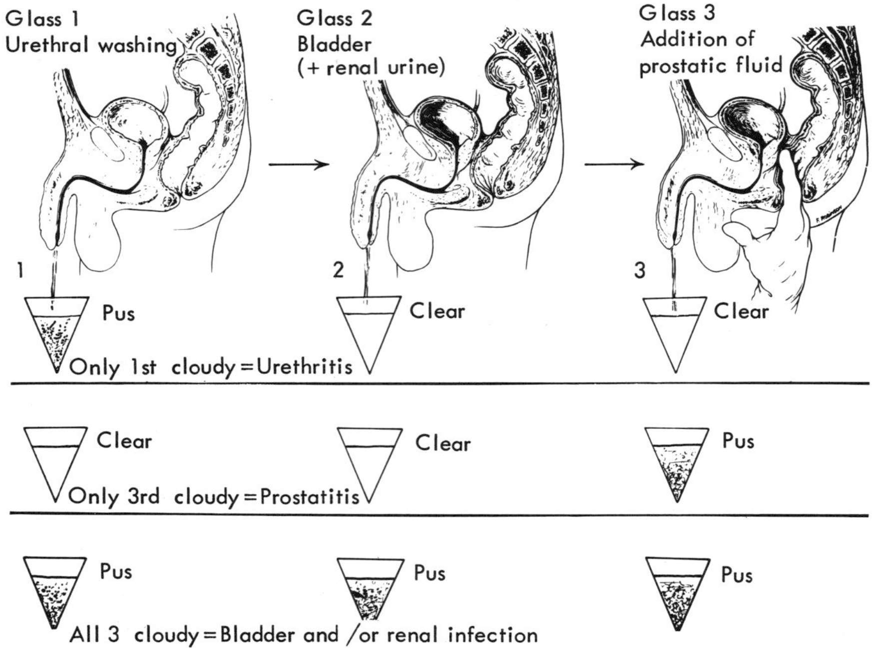

FIGURE 9-1. Three-glass test. (Reproduced by permission from Marshall, Victor F.: *Textbook of Urology*, 2nd ed. Hoeber Medical Division, Harper & Row, New York, 1964.)

structed to void about 60 ml into the first specimen bottle and then a similar aliquot into the second container. The physician then massages the prostate, and a third voided specimen is obtained.

The first-glass specimen will contain bladder urine and washings from the urethra. The second glass will consist of urine from the bladder and the upper urinary tract, but minus the urethral washings. Prostatic fluid will be added in the third-glass specimen. If many cells are present in the first glass only, one would suspect that they come from the urethra. If cells appeared only in the third glass, a prostatic source would be shown. Equal quantities of cells in all three glasses would suggest a source in the bladder or higher up in the urinary tract. A simple fractionated urinalysis may help greatly in initial localization of the site of trouble (Fig. 9-1).

Catheterized Specimens

When the abnormal findings of a clean-catch urinalysis are clinically questionable, a more accurate specimen can be obtained by urethral catheterization. Catheterization of the male urethra is usually not necessary to obtain an accurate specimen. Such catheterization is more often performed for other diagnostic reasons, such as in evaluating residual urine and calibration of the urethra. The nurse, in preparing the female patient for catheterization, must have all the necessary materials on hand and should review the procedure until it is so familiar that her actions are almost automatic. At best, catheterization is not a comfortable experience. The nurse who is unsure of herself or must stop to obtain a forgotten piece of equipment not only adds to the patient's discomfort and apprehension but also increases the probability of a break in aseptic technique.

The catheter and materials used must be sterile, and scrupulous aseptic technique must be used even though many of the catheterizations are performed in the presence of existing infection. The major hazards are introduction of a new infectious organism and trauma to the urethra. Great care must be taken not to transfer organisms from one patient to another. A standard setup for catheterization is shown in Figure 9-2.

Once the nurse has prepared herself, she should next prepare the patient. The "uncooperative" patient is often the apprehensive, frightened one who changes position at the most inopportune time. No amount of explanation will allay the fear and apprehension of some patients. The large majority, however, if told beforehand of why and how the procedure is to be done, will cooperate fully.

Probably the most important prerequisites for a successful and uncomplicated catheterization are adequate explanation, proper positioning, and good lighting. Ideally catheterization should be performed with the patient in the lithotomy position on a treatment table. It is often necessary, however, to catheterize the patient in bed. In such an instance, the bed

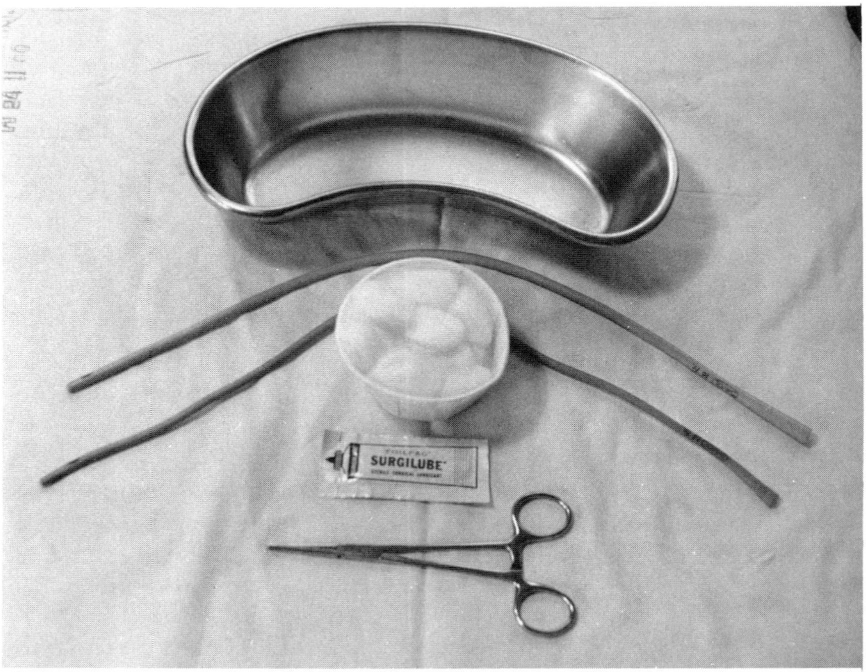

FIGURE 9-2. Standard setup for catheterization.

should be flat with the patient lying in the supine position. Adequate exposure is achieved by having the patient place the plantar surfaces of her feet together and drawing her legs toward her buttocks. Pillows may be used to support the knees in the abducted position. The nurse should make certain that the patient is comfortable enough to maintain this position for the anticipated length of the procedure. Following positioning, the patient should be draped so that only the genitalia are exposed.

Light must be sufficient to illuminate the area without shadows. An adequate source is a gooseneck lamp. If this is not available, a flashlight can be used, although it is not as satisfactory. Adequate lighting is particularly important when catheterizing the female patient because of individual anatomic variations. The urethral meatus may be quite anterior, just below the clitoris, or it may be farther posterior at the vaginal orifice. Folds of the inner labia can look deceptively like a urethral meatus, and without adequate exposure and lighting an inordinate amount of time can be spent looking for the meatus.

After position and lighting are satisfactory, the sterile catheterization set is placed between the patient's legs and opened. The wrapper of the

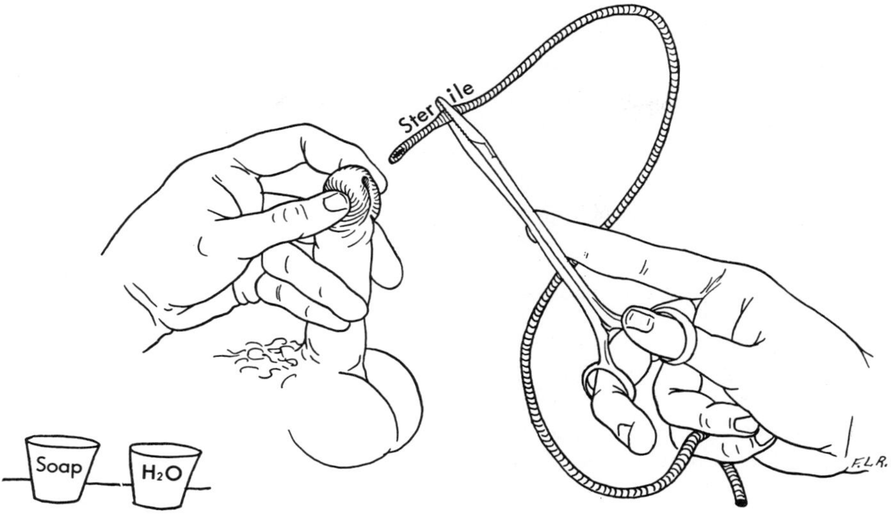

FIGURE 9-3. A practical technique for the clean and gentle catheterization of male patients. (Reproduced by permission from Marshall, Victor F.: *Textbook of Urology*, 2nd ed. Hoeber Medical Division, Harper & Row, New York, 1964.)

set acts as the bottom drape. Using sterile technique, the equipment is then arranged on the drape so that it is ready for use. Two dry cotton balls are applied with the thumb and forefinger to separate the labia. It is important that the fingers be placed deeply in the labial folds in the area of the vaginal introitus. Cleansing and catheterization should proceed only after the nurse has a secure hold on the labia to ensure maintenance of position and exposure throughout the remainder of the procedure. The area is cleansed using front-to-back strokes. The lubricated catheter is introduced gently into the urethra using either a hemostat or the sterile gloved hand. After the initial aliquot has been discarded, the remainder of the specimen is collected in the sterile basin that comes with the set. The specimen can be transferred to a sterile test tube for bacteriologic study and to other clean, dry containers for other studies. Sterile disposable plastic catheterization sets are now available and very convenient. The necessary components, including catheters, drapes, lubricant, gloves, and antiseptic, are neatly packaged. These sets have the advantage of assured sterility and they save time and labor, since the articles are discarded after use.

Although catheterization of the adult male patient is not usually the nurse's responsibility, knowledge of the techniques and equipment used certainly is. A set similar to that used for the female patient should be available. Most adult male urethras will tolerate a No. 14–16 F catheter with ease. Both the Robinson and coudé type catheters should be available, particularly the latter for older patients. The curvature in the posterior urethra from prostatic hypertrophy may make it impossible to insert a straight catheter, whereas the coudé may slip in very easily. Catheterization using the "no-touch" technique, wherein sterile gloves are not necessary, is often employed. An illustration of this technique while catheterizing a male patient is shown in Figure 9-3.

Collecting Urine Specimens from Children

The degree of difficulty in collecting urine specimens from children depends largely on the age and size of the child. If he is toilet-trained and also able to follow instructions, voided and clean-catch specimens can be obtained in the same manner as from the adult.

Coming into wide use today are sterile, disposable, plastic pediatric collection devices. These are small pouches with an appropriate opening and an adhesive surface for attachment to the skin of the pubic area. Two types of pouches are available—a closed type for collection of a single voided specimen, and an open type with an outlet and tubing for studies requiring prolonged collections. While no pediatric collection device is entirely foolproof, these disposable units are the most satisfactory in the opinion of many pediatric nurses.

To apply a disposable pouch, the opening is tailored to allow unobstructed inclusion of the meatal area. With girls, the adhering surface is secured to the labia majora with the opening extending from just above the clitoris to below the vagina. For boys, the opening is fitted to accommodate the penis. With small male infants, it is often possible to include the penis and scrotum together through the opening. If this is possible, the pouch will usually adhere more effectively.

Before applying the pouch, the external genitalia and perineum are thoroughly washed and dried. Compound tincture of benzoin applied to the skin will improve adhesion, particularly if the pouch is attached while the benzoin is "tacky" and before it has dried completely. Once the receptacle is in place, a loosely applied diaper will give additional support. If the diaper is snug, the flexible pouch cannot expand as the urine accumulates. This will often cause loosening of the pouch with leakage, loss, and contamination of the specimen. The receptacle can be applied more effectively if the nurse has an assistant who can distract the child while helping with application. Once the pouch has been secured, the child should be examined every twenty minutes or so in order to take the specimen soon after voiding.

A time-honored method for collections from infants and toddlers is the use of the birdcage feeder. The device is exactly that—the glass feeder from a birdcage. After cleansing and drying, the feeder is placed over the urethral meatus and held in place using a T binder and an overlying, snugly applied diaper. Another apparatus useful for small male infants or toddlers is a glass test tube of appropriate size. To apply the tube, a finger cot is placed over its opening and secured to the sides with adhesive tape. An adequate hole is made in the cot, and the washed and dried penis is inserted. The tube is anchored with a T binder with a hole cut large enough to accommodate the diameter of the tube.

The routine use of adhesive tape to the skin of little children for anchoring purposes is to be avoided whenever possible. If it is necessary, the porous "nonallergic" variety is more suitable, since the skin is so sensitive and easily abraded. Restraining measures are not often necessary for the very young infant. With older ones, restraints using the frog-leg position may be helpful. Elevation of the head of the bed reduces the likelihood of backflow and spillage. Offering the child oral fluids will speed urine flow and cut down the waiting time for the specimen. Five to ten milliliters of urine should be sufficient for analysis and cultures. Glass receptacles are inexpensive, are easily cleansed and sterilized, and are reusable. However, being rigid and breakable, they should be used with care. All edges are covered with adhesive tape to make them smoother and avoid cutting into the child's delicate skin.

Adaptation for prolonged urine collections such as Addis counts, 12- and 24-hour chemical determinations, and simple output measurements requires ingenuity and care on the part of the nurse to ensure accurate collections. Disposable receptacles for prolonged collections are similar to single-specimen bags except that the open outlet must be attached to an appropriate set of tubing and a drainage container. An alternate method for urine collection is the use of a special mattress, frequently called a metabolic mattress, constructed with an opening in its center and with a urine collection device under the opening.

On many occasions it may be necessary to obtain urine from the female pediatric patient by catheterization. This may be needed not only for a specimen but also to measure the vesical residuum. With older children, the key to success is cooperation from the child accompanied by ability and dexterity on the part of the nurse. Sometimes, allowing the child to play with the equipment to be used and acting out the procedure on a doll may minimize the child's fear. Body and extremity restraints may be necessary if the child remains uncooperative or is unable to understand or follow instructions. An aide or a second nurse should be present to assist. It is preferable not to have the parents in the room. Catheterization of male children, particularly older ones, is a physician's responsibility in most instances.

The equipment needed is the same as for the standard adult catheterization setup, except for the use of smaller-diameter catheters. Several sizes from 8 to 14 French should be available. Most infant urethras of both sexes can easily accept a size of 10 to 12 if no anatomic abnormality is present. Both Robinson and coudé types should be available. The same principles and technique as for the adult are followed. Since the structures in the female child are smaller and visualization may be more difficult, it is particularly important that separation of the labia and lighting be adequate.

The Urinalysis

Color

Normal urine may vary in color from a pale yellow to a dark amber, simply from variations in concentration (Table 9-1). The color of urine is

TABLE 9-1
NORMAL URINALYSIS FINDINGS

Color	Pale yellow to dark amber
Turbidity	Usually clear (cloudiness not always abnormal)
Specific gravity	1.005 to 1.025
Acidity	pH 4.8 to 7.5
Protein	None to trace ($<$200 mg/24 hr)
Glucose	None to trace
Red blood cells	None to three/high-power field
White blood cells	None to four/high-power field
Casts	Rare/high-power field

normally due to the presence of pigments known as urochromes. Certain foods, many drugs, and various disease processes can change the color of urine. Red urine usually means blood. However, the ingestion of large amounts of beets, use of the drug pyridium, or injection of phenolphthalein can cause red urine. Methylene blue tablets can produce green or blue urine. A dark yellow color suggests the presence of bile. Variations in the gross appearance of urine are summarized in Table 9-2.

Turbidity

The majority of normal urine specimens are clear. A cloudy urine, however, does not necessarily imply the presence of pus cells or disease. In fact, mostly cloudy urines are due to the precipitation of amorphous phosphates in alkaline urine, a normal condition. A similar reddish-brown precipitate is occasionally seen in acid urine with amorphous urate crystals.

TABLE 9-2
VARIATIONS IN GROSS APPEARANCE OF URINE

COLOR	SOURCE	COMMON CAUSE
Colorless	Dilute urine	Excessive fluid intake, chronic renal disease, diabetes insipidus
Yellow to amber with pinkish sediment	Acid urine with excessive urates	Hyperuricemia and gout; may appear normally
Yellow to amber with white sediment	1. Alkaline urine with excessive phosphates 2. Pus in urine	1. Normal variation 2. Innumerable causes
Milky	Lymph in urine (chyluria)	Parasitic diseases
Deep orange to mahogany	1. Bile in urine 2. Certain cathartics	1. Jaundice, usually obstructive 2. Cascara, rhubarb, and senna
Orange-red to red	1. Gross blood 2. Hemoglobin breakdown 3. Porphyrins 4. Certain medications	1. Innumerable causes 2. Various hemoglobinurias, malaria, injuries 3. Porphyria 4. Pyridium, phenolphthalein, and PSP dye
Green	Methylene blue	
Black	Melanin	Melanoma

Specific Gravity

The specific gravity is a measure of the concentration of urine as compared with water. It is measured by floating a hydrometer (urinometer) in the specimen. A normal random sample of urine may vary from a specific gravity of 1.005 to 1.025, depending on the patient's state of hydration. In certain disorders the kidney loses its ability to dilute or concentrate urine, particularly the latter. Large amounts of dilute urine are then produced daily with obligatory loss of body electrolytes. Large amounts of pus or albumin will falsely raise the specific gravity, as will intravenously injected contrast media.

pH

Urine acidity is measured as pH (the inverse logarithm of the hydrogen ion concentration). The normal urine specimen will be on the somewhat acid side with a pH of 5.5 to 6.5 but may vary from 4.8 to 7.5. The pH of normal urine will vary during the day, with a tendency to become more alkaline after meals. Acidity becomes of some importance in patients with urinary calculi and in the control of urinary infections.

Protein

The urine is checked for the presence of protein, mostly albumin. A normal urine will have little or no protein on testing. The presence of persistent proteinuria suggests a serious disorder of the urinary tract, unless proven otherwise. The "pores" in the glomeruli of a normal kidney usually do not allow protein molecules to pass through in any significant quantity. Under normal circumstances if any protein does leak through, it is resorbed in the proximal tubule. Beside a rough estimate (1 to 4 plus), accurate quantitative measurements in the form of a 24-hour collection may be obtained. The maximum normal amount of albumin within a 24-hour period should be no greater than 0.2 g. When the excretion is greater than 4 g over 24 hours, the patient is considered to have a nephrotic syndrome.

Sugar

Under normal conditions, there will be no glucose in the urine. The kidney has a "threshold" for glucose which will vary from person to person. When the blood level of glucose exceeds the threshold for that specific individual, glycosuria is present. The appearance of glycosuria, except in the rare individual with a very low renal threshold, will usually indicate diabetes mellitus, for which further studies are indicated. Glycosuria may also appear in the nondiabetic patient receiving intravenous infusion of dextrose.

Microscopic Sediment

The microscopic sediment represents all the insoluble elements that have accumulated in the urine beginning from the glomerulus and ending with its passage through the entire urinary tract. Cellular elements include red blood cells, white blood cells, casts, desquamated epithelium, and microorganisms. More than three or four red or white blood cells from a centrifuged specimen in a high-powered microscopic field are considered abnormal. Studies have shown that 50 per cent of urines with three to four pus cells per high-powered field will have significant bacterial infection. In the presence of such findings in a routinely obtained urine specimen, contamination must be suspected, thus indicating the need for a catheterized or "clean-catch" specimen. Furthermore, although the urine findings may be abnormal, no serious abnormality of the urinary tract may be uncovered on further evaluation.

Casts, as the name implies, are casts or molds of the renal tubules which appear in the urine. Their size will vary with the diameter of that portion of the nephron from which they arise. Their description depends on their component cells and microscopic appearance. Red blood cell casts will usually pinpoint microscopic red blood cells as originating within the kidney itself, as in glomerulonephritis. White blood cell casts usually indicate infection. Hyaline, granular, waxy, and fatty casts in large numbers are desquamated tubular cells seen in various forms of nephritis.

Bacteria are not normally seen in fresh urine. If bacteria are noted, one must first inquire as to the time the urine specimen was obtained. If a urine specimen is allowed to stand several hours at room temperature before analysis, the appearance of bacteria in the specimen may be of no significance. Consequently, it is important to record the time of collection on the specimen label. If there must be a delay before the specimen is delivered to the laboratory, it should be kept in the refrigerator. Also one must determine whether any contamination be present, such as with a voided specimen from a woman with a heavy vaginal discharge. After these considerations have been eliminated, the presence of bacteria in a fresh centrifuged specimen usually indicates significant infection. Further identification can be obtained immediately by staining the smear with gram stain. Specific bacterial cultures are usually indicated. Various fungi and the parasite *Trichomonas vaginalis* are rarely encountered in a urine specimen directly from the bladder. Tubercle bacilli are almost never found in a routine urinalysis but usually require identification by painstaking staining and culture techniques.

Crystals are frequently identified as normal findings in a routine analysis. Those commonly found are the varieties of calcium oxalate, calcium phosphate, uric acid, and urates. Certain crystals such as cystine are abnormal and indicate a definite disorder—cystinuria in this instance. Certain drugs can occasionally be identified by the recognition of their specific crystals in the urine.

Addis Count

An Addis count is a quantitative determination of the cellular elements in the urinary sediment. Coffee, milk, soup, and tea are omitted for 24 hours beginning after breakfast on the day before urine is to be collected. The patient should void before retiring. This specimen is discarded and the time recorded on the bottle. All urine is then collected during the night and also the first voided morning specimen. The exact time of the morning specimen should be recorded.

Normal values per 24 hours are 2000 casts (all hyaline), 130,000 red blood cells, and 650,000 white and epithelial cells.

Quantitative Urine Cultures

A useful tool for evaluating bacteriuria is the quantitative urine culture. This figure is obtained by the *colony count*, determined by counting the number of bacterial colonies per milliliter of urine on a culture plate, the assumption being that each colony initially represents a single bacterium. This is accomplished by diluting a known volume of urine in multiples of ten and culturing on separate plates according to dilution. A count of 10^5 or greater (more than 100,000 organisms) grown from a properly obtained culture implies a clinically significant urinary infection. A lower count does not rule this out, and the physician's judgment must be the ultimate guide. Certainly, an acutely ill patient with a tender kidney, chills, and fever usually has a urinary tract infection, regardless of the colony count. It is also important to know if the patient had been receiving antibiotics at the time of the culture for this may suppress the true picture. Finally, the aforementioned considerations in properly obtaining the culture specimen and its prompt delivery to the bacteriology laboratory are important.

Cytologic Studies

Urothelial neoplasia can often be recognized early by cytologic study of the urinary sediment. The method is relatively useless for hypernephroma and prostatic cancer. The technique requires fixation of the urine in equal parts with 95 per cent ethyl alcohol. The cells are stained with the Papanicolaou stain and studied microscopically for characteristic changes of neoplasia. The results are reported as Class I through V; The higher the classification, the greater the likelihood of malignant neoplasm. Classes I and II mean that neoplastic cells are not recognized; Class III indicates some suspicion; and Classes IV and V mean that neoplastic cells are present.

An aliquot (at least 30 ml) of a single voided specimen is usually adequate in the male, whereas in the female a catheterized specimen is preferable to avoid admixture of vaginal contents. The specimen should not be allowed to stand for more than 10 to 15 minutes, since the cells degenerate on standing. Interpretation of the findings in the urinary sediment is more difficult than with cells of other body secretions, particularly because of the changes from variations in osmolality of the urine on normal cells. In the laboratory at The New York Hospital–Cornell Medical Center, demonstrable urothelial neoplasia were present in more than 95 per cent of those patients with a urine sediment reported as Class V. The number of false-positive and false-negative results is few.

24-Hour Urine Collections

Urine can be studied for innumerable chemicals and compounds. These include the various electrolytes that are normally present, foreign materials such as drugs and ingested toxins, products of endocrine glands, and body metabolites. Often these materials are present in minute quantities, and assay requires specialized techniques, not all of which are available in the average clinical laboratory. Furthermore, since the quantities present may be minimal, an analysis of a 24-hour urine collection may be needed. Finally, a total amount of any compound excreted within a 24-hour period can be compared with known normal values.

A large bottle which can hold at least 2500 ml should be provided for the adult patient. Usually a preservative is added to the bottle in the form of thymol crystals or several milliliters of toluene. Dietary restrictions, avoidance of medications, and requirement for refrigeration depend on the test desired. Generally, the patient is instructed to void and discard a specimen on the morning the collection is to begin. The time of voiding must be recorded. All urine voided during the ensuing 24 hours, including the first voided specimen on the following morning, is saved; this must be obtained at the same time as the collection was started on the previous day. The time of the last voiding is also recorded.

Certain urinary assays are of particular value to the practice of urology, and their rationale will be discussed.

Calcium, Phosphorus, and Creatinine Excretions

These values can be determined from a single 24-hour collection and are useful in evaluating patients with recurrent urinary tract calculi. The creatinine output is measured because this is a fairly constant figure and thus permits determination of whether the sample is a true 24-hour collection or not. The physician is looking for an excessive excretion of calcium (hypercalciuria). If this is demonstrated, the causes for increased calcium output are then explored. The 24-hour calcium and phosphorus excretion is also the only way to check on the efficacy of low calcium-phosphorus dietary regimens in the prophylaxis of urinary calculi.

Other Studies

Twenty-four-hour steroid excretion studies are useful to the urologist in evaluating hypertension and certain forms of ambiguous sexuality, as well as in diagnosing certain tumors. Two potentially curable causes of hypertension are pheochromocytoma and aldosterone-producing adenomas of the adrenal cortex.

Pheochromocytomas excrete the *catecholamines* epinephrine and norepinephrine in large amounts, whereas under normal conditions these compounds are barely detectable. The increased amount of catecholamines will produce the vasoconstriction and hypertension seen with this tumor. *Aldosterone* is an electrolyte active hormone which in excessive amounts causes hypertension. Increased excretion may derive from a primary tumor or be secondary to chronic renal disease. *Vanilmandelic acid* (*VMA*) is a metabolite of norepinephrine. Increased excretion is therefore seen with pheochromocytoma. VMA excretion is occasionally increased with neuroblastoma, which is the childhood malignancy of the adrenal medulla.

The various hormonal assays useful in problems of intersex are those of the adrenal androgens (17-ketosteroids) and pituitary gonadotropins. For example, in congenital adrenocortical hyperplasia there is a markedly increased excretion of 17-ketosteroids, particularly the compound pregnanetriol. A suppressed excretion of this compound after cortisone therapy completes the diagnosis. The normal values for 24-hour urine excretions will vary from laboratory to laboratory, since different techniques may be used in the determinations.

REVIEW QUESTIONS

1. Describe the various techniques used in the collection of urine specimens for the following studies:
   - Routine urinalysis
   - Bacterial culture and sensitivity
   - Papanicolaou smears
   - Tubercle bacilli
   - 24-hour collections
2. What is a three-glass urinalysis? What information can be obtained with this technique?
3. Discuss in detail a procedure for catheterization of the female patient using either the "no-touch" or sterile-glove technique. Identify those factors that are crucial in maintaining aseptic technique.
4. Describe several techniques used in collecting urine specimens from infants and toddlers. Explain any special considerations related to each.
5. Describe the findings in a normal urinalysis. If the urine is allowed to stand for an hour at room temperature, which of these normal values may be altered and why?
6. What may be the significance of the following changes in the appearance of the urine?
   - Red color
   - Mahogany or deep amber color
   - Green color
   - Black color
   - Milky appearance
   - Air bubbles

7. What are acid-fast bacilli? Why may it be important to collect a midstream specimen for this examination?
8. Explain the classification of Papanicolaou urine smears and the significance of each class. Why should such specimens be collected by catheterization from the female patient?
9. Describe six 24-hour urine collections useful in urologic practice and the reasons for each. What are the nurse's responsibilities to ensure accuracy of the test in relation to the patient, collection of specimens, and all nursing personnel?

CHAPTER 10
Blood Studies

CERTAIN blood and serum determinations are of particular importance to the practice of urology. The significance of those most commonly performed will be discussed. Although not always mandatory, it is preferable to obtain fasting specimens for more accurate results. The normal values for these studies are listed in Table 10-1. The types of specimen (clotted, heparinized, etc.) are also listed in the table.

The blood urea nitrogen (BUN) is a rough index of renal function, as are the nonprotein nitrogen (NPN) and creatinine. Inability of the kidneys to eliminate adequately these breakdown products of protein metabolism will result in a rise of their blood concentration. However, a 60 to 70 per cent decrease in renal function is needed before these values rise. Consequently, elevation indicates deterioration of renal function, but normal values do not necessarily mean normal function.

Serum calcium, phosphorus, and uric acid concentrations are usually obtained in patients with calculous disorders. An elevated serum calcium and lowered phosphorus are starting points in the search for hyperparathyroidism and other causes of hypercalcemia. An increased blood level of uric acid (hyperuricemia) in patients who form uric acid calculi suggests a disturbed metabolism which may be controlled with dietary measures and the use of drugs to lower the body uric acid by either excretion of the excess or prevention of further formation.

Serum sodium, potassium, chlorides, and carbon dioxide–combining power are frequently obtained, since the kidneys and adrenals have much to do with regulation of body acid-base balance. These levels are of particular importance in following patients with severely decreased renal function wherein the normal ability to maintain this balance is lost.

Acid and alkaline phosphatase determinations are obtained in patients who may be suspected of having prostatic cancer. Acid phosphatase is an enzyme occurring only in the prostate gland. Normally a small amount of this substance is present in the blood. The blood level is elevated in about 75 per cent of cases where the cancer has extended beyond the prostatic capsule. Consequently, normal blood values do not rule out metastases or extracapsular extension. Rarely, an acid phosphatase can be elevated by nonmalignant prostatic conditions such as large infarcts. Alkaline phosphatase is a nonspecific enzyme which is produced by bone and excreted via the liver. Elevations may suggest increased bone activity, as with prostatic metastases. Biliary obstruction can also raise this value. Determining the blood level of lactic acid dehydrogenase, a recently studied enzyme, seems to be of limited value in urologic diagnosis. Elevation in

TABLE 10-1
NORMAL BLOOD VALUES

DETERMINATION	NORMAL RANGE	METHOD OF COLLECTION	MINIMUM VOLUME OF SPECIMEN
Calcium	9–11 mg %	Clotted	6 ml
Chlorides	97–106 mEq/L	Under oil	3 ml
CO_2 content	22–29 mM/L	Under oil	5 ml
Creatinine	0.5–1.0 mg %	Clotted	6 ml
Phosphorus	2.5–4.5 mg %	Clotted	3 ml
Phosphatase, acid	0–1.1 Bodansky units	Clotted	3 ml
Phosphatase, alkaline	1.5–5.0 Bodansky units	Clotted	3 ml
Protein, total	6.0–8.0 g %	Clotted	3 ml
Albumin	3.8–5.0 g %	Clotted	
Globulin	1.8–2.8 g %	Clotted	
Potassium	4.0–5.5 mEq/L	Under oil	2 ml
Sodium	130–150 mEq/L	Under oil	2 ml
Uric acid	2–5 mg %	Clotted	4 ml
Sugar (fasting)	60–90 mg %	Oxalated	2 ml
Urea nitrogen (BUN)	8–18 mg %	Oxalated	2 ml
Dehydrogenase, lactic	150–350 units	Clotted	2 ml
Fibrinogen	200–500 mg %	Citrate 0.5 ml	4.5 ml (exactly)
Fibrinolysin activity	>120 sec	Citrate 0.5 ml	4.5 ml (exactly)
Prothrombin time	Relative to control value	Citrate 0.5 ml	4.5 ml (exactly)
Clotting time (Lee-White)	5–16 min		
Bleeding time	2–7 min		

the urinary output has been frequently found with urinary tract neoplasms, but this is too nonspecific and its value to the urologist is unresolved.

Studies of factors affecting blood coagulation are frequently necessary in urologic practice. Hematuria may be a reflection of generalized clotting disorders. Measurements of the *bleeding time*, *clotting time*, *prothrombin time*, and other parameters are often obtained. More esoteric studies of blood coagulation may be ordered by the consultant hematologist if they are considered necessary. *Hemoglobin electrophoresis*, a study of the various kinds of hemoglobin present, is occasionally done. Abnormal hemoglobins may be present, for example, in patients with sickle-cell anemia or sickle-cell trait which can be accompanied by hematuria. Studies for blood *fibrinolysin* activity are often obtained in patients with prostatic carcinoma. On rare occasions, men with such a cancer may have an increased amount of this substance in the bloodstream, which can cause severe bleeding during and after surgery. A simple, useful bedside test for fibrinolysin activity can be performed by drawing 5 ml of blood, which is allowed to clot in a specimen tube placed at the bedside. If the clot remains firm 24 hours later, the blood fibrinolysin activity is probably within normal limits.

Renal Function Studies

Studies of total renal function, i.e., the function of all the available nephron units, are useful, usually painless, and easy to obtain. Studies of each kidney separately may involve cystoscopic catheterization of the ureters, although numerous indirect methods, many quite ingenious, have been described. The main renal function tests most often used clinically are those that test the ability of the kidneys to "clear" a substance from the blood, those that measure the ability to excrete an injected foreign substance in a certain period of time, and those that test the power to concentrate and dilute urine.

The Clearance Concept

At this point, a discussion of the "clearance" concept is appropriate. As mentioned in Chapter 2, only a fraction of the blood coursing through the kidneys is filtered at any one time. This is normally 20 per cent of the renal blood flow and is known as the filtration fraction. From this filtration fraction a certain quantity of a substance in the blood is removed per unit time. The number of milliliters of plasma from which a substance is completely removed from the plasma is known as the "clearance" of this substance, which clearance can be assayed in any one patient and compared with known normal values. The clearance of different substances may be accomplished by the glomeruli alone, tubules alone, or in combination. For example, inulin is cleared by the glomeruli alone. Para-aminohippurate is essentially all cleared by the tubules, and this clearance is a test of tubular function. On the other hand, urea is filtered by the glomeruli but partially resorbed in the tubules at a fairly constant ratio, whereas creatinine is cleared by both glomerular filtration and active tubular excretion, again at a fairly constant ratio.

The clearance may be expressed either in absolute values, such as milliliters cleared per minute, or as a percentage of a known normal value. To determine a clearance, one must know the concentration of the substance in the urine (U), the concentration in the blood plasma (P), and the volume of urine excreted in milliliters per minute (V). The formula can thus be written:

$$\frac{U \times V}{P} = \text{clearance}$$

Glomerular Filtration Studies

UREA CLEARANCE. A commonly used study of glomerular filtration is the urea clearance. Actually one measures glomerular filtration with the constant ratio of partial resorption within the proximal tubule. For practical purposes, however, the test is simple to obtain and simple to perform in the laboratory. The test has the added advantage that urea, an end product of protein metabolism, is endogenous and does not have to be injected into the patient.

Several factors are necessary for an accurate test. First, the patient must be well hydrated to give an adequate urine flow, since the glomerular filtration affects the clearance of urea. Second, the patient must empty his bladder completely for each collection to correctly measure the urine flow per unit time. A blood sample for urea nitrogen determination must be obtained during the collection of the urine specimens. This is usually done at the end of the first hour's collection. Last, in order to calculate the clearance, the laboratory must know the exact time of the discard specimens as well as the closing time of each of the urine collections.

The test is usually begun in the morning with the patient in the fasting state to avoid variations in the blood urea nitrogen levels. If breakfast is allowed, foods containing protein are omitted, as well as coffee and tea. The patient may be up and about and may smoke. With adequate explanation, most patients, if given specimen containers, pencil, and wristwatch, can collect the specimens with minimal supervision. If the patient has an indwelling catheter from which the specimens are to be collected, it should not be clamped between specimens. Usually the indwelling catheter is in place to provide continuous drainage of the urinary tract. It should never be clamped except on specific instruction from the physician. To collect specimens from catheters, the drainage tubing is taped to the side of the collection container. At the completion of each specimen, the tubing is transferred to a clean, dry container. This process is repeated until the desired number of specimens is collected.

The test may be carried out in the following manner:

1. 7:00 A.M. Hydrate the patient by giving him 1000 ml of water (it is preferable that he drink this within the first 30 minutes).
2. 8:00 A.M. Have the patient void and discard this urine. Write the exact time of the discarded specimen on the label of the No. 1 specimen bottle. If the patient has a catheter, place the drainage tubing in a clean, dry bottle and note the time, as above.
3. 9:00 A.M. Have the patient void in a clean, dry specimen bottle. If a bedpan is used, make certain that it is dry before using and that the *entire* specimen is transferred to the specimen bottle. Transfer the catheter drainage tubing to specimen container No. 2. The label of the No. 1 specimen container should carry the time of the discard specimen and the time the No. 1 specimen is completed.
4. Draw a blood sample for urea nitrogen determination.
5. 10:00 A.M. Have the patient void into specimen bottle No. 2. Connect the drainage tubing of patients with catheters to the regular collection container. Label specimen bottle No. 2 with the exact time of ending of the second collection.

During the test the patient should drink at least one glass of water every 30 minutes to ensure an adequate volume of urine. If the patient wishes, fruit juices may be substituted. Urea clearance is optimal when urinary output is at least 2 ml per minute (120 ml per hour). If the patient is on measured output, the volume of the specimen can be determined by taking an identical container, filling it with an equal volume of water, and measuring the water. This avoids the possibility of accidental loss of any part of the specimen. If fluids are being restricted for any reason, the doctor should be consulted as to the amount of fluid to be used for hydration. If the patient has bilateral nephrostomy or ureterostomy tubes, a "divided" urea clearance may be done, thus evaluating each kidney separately. The test is performed in the same manner as described, except that specimens are collected separately from each catheter. In this instance it is important to record not only the time but also the site of specimen collection on the label of the container. If the patient has residual urine, the doctor may order an indwelling catheter to be inserted for the duration of the test to ensure collection of the entire specimen.

The range of normal for the urea clearance is 60 to 90 ml per minute, with 75 ml per minute being the average.

CREATININE CLEARANCE. Creatinine is a substance derived from muscle creatine and phosphocreatine. It is filtered by the glomerulus and also excreted by the tubules. Because its rate of excretion is almost constant and relatively unaffected by diet or hydration, a 24-hour creatinine clearance can be simply obtained and is really not influenced by residual urine. The greatest sources of error are the low blood concentration of creatinine and difficulties in accurate laboratory determination. However, the test is a useful index of glomerular filtration. The normal creatinine clearance is between 130 and 140 ml per minute.

The test is conducted simply by collecting urine for 24 hours in a chemically clean container to which a small amount of a preservative, such as a few milliliters of toluene, has been added. At a convenient time during the collection period, a blood sample for creatinine level is obtained.

INULIN CLEARANCE. Inulin clearance is the most accurate measure of the true glomerular filtration rate. Inulin is a polysaccharide excreted exclusively by the glomeruli. The test is not often obtained clinically for several reasons. The blood and urine assays are complicated. In addition, after a priming dose, the inulin must be given intravenously at a very constant rate to maintain a constant blood level. The infusion must be monitored carefully. The average glomerular filtration rate is 132 ml per minute in men and 117 ml per minute in women. This value is greater than the urea clearance but less than the creatinine clearance, for the previously outlined reasons.

Tubular Function Studies

PHENOLSULFONPHTHALEIN EXCRETION (PSP TEST). This test is a simple and accurate way to assess tubular function. One milliliter (6 mg) of phenolsulfonphthalein is injected intravenously, and the amount excreted in the urine over the next two hours is measured. The appearance of 25 to 35 per cent of the amount injected in the first 15 minutes indicates good function. Within 2 hours, 65 to 85 per cent should be recovered. An adequate urinary flow of at least 50 ml per specimen predicates an accurate study.

The test may be carried out in the following manner:

1. The patient is hydrated with water by mouth, beginning one hour prior to the injection of the dye. Preferably he should drink a quart to ensure a good urinary flow during the test. Thereafter he should drink at least one glass every half hour until the test is completed. Any urine voided during the first half hour of the hydration period can be discarded with impunity.

2. Following the hydration period, 1 ml (6 mg) of phenolsulfonphthalein dye is injected intravenously. The test will be inaccurate if the dye infiltrates into surrounding tissues. The time of the injection is recorded on the label of the No. 1 specimen bottle.

3. Urine specimens are collected 15, 30, 60, and 120 minutes after the injection of the dye.

The nurse may note that the urine of some patients appears pink or red after the dye injection. Such a color simply means that the urine is alkaline. If the color does not appear in the specimen, this does not necessarily imply poor renal function. The patient must also be forewarned that the urine may be red during the test and that this is not due to blood in the urine. The test can be accurate only if the patient can void adequately without residual urine. Should residual be present, a more realistic result can be obtained by using an indwelling catheter during the collection period. When circumstances are such that urine is collected from either kidney separately, individual renal function can be assayed. The sum of the results from either side will then give a value for total renal function.

Sulfobromophthalein (Bromsulfalein), a dye used to study liver function, interferes with PSP determination. At least 24 hours should elapse between the performance of these two tests. The PSP excretion test cannot be optimally performed while the urine is grossly bloody or discolored by the presence of medications which interfere with the determination, such as Pyridium or methylene blue.

The urea clearance and PSP excretion tests should not be obtained if the patient is vomiting or dehydrated. It is also better not to schedule them immediately following other diagnostic studies that require the previous omission of food and fluids. When both studies are ordered, they can be obtained in sequence. The urea clearance is obtained first. The second specimen is considered the discard specimen for the PSP study. The latter is then performed in the usual manner. Both the urea clearance and PSP excretion are considered estimates of renal function but are clinically useful and easily obtained.

Urine Concentration-Dilution Tests

A simple test of renal functional impairment is the ability of the kidneys to concentrate or dilute urine beyond a fixed specific gravity of 1.010. The test has not been used too widely in recent years, having been supplemented by the more accurate clearance studies.

The concentration test is usually performed first. The patient receives his usual evening meal except that fluids are limited to one glass. Thereafter, the patient remains in bed as much as possible, and fluids are withheld until the test is completed. On retiring, the patient empties his bladder, and the specimen is discarded. When the patient awakens, the first specimen is collected and saved. Second and third specimens are collected one and two hours later. Each specimen is collected in a separate bottle labeled with the exact time of voiding. Normally, the specific gravity of at least one of these specimens will be greater than 1.025. Failure to reach this concentration indicates renal damage. Concentration tests are usually not performed where the patient is known to have severely impaired renal function, because of the danger of dehydration and of exacerbation of uremic symptoms. The reliability of test results in the edematous patient is also questionable because of the possible occurrence of spontaneous diuresis.

The dilution study is begun by giving the patient his usual evening meal, including fluids. Thereafter, the patient remains in bed as much as possible and fluids are withheld until the following morning. When the patient awakens, the first specimen is collected and discarded. Immediately after voiding, the patient begins the drinking of 1000 ml of water (weak tea or lemonade may also be used) over the next 30 to 45 minutes. No other food or fluid is allowed until the test is completed. The patient voids and specimens are collected at 1-, 2-, 3-, and 4-hour intervals. Each specimen is collected in a separate bottle labeled with the exact time of voiding. Normally, the specific gravity of the first specimen will be about 1.003 and will gradually increase. Failure to dilute also indicates renal damage. On explaining the test to the patient, the nurse should emphasize and make certain he understands the fluid restrictions, the need for rest, and the hours when specimens are to be collected. The normal values of the commonly used renal function studies are listed in Table 10-2.

Differential Renal Function Studies

Differential function studies are sometimes done when one wishes to determine the absolute function of one kidney, such as in situations requiring a decision as to whether a kidney should be removed or an attempt made to save it. A different type of divided renal function study is sometimes used when one wishes to decide whether a given kidney is a cause for hypertension.

Divided function studies usually require separate urine collections simultaneously from each kidney. If a patient has a nephrostomy tube in place or a separate cutaneous ureterostomy opening, this can be done with minimal difficulty. If the urinary tract is intact, catheters will have to be inserted up the ureters to obtain separate specimens cystoscopically. Studies for urea clearance, PSP excretion, and so forth can then be obtained. The sum of the divided specimens will give total renal function.

Numerous indirect methods of divided study have been devised, but none is too reliable. The intravenous pyelogram can give some idea of divided function, but this is only a very gross differential. With the refinement of present-day intravenous contrast media, many very poorly functioning kidneys may seem to be working well when in actuality they are not. One may try to get urine only from one kidney in the intact patient by considerable extrinsic pressure over the opposite ureter by means of wooden blocks, inflated cuffs, and so forth, but the technique is not always reliable. Another method is the assay of urinary excretion of radioactive isotopes (radiorenography), which will be discussed later

TABLE 10-2
NORMAL VALUES FOR COMMONLY USED RENAL FUNCTION TESTS*

	NORMAL RANGE
Glomerular function	
Inulin clearance: Male	132 ml/min
Female	117 ml/min
Urea clearance	
Maximum clearance at flows >2 ml/min	75 ml/min
Standard clearance at flows <2 ml/min	57 ml/min
Creatinine clearance: Endogenous	Similar to inulin clearance
24 hour: Male	140–200 L/day
Female	120–180 L/day
Tubular function	
PSP excretion: 15 minutes	35%
60 minutes	65%
Concentrating power (24 hr dry regimen) specific gravity	>1.026
Diluting power (after 1 liter of water) specific gravity	<1.003
Renal plasma flow	
Clearance of para-aminohippurate where blood level PAH is less than 2 mg %	680 ml/min

* After R. F. Pitts in Meredith F. Campbell, ed.: *Urology*, Vol. I. W. B. Saunders Co., Philadelphia, 1954, p. 48.

in this chapter. Differential urine collections, besides assaying individual function, are also useful to track down the exact source of a total urine abnormality such as pus cells, tubercle bacilli, protein, and cancer cells.

Studies for Hypertension

These studies are basically differential and comparative rather than absolute. They are predicated on certain changes in renal function associated with a decreased renal blood flow and are useful in evaluation of patients suspected to be hypertensive on a renovascular basis. When there is decreased blood flow to a kidney and relative ischemia (but not necrosis) of subtended renal parenchyma, certain functional changes follow. There is a substantial drop in urine volume from the involved kidney because of increased reabsorption of water back into the circulation. Sodium is passively reabsorbed with this water and, consequently, its concentration falls. Substances excreted by the glomeruli or proximal tubules which cannot be reabsorbed distally in the nephron will then become more concentrated. Among such compounds are inulin, creatinine, and para-aminohippurate.

This type of differential function study is most useful in evaluation of a renal artery obstruction as shown on arteriography. The cross-sectional area of an artery must be decreased 80 per cent before there is a significant fall in flow rate. Consequently, the divided study determines the functional significance of the lesion.

The original test was the Howard test. Using oral water diuresis, the divided urine volumes and sodium concentrations were compared. A fall in volume of 50 per cent and in sodium of 15 per cent concentration from the affected side was considered diagnostic of a unilateral main artery lesion. In general, the test has not been as accurate as its new version, the Stamey modification. This variation results in an enhancement of the functional changes. Urea, as an osmotic diuretic, is infused to promote maximal urinary output in the well-hydrated patient. A small aliquot of para-aminohippurate is added to the infusate. The urine volume and divided para-aminohippurate concentration are measured. The test is positive when the urinary volume is down at least 50 per cent from the affected side and para-aminohippurate concentration at least doubled. The large urinary output and carefully monitored rate of infusion give reliable and reproducible results.

The patient is instructed to drink at least 1500 ml of fluids on the morning of the test. Prior to urine collection, he is prepared with an intravenous infusion of an 8 per cent urea-saline solution given at 10 ml/min for 30 minutes prior to cystoscopy. A calculated amount of para-aminohippurate and vasopressin (Pitressin) for maximum antidiuretic activity is added. Cystoscopy is performed with either local or spinal anesthesia, and large ureteral catheters are passed up midway to the kidneys on either side. After a 15-minute waiting period for subsidence of ureteral reflex activity, three divided 10-minute specimens are collected. The infusion continues at a constant rate throughout the entire study.

The reason for the test should be outlined to the patient. He should be advised that the urine may be bloody for up to 24 hours owing to the large ureteral catheters necessary for accurate volume collections. He should know that he may have a temporary mild headache from the dehydrating effects of urea on the brain. Both the hematuria and headache will usually clear readily on a continued forced-fluid intake at the conclusion of the test.

Radioactive Renography

The radioactive renogram has been enthusiastically received in some clinics as a test of individual renal function. The test involves measurement of radioactivity over either kidney by use of scintillation counters placed on the patient's back overlying the kidney. A small aliquot of radioactive substance which will be excreted by the kidneys is injected intraveneously. Favorite compounds are those containing radioactive iodine. Most commonly used is ^{131}I Hippuran.

The normal renogram presents as a graph of three parts: a vascular spike, a tubular secretion phase, and a drainage phase. These phases are recorded on a direct writing graph at "counts per second." The short-lived vascular spike records the arrival of the radioactive material at the kidney. As tubular secretion occurs, the counts per second taper off at a fairly rapid rate. The curve then gradually flattens as drainage out of the kidney occurs and may be prolonged in obstructive uropathies. Renal artery obstructions may show a low vascular spike.

The amount of radiation exposure is minimal—much less than that of a single diagnostic chest film. The risk and discomfort to the patient are not greater than that of any intravenous injection. However, the initial cost of the necessary equipment is high, and the results, using scrupulous technique, are probably not more than 80 per cent accurate.

REVIEW QUESTIONS

1. Explain the significance of abnormalities of the following blood determinations:

   Urea nitrogen
   Calcium
   Phosphorus
   Uric acid
   Acid phosphatase
   Alkaline phosphatase
   Fibrinolysin activity

   Why might these abnormalities be of practical importance to the nurse in planning patient care?
2. Discuss the clearance concept. What information must the laboratory have to calculate the clearance of a substance? How is this value reported?
3. Define the following renal function tests and what they measure:

   Urea clearance
   Creatinine clearance
   Inulin clearance
   PSP excretion
   Concentration-dilution tests
4. Describe the protocol of each study as related to the nurse's responsibility in preparing the patient and collecting specimens.

5. Discuss the rationale for divided renal function studies for renovascular hypertension. What simple nursing measure is of importance in the aftercare of these patients?
6. What is a radioactive renogram?
7. What factors will cause the results of a PSP test to be invalid?

CHAPTER **11**

Roentgenographic Examination of the Urinary Tract

THE adaptation of radiographic techniques to the study of the genitourinary system is in large measure responsible for the high degree of accuracy in urologic diagnosis. Since many of these studies require the parenteral administration of radiopaque contrast media or instrumental manipulations such as cystoscopy or catheterization, they are not without some associated risk. This risk is usually not great but, regardless, signed permission by the patient (or parents in the case of minors) is required. Consequently, adequate medical indications for such studies are necessary. Rarely, however, is the risk of an indicated study great enough to prevent one from obtaining the needed information.

The development of optical instruments for the examination of the bladder interior, the discovery of the physical properties of the rays emitted from the Crookes tube by William Roentgen, and the development of radiopaque contrast media by the chemical industry go hand in hand in the history of radiographic study. Toward the end of the nineteenth century, it was shown that the shadows of radiopaque calculi could be demonstrated on a simple roentgenogram of the abdomen. Early in the twentieth century, it was shown that the renal pelves could be outlined with contrast media such as sodium iodide injected through catheters inserted up the ureters through the cystoscope. In the late 1920s, Rowntree, Swick, Von Lichtenberg, and Lichtwitz, demonstrated that intravenously injected iodine-containing contrast media would be excreted by the kidneys, during which time the upper urinary tract could be delineated. Subsequently, these contrast media have been used to demonstrate all the blood vessels of the body, including those of the urinary tract, and to the study of the lymphatic system.

Plain Film

Much information can be gained from a single plain film of the abdomen (Fig. 11-1). Synonyms are flat plate, scout film, and KUB film (kidneys, ureters, bladder). One may determine the size, shape, and location of the kidneys. In 85 per cent of patients, the right kidney is lower than the

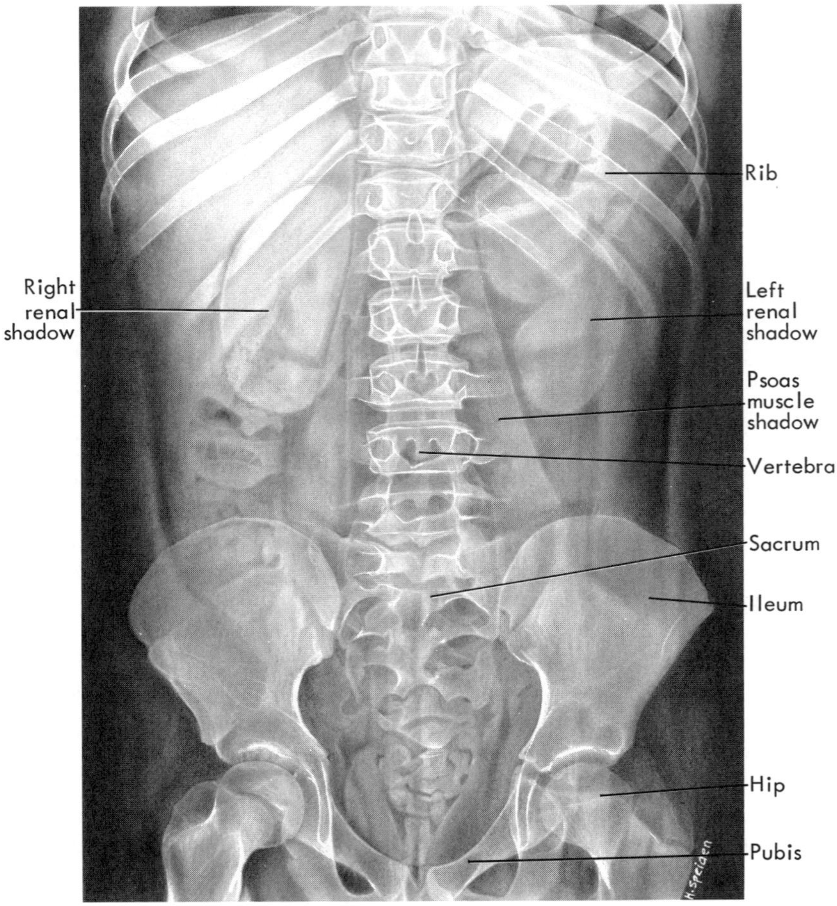

FIGURE 11-1. Plain film of abdomen.

left one. Abnormal position may suggest renal ectopia or pressure from an extrinsic mass such as an enlarged spleen or an adrenal tumor. Abnormalities of renal contour or size may suggest the presence of a mass lesion of the kidney such as neoplasm, cyst, or hydronephrosis. A small kidney, either congenital or acquired, may be shown. Radiopaque stonelike shadows may be present overlying the kidney, course of the ureters, bladder, or prostatic region. The bony shadows may show metastatic lesions, such as the characteristic osteoblastic spread from carcinoma of the prostate. The psoas muscle margins may be obscured, such as is seen with a perinephric abscess. A communication between the urinary and intestinal tracts may be suspected by demonstration of air outlining a renal collecting system. All of this information can be obtained on a simple plain film of the abdomen wherein no contrast material is used, no instrumentation is necessary, and the only risk is that of the minimal radiation exposure required to obtain a picture. Consequently, not only is the plain film worthwhile on its own merits but should be obtained as the baseline first step in all of the subsequent, more sophisticated studies to follow.

Laminography

Additional risk-free information can be obtained using laminography or tomography. This study is performed with the x-ray tube and film cassette in motion during the exposure. The purpose of this technique is to keep only one section of the body in sharp focus, all other levels being blurred. By appropriate calculation, "cuts" of the body can be obtained at 1-cm intervals to better delineate the contours and appearance of the kidneys. Again, the risk of this study is only that of the radiation exposure. In practice, however, this technique is usually combined with intravenously injected contrast media or perirenal gas insufflation to better outline mass lesions.

Retroperitoneal Gas Studies

The retroperitoneal insufflation of gas, often combined with intravenous pyelography and/or laminography to delineate the renal and adrenal contours and other retroperitoneal mass lesions, enjoys varying degrees of popularity in many medical centers. It is seldom used at The New York Hospital–Cornell Medical Center, since it is our opinion that the needed information can usually be obtained with less risky procedures. However, the method, materials, and possible complications will be described.

Basic essentials of this technique involve the retroperitoneal injection of a gas which will appear radiolucent in contrast to the solid structures in this area, thus rendering the contour of these structures more prominent. Room air, nitrous oxide, and oxygen have been used. Since the gas must be injected under pressure, the ever present risk of embolism must be seriously considered. Consequently, the most soluble gas, 100 per cent carbon dioxide, is now used by most institutions.

Although it is a painful procedure, most patients can be handled under local anesthesia if they are heavily sedated beforehand. The patient should be fasting for at least 12 hours, and a simple cleansing enema should be given several hours before the study. In the usual position for injection, the patient lies on his side with the knees drawn up on the abdomen or in the knee-chest position. After appropriate sterile preparation and draping of the skin of the buttocks and perianal regions, a large needle is inserted anterior to the coccyx and behind the rectum using local anesthesia. A catheter is threaded through the needle and the needle withdrawn. Frequently two separate catheters are inserted so that more gas may be introduced at one time. Usually 1500 to 2000 cc of carbon dioxide is introduced, and x-rays are obtained from 5 to 15 minutes after injection, or later if the gaseous diffusion is slow.

Radiopaque Contrast Media in Urology

The following studies to be described involve the use of radiopaque contrast media. A discussion of the media available and the reactions secondary thereto is pertinent. Although many elements are opaque to x-ray, iodine-containing compounds have proven to be the most suitable contrast media. The simplest compound is inorganic sodium iodide, which is excellent except that it is quite toxic on entering the bloodstream and is locally irritating to tissues. Consequently, various organic acids containing iodine have been developed over the years with progressively improving visualization of the kidneys and less toxicity to the patient. Commonly used compounds for parenteral injection presently include sodium diatrizoate (Hypaque), methylglucamine diatrizoate (Renografin), and n-methylglucamine iothalamate (Conray). These materials are colloquially known as dyes, although they are clear, colorless solutions. The term *dye* is a throwback to the German dye-chemical industry which pioneered in the early development of these materials.

Reactions to Contrast Materials

Reactions to these media occur in one of two forms. The first is an obvious allergic response consisting of urticaria. The more severe allergic manifestations are periorbital edema, laryngeal edema with obstruction of the airway, and asthmatic breathing. The second, and fortunately much rarer, reaction is a sudden cardiovascular collapse. The patient complains of a weak feeling and becomes obviously quite gray with marked hypotension and a slow, weak pulse.

The milder allergic reactions are the most common. They may require no treatment at all, but if facial edema or severe urticaria seems to be progressing rapidly, intravenous or intramuscular injection of 25 to 50 mg of diphenhydramine (Benadryl) or other antihistamines is useful. The subcutaneous injection of 0.2 to 0.5 ml of 1:1000 aqueous epinephrine solution is helpful, particularly if signs of respiratory distress such as wheezing or stridor appear. Oxygen should be available as well as oral airways and equipment to perform simple tracheotomy.

Cardiovascular collapse requires prompt attention. The patient should be placed immediately in the Trendelenburg position with lowered head.

Should he lose consciousness, some type of oral airway must be introduced and oxygen administered. The blood pressure must be maintained by solution of phenylephrine (Neo-Synephrine) or metaraminol (Aramine) in an intravenous drip at a rate determined by monitoring the blood pressure. One must be prepared to institute closed cardiac massage. In the more severe forms of this reaction, the blood pressure may have to be supported by vasoconstrictor agents for as long as 24 hours.

Reactions of the more severe type are usually not preventable unless the patient gives a specific history of similar reactions to previous intravenous pyelograms or a history of severe allergy to iodine, which is quite rare. If a patient gives a history of multiple allergy, the minor types of reaction might be prevented by preliminary or simultaneous administration of antihistamines with the contrast media. Testing for sensitivity is notoriously inaccurate—the only reliable method is to inject a very small aliquot, such as 0.5 ml, intravenously and then to wait for five to ten minutes. A serious anaphylactic reaction will probably not occur with this small dose. Skin testing often means nothing since the compounds can be locally irritating. Ocular tests are dangerous since if a true allergic reaction develops in the eye, it may be placed in jeopardy. The severity of reaction seemingly is not related to the rate of injection. In our experience, fatalities following the injection of modern intravenous contrast media are exceedingly rare (in about 1 of 150,000 or more injections).

In the case of patients with a known severe idiosyncrasy to iodide compounds wherein visualization of the renal pelves and ureters is important, other materials are available to the urologist. This involves instillation of these other materials by means of ureteral catheters inserted through a cystoscope. Such media include dilute solutions of barium, very dilute silver nitrate, and finally the simple injection of air as a contrasting agent.

Intravenous Pyelography

An intravenous pyelogram is a study that utilizes the radiopacity of injected contrast media to visualize the urinary tract. These media are injected intravenously and are excreted primarily by the tubules. Within 2 minutes of the completion of the injection, the entire renal contour will take on a hazy appearance, the nephrogram effect, as the material circulates throughout the kidney. At the same time, wisps of contrast material can be seen in the calyces. By 5 minutes after injection, the renal pelves should visualize well. Additional films can be exposed at intervals up to 30 minutes to show progression of contrast down the ureters and into the bladder. A film can be taken immediately after voiding to estimate the efficiency of bladder emptying.

Synonyms for this study are intravenous urogram and excretory urogram. Other routes of administration are available but not recommended. A contraindication to the oral route is dispersion of contrast material throughout the intestinal tract which obscures the pyelogram. The intramuscular and subcutaneous routes are not recommended, since the rate of absorption of the media is variable and the compounds are locally irritating to the tissues. The adult dosage of medication varies from 20 to 30 ml, depending on the product. Correspondingly smaller volumes are used for children (Table 11-1).

TABLE 11-1
VOLUME OF CONTRAST MATERIAL FOR INTRAVENOUS PYELOGRAPHY

AGE	VOLUME
Newborn premature	6–8 ml based on weight*
Newborn full term	10 ml
1–6 months	12–15 ml
6–12 months	15–18 ml
12–24 months	18–22 ml
2–5 years	22–26 ml
Over 5 years	30 ml

* For infants 3–5.6 ml/kilogram of weight; 4.5 for smaller infants.

Contraindications to the study are relatively few. A previous history of an anaphylactic response should make one proceed cautiously. Severe reactions and death have occasionally occurred in patients with multiple myeloma. The likelihood of adequate visualization when the renal function is depressed sufficiently so that the blood urea nitrogen is 40 mg per cent or higher is poor, but even so the risk under these conditions is low enough that an attempt can be made. Contraindications are always relative, and one must weigh the risks in these rare situations against the need for the information to be gained and against other methods available. Intravenous pyelography, in a sense, is a test of renal function. One may assay the rapidity of appearance and the density of the contrast material in either kidney. In fact, the excretion of iodopyracet (Diodrast), a presently outmoded medium, was once used as a test of renal tubular function. The present media, however, are so well excreted and so opaque that this aspect of the study is no longer useful except when there are drastic differences between the two kidneys.

Since the intravenous pyelogram depends on urinary excretion of media, the patient should be well dehydrated so that the urine will be concentrated. The patient is instructed not to eat or drink anything from the evening prior to the examination. An intestinal cleanout using oral cathartics is begun the night before. Laxatives used include Dulcolax (15 to 20 mg), senna powder (12 ml), or castor oil (30 to 60 ml). A written consent is necessary. On the morning of the study, a preliminary film is taken in the supine position. This film is reviewed to check on the adequacy of intestinal preparation, radiographic technique, and the presence or absence of barium from previous studies which may confuse the picture. In general, if multiple x-ray studies are planned for a patient, the studies requiring the introduction of barium should be withheld until intravenous pyelography and the necessary urologic studies are completed, since all the barium may not be removed easily and the work-up will be delayed unnecessarily. Following the plain film, the contrast material is injected intravenously. The patient should be forewarned that he may experience a hot sensation or a wave of nausea as the material travels through the circulation. He is observed for an untoward reaction; and should nausea occur, he should be advised to take slow deep breaths through his mouth and that this sensation will leave him almost as quickly as it came. An emesis basin should be handy, although the nausea produced by modern media is much less than in bygone days.

Films are exposed 7 and 15 minutes after the injection of the contrast media. The patient is then sent to the bathroom to empty his bladder and another film is exposed at 25 minutes. This will serve as a "postevacuation" film, giving the doctor an approximate idea of the efficiency of bladder emptying and the vesical residuum. Figure 11-2 represents a typical film from a normal intravenous pyelogram. The renal parenchyma has taken on the hazy "nephrogram" effect. The calyces, infundibula, and renal pelves are well outlined. It must be emphasized that this is a split-second exposure of a living system and that the nonvisualized segment of ureter represents a peristaltic wave. Contrast material can also be seen in the bladder.

The pyelogram should be monitored as it is being performed so that the maximum information be obtained from the study. If a shadow is suggestive of a renal calculus, an oblique film can be taken to further localize this calcification. If there is a suggestion of a perinephric abscess with fixation of the kidney by inflammation, a film can be exposed while the patient is breathing. The normal kidney shadow will be blurred during the motion, but the "fixed" kidney will remain sharply outlined. Should there be a question of unusual mobility of a kidney which "drops" and causes pain, a film can be exposed in the upright position. Finally, if a hydronephrosis is present with poor function, delayed exposures up to as long as 24 hours after injection may be necessary to get complete information.

Variations of the Standard Intravenous Pyelogram

There are many variations to this standard pyelographic technique, a few of which will be described briefly. A "double-dose" pyelogram is used where renal function is known to be depressed or renal concentrating

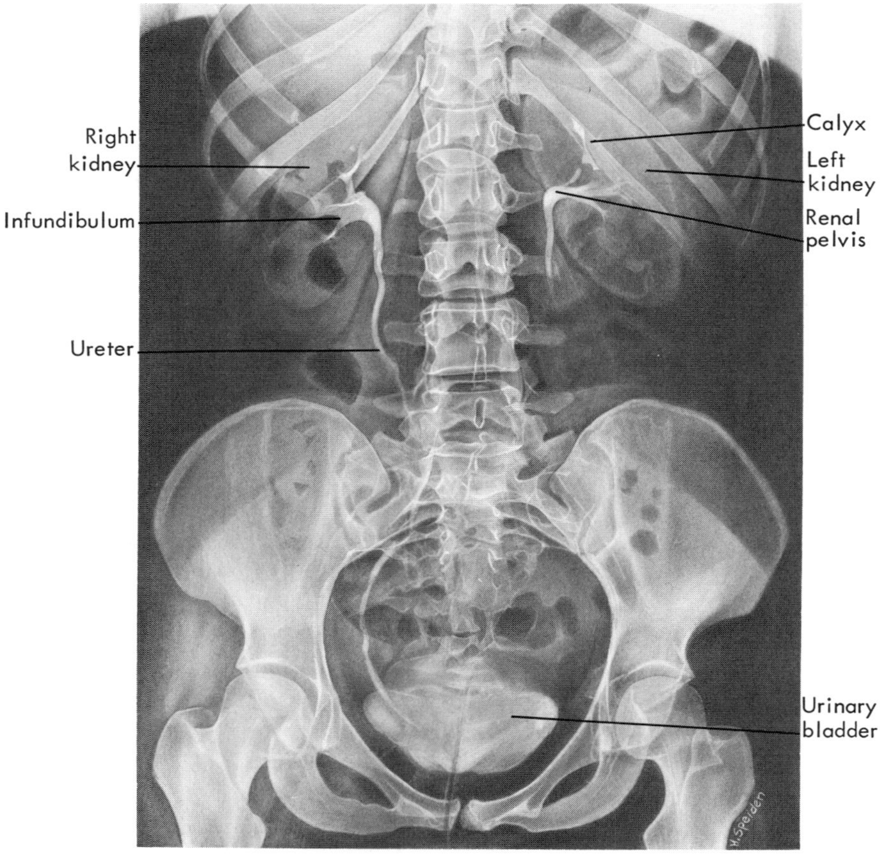

FIGURE 11-2. A normal intravenous pyelogram.

ability is impaired. As the name implies, twice the usual volume is injected. This can be done initially, or two regular injections can be given 10 to 15 minutes apart.

A further technique is the "drip infusion pyelogram," of which there are many variations. This study is used when renal function is very poor and when the doctor does not wish to risk excessive dehydration of the patient as for a routine study. The main feature of this approach is the instillation of an unusually large amount of contrast material. There are many ways to accomplish this goal. One technique is the direct intravenous injection of twice the usual adult injection (60 ml). This is immediately followed by an infusion of a solution containing an additional 90 ml of contrast material diluted with 250 ml of 5 per cent dextrose in water given over the ensuing 10 or 15 minutes. Although the volume of contrast material is large (five times the usual dose), most seriously ill patients who need the study seem to tolerate it well.

To better visualize the upper tracts one may also utilize external ureteral compression. This is accomplished either by sandbags or by a pneumatic cuff surrounding the lower abdomen. This pressure is then transmitted to the ureters and effectively accomplishes a partial obstruction so that the contrast medium is trapped in the kidneys temporarily.

Another variation of the intravenous pyelogram can be used as a screening test for renovascular hypertension. This is predicated on the functional changes that occur in a kidney when there is a partial obstruction to renal blood flow. These changes consist of a markedly reduced output of highly concentrated urine by the ischemic kidney. This can be shown frequently by the use of the "rapid series pyelogram." Following the injection of the contrast material, films are exposed at one-minute intervals up to five minutes. Subsequent routine exposures are taken. A positive result will be a delay (often only a minute or two) in the appearance of renal contrast on the affected side. Later films may show an overly dense appearance owing to less volume and more concentration. Another variation of this technique is to perform the pyelogram on a well-hydrated patient (the "washout" pyelogram). The normal kidney will visualize poorly, but the ischemic one may show up well, as one would expect under dehydrated conditions.

Nephrotomography

Nephrotomography is a more sophisticated form of intravenous visualization which is used to delineate mass lesions of the kidney. The study is a combination of intravenous pyelography and laminography (tomography).

The preparation of the patient is the same as for intravenous pyelography. A large bolus (usually 50 ml) of contrast material is injected rapidly into an antecubital vein. A film taken immediately after injection will often visualize the abdominal aorta and renal arteries. During the pyelographic phases, plates are exposed obtaining laminographic cuts at 1-cm intervals. The depth and location of a mass lesion can then be determined on a composite of all films. A renal cyst will appear as a sharply delineated smooth lesion with a central lucency due to the fluid contained therein. A solid tumor, on the other hand, will appear hazy and dense but may have scattered lucencies if there is a cystic degeneration. Interpretations are about 90 per cent accurate in experienced hands.

Retrograde Pyelography

A retrograde pyelogram, as the name implies, is a radiographic study of the upper urinary tract obtained by a retrograde (or backward) instillation of contrast media into the upper tract. This is accomplished by means of suitable cathethers introduced into the ureteral orifices via the cystoscope. Since urethral instrumentation, injection of material directly into the collecting system, and varying degrees of patient discomfort are involved, a retrograde pyelogram is obtained only on certain indications. The most common indication is the failure of intravenous techniques to deliver all of the necessary information. A much less common indication, mentioned earlier, is hypersensitivity to the intravenous media.

Retrograde pyelograms can be obtained in one of two ways. The first method requires insertion of a ureteral catheter into the renal pelvis. After a plain abdominal film is obtained, the renal pelvis is filled with contrast medium either injected through a syringe or allowed to flow in by gravity. The latter method is preferable, since there is less likelihood of unintentional overdistention with possible extravasation into the renal parenchyma by backflow. After an anteroposterior film is exposed, a second view in the form of an oblique projection can be obtained. The oblique projection will give the examiner a further opportunity to localize lesions in a three-dimensional sense. To visualize the ureters, contrast material is injected as the catheters are slowly withdrawn and another exposure is made. Subsequent delayed or "trapping" films are taken following removal of the catheters to ascertain the rapidity of emptying of the upper tracts. Within 10 to 15 minutes, the normal, unobstructed, upper urinary tract should have emptied itself.

An advantage of this method of retrograde pyelography is that differential urine specimens can be obtained from either kidney separately, particularly when one is interested in the source of malignant cells, pus, bacteria, or tubercle bacilli. The function of each kidney can be separately assayed. A disadvantage is that local reaction may occur from the trauma of the catheterization. These reactions include subsequent acute obstruction to the flow of urine from ureteral edema, the painful passage of small blood clots, or occasionally an acute pyelonephritis following instrumental examination of an already obstructed or infected upper tract. To obviate this complication, an antibiotic is frequently added to retrograde contrast media.

The disadvantages of direct ureteral catheterization can often be avoided by employing the second method, the obstructive pyeloureterogram. One of several types of catheters with bulb-shaped tips is inserted into the ureteral orifice, plugging it like the cork in the neck of a bottle. The opaque medium is injected into the catheter, progressively filling the ureter and renal pelvis. Injection films are exposed in various projections, the catheter removed, and delayed films obtained. Retrograde pyelography is the best method to visualize the degree of obstruction to an upper urinary tract by observing the length of time for the contrast material to empty out. Because of the catheters used, this method is often referred to as "bulb" pyelography. Meticulous technique is necessary, since air bubbles inadvertently introduced into the system may be mistaken for other radiolucent defects such as nonopaque calculi or papillary tumors.

Contrast media used for retrograde pyelography need not be parenterally injectable. Sodium iodide (10 per cent) and methiodal (Skiodan) (20 per cent) provide sharp contrast but tend to be irritating, while the newer compounds are much less so. A truly major disadvantage of sodium iodide is that it may be inadvertently confused with sodium hydroxide solution which may be available (for alkalinization of the urine in the PSP test). Organic compounds, frequently with added antibiotics, are more commonly used nowadays because reactions are less frequent. The intravenously injectable contrast media can also, of course, be used for retrograde study. Since these retrograde visualizations do not depend on kidney function, the preparation of the patient is that for the cystoscopic examination itself.

Cystourethrography

A cystourethrogram studies the structure and function of the bladder and the urethra. One standard technique will be described, but other methods exist in various centers. A plain abdominal film is obtained, usually in the oblique position. The bladder is subsequently filled with contrast medium allowed to flow in through a catheter at 15 cm of gravity pressure. This can be roughly approximated by holding an Asepto syringe without the bulb with its outlet 15 cm above the level of the bladder neck. A film is exposed followed by another at 30 cm of pressure using a similar technique. The purpose of these pressures is partly to quantitate when vesicoureteral reflux first appears. Another film is taken while the patient is urinating. The patient is then instructed to empty his bladder as well as possible, following which a final "post-evacuation" film is obtained to permit estimation of vesical residuum. Should diverticula be present which remain full, the doctor may wish to take an additional film after a catheter has been reintroduced into the bladder to determine whether the diverticula are retentive of themselves. A cystogram can be similarly obtained under general anesthesia in children. The anesthesiologist can lighten the plane of anesthesia after the filling films, and often the child will void unconsciously, although the postevacuation film under these conditions is not accurate.

Information that can be obtained includes the size and configuration of the bladder, demonstration of trabeculation or diverticula, opening and descent of the bladder outlet during micturition, and bladder emptying. The competency of the ureterovesical junction can be evaluated by the presence or absence of vesicoureteral reflux at different intravesical pressures. The caliber of the urethra can be seen during the voiding film. If this is not well outlined, a catheter can be inserted into the urethral meatus and a "retrograde urethrogram" can be obtained by rapidly injecting 50 ml of contrast medium. Figure 11-3 is an example of a cysto-urethrogram of a normal male voiding.

Methiodal (Skiodan) and sodium iodide are commonly used cysto-

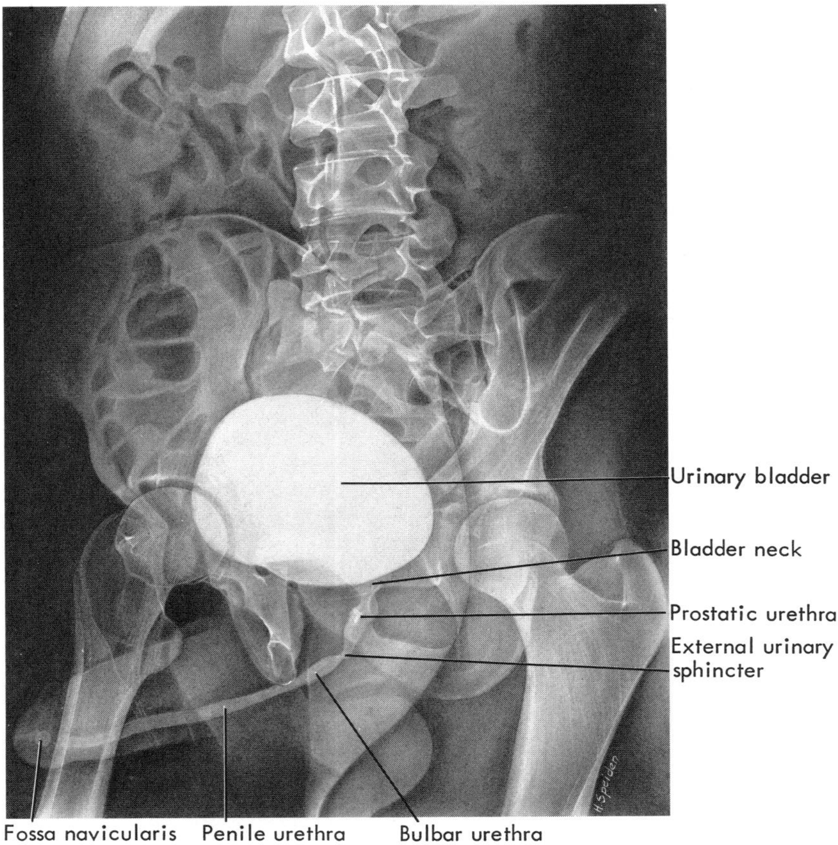

FIGURE 11-3. A normal male voiding cystourethrogram.

graphic media. For special purposes, one can use air or thin barium, but these are rarely valuable. Special precautions must be taken if there is any suspicion of bladder injury such as laceration or rupture, as in patients with fractures of the bony pelvis. Under these circumstances, an intravenous type of medium should be used so that inadvertent absorption of material into the general circulation would be better tolerated.

Cinecystography is an x-ray motion picture study of the bladder. Such special equipment as needed has been available for years but was never used widely because of the large amount of radiation exposure necessary for these studies. The development of the image intensifier, wherein a weak x-ray beam is intensified after it has gone through the patient to produce an acceptable picture, has renewed interest in all cine studies. With relatively little exposure to the patient, the act of voiding and bladder function can be studied in motion.

Renovascular Studies

Techniques are now available for the study of the arteries, veins, and lymphatics of the urinary system.

Arteriography

A renal arteriogram depicts the arterial blood supply of a kidney. These techniques have added considerably to the preoperative fund of information available to the surgeon, information that previously was obtainable only at the time of operation, and often not even then. An arteriogram can give information as to the size and configuration of the main arterial supply. One can evaluate the patency of the arteries, demonstrate blockage to flow by constrictions, thromboses, atherosclerotic plaques, and other obstructions to arterial flow, especially those that may cause surgically correctable renovascular hypertension. Arteriography can usually delineate the nature of a space-occupying lesion of the kidney. Often, a solid neoplasm will show numerous abnormal blood vessels giving rise to a characteristic "tumor stain," whereas a cystic lesion will show a spread of blood vessels around a lucent cavity. When a large tumor mass is present, the surgeon can be aided by knowing the number and location of the renal arteries, since variations from the normal may occur in fully one third of patients.

There are various techniques available to demonstrate these vessels. Three of them will be described briefly. The *transfemoral renal arteriogram* is becoming increasingly popular, particularly since the risk of the examination is low and since exquisite detail can be demonstrated. A delicate catheter is introduced through one of the femoral arteries in the groin and threaded retrograde up the abdominal aorta until the eyes of the catheter are opposite the orifices of the renal arteries. This catheter can be inserted either through a direct open arteriotomy or more frequently through the inner bore of a large needle inserted into the artery percutaneously. Open arteriotomy may be necessary in children, and the percutaneous technique can usually be performed in adults. Obviously, if the arteries distal to the renal arteries are obstructed by thromboses or plaques which mechanically prevent the introduction and placement of the catheters, some other technique must be used.

Once the position of the catheter is determined by fluoroscopic image-intensifier control, radiopaque contrast medium is rapidly injected into the catheter, and a sequence of rapidly exposed films is taken showing the entrance of contrast medium into and through the kidney tissue. In capable hands, the technique can be further modified so that the catheter tip is actually inserted into one renal artery alone, and detailed selective films can be taken of one or even a portion of one kidney alone.

After the study the patient is kept on bed rest until the following morning. A tight pressure dressing is applied to the groin reinforced with an overlying sandbag to give added pressure. During this time, frequent observations should be made and recorded of the pulses and color of the extremity and of any bleeding on the dressing. Any abnormality should be reported to the doctor immediately since, in rare cases, serious complications such as hemorrhage, interference with the circulation of the foot, or false aneurysm formation can occur. Except for children, this technique is usually performed under local anesthesia. Figure 11-4 illustrates a normal renal arteriogram.

A second method of visualization is the *translumbar aortogram*. This method involves direct needle puncture of the abdominal aorta at the level of the renal arteries through the back with injection of contrast medium. The examination is usually performed under local anesthesia with the patient in the prone position. The needle is inserted alongside the left lower border of the first lumbar vertebra until the aorta is entered. The abdominal aorta travels downward just in front and slightly to the left of the lumbar vertebrae. After injection of 10 to 20 ml of contrast medium, films are sequentially exposed, developed, and seen, following which the needle is removed and the patient observed on bed rest until the following day.

Intravenous abdominal aortography is a third method useful more for visualization of the entire abdominal circulation and less likely to give the details of the renal circulation of interest to the urologist. It is a useful study when the abdominal vessels are known to be bad, as with aneurysms. A large bolus of contrast medium (1 ml/kg of body weight) must be injected rapidly into the veins of the arm. This usually requires large needles (No. 12) in each arm and very rapid injection by means of a pressure injector. Using a previously determined circulation time, radiographs are obtained as the bolus reaches the abdominal aorta. The

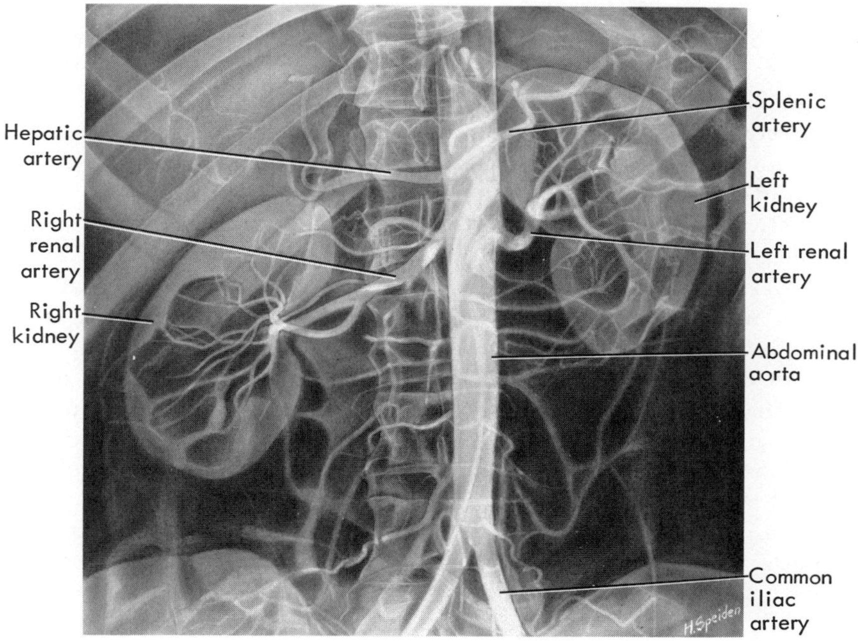

FIGURE 11-4. A normal renal arteriogram.

technique must be precise, since split-second timing is necessary. If the arrival of the bolus is missed, a second injection of large amounts of contrast is necessary, and opacification of the entire abdominal vasculature at once may make subsequent interpretation of films difficult. At least two deaths from pulmonary edema have been reported by this technique.

One can surmise from the preceding paragraphs that arteriograms are a very useful adjunct in the diagnostic armamentarium but that regardless of the technique employed they are not risk-free procedures. Such studies are best performed on an inpatient basis at the hospital so that the patient can be observed carefully by nursing personnel for at least 24 hours following such studies.

Venography

Venous studies are also available to the urologist but are less frequently indicated clinically than arterial ones. The usual indications are to visualize any indentation or distortion of the inferior vena cava, such as from lymph node metastases from testicular neoplasia, or to determine the patency of the renal veins. An injection is made directly into the femoral vein or by means of a catheter threaded percutaneously up the inferior vena cava, and contrast medium is injected.

Lymphangiography

Lymphangiography is a study wherein cannulated lymphatic channels are injected with an oily contrast medium which ultimately settles in the lymph nodes draining the cannulated area. It is used in urology to locate retroperitoneal lymph node metastases, to study retroperitoneal inflammatory disease, and to evaluate the thoroughness of retroperitoneal lymph node dissection preoperatively and postoperatively.

Briefly the technique requires the visualization of dye-filled lymphatic channels in the dorsum of the foot after intradermal injection of Evans blue dye. One of these channels is isolated through a small dorsal skin incision made under sterile conditions using local anesthesia. A small needle in the order of size 23 to 27 is used to cannulate the lymphatic, through which warmed oily contrast medium is slowly injected at a rate of less than 1 ml/min. A faster rate of injection often will cause rupture of the lymphatic. Roentgenograms are obtained after injection and 24 hours later. By that time, contrast material will have left the lymphatics but will be well embedded in the lymph nodes.

There are few complications from such a study. These would include technical inability to cannulate the lymphatics, later infection in the cutdown site, and rarely a pneumonitis caused by a diffuse accumulation of the oily substance in the peribronchiolar lymphatics. The last complication can usually be prevented if the volume of contrast material is kept below 20 ml.

REVIEW QUESTIONS

1. Discuss the information obtainable in relation to the urinary tract from a plain film of the abdomen.
2. Describe the radiopaque media used in urologic x-ray studies. What reactions may occur to these, and how are they treated?
3. What information is provided by the normal intravenous pyelogram? Explain the preparation of the patient for this study and the reasons for same.
4. Define these variations of standard intravenous pyelography and why they may be requested by the doctor:
   - Double dose
   - Drip infusion
   - Rapid series
   - Washout
   - Ureteral compression
5. What is a retrograde pyelogram? How and why is it done? Describe the nursing considerations in patient care after such a study.

6. Define the following studies and discuss why they may be ordered:
   - Nephrotomogram
   - Renal arteriogram
   - Inferior venacavogram
   - Cystourethrogram
   - Lymphangiogram

CHAPTER 12
Instrumental Examination of the Urinary Tract

THE precision and accuracy of urologic diagnosis and treatment would not be possible if it were not for the highly specialized group of catheters, sounds, and optical instruments available. Many of these instruments are of delicate construction, are expensive to buy and repair, and require special handling and methods of sterilization. Since the care and preparation of this equipment are usually the nurse's responsibilities, there are some basic facts with which she must be familiar if she is to do her job well.

Calibration of Urologic Instruments

Tubular instruments that are to be inserted into the urinary tract are graded according to their outer diameter. Although there are both American and English scales of measurement, the Charrière or French (F) scale is most commonly used. With the French scale, the size is determined by multiplying the diameter in millimeters by 3. Thus a diameter of 8 mm is equal to No. 24 F. Or, conversely, No. 24 F is 8 mm in diameter. For the adult, the sizes most often used for urethral catheterization vary from 12 to 24 French and for ureteral insertion from 4 to 8 French. Sizes for children will vary according to age and physical development.

Catheters

Catheters are hollow, tubular instruments used for drainage of fluid media, usually urine. They may be constructed of various materials, including rubber, latex, plastic, woven silk (stiffened by shellac), glass, or metal. They vary from a single straight tube for a single insertion to tubes of varying shapes, curves, and diameters for specific situations. They may be constructed so as to remain within a cavity for more or less permanent drainage. If properly used, cleaned, and sterilized, they may be used many times.

The actual variations in size, shape, and construction of catheters are almost as great as the number of urologists. A description of every catheter

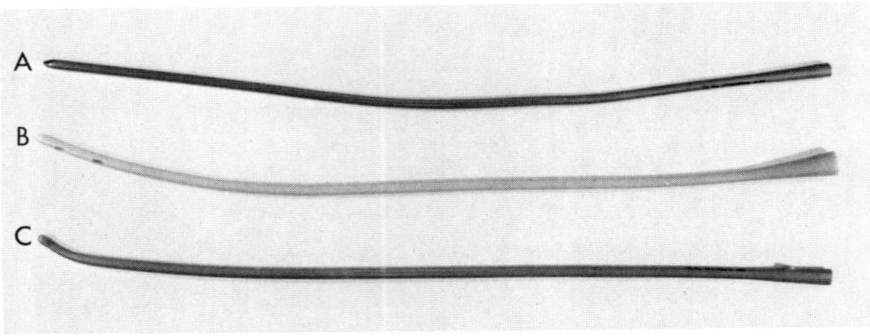

FIGURE 12-1. *A*, whistle-tip catheter; *B*, Robinson catheter; *C*, coudé catheter.

ever manufactured would be impossible. For more complete descriptions, the reader is referred to the catalogues of the various manufacturers.

The most frequently used straight, nonretentive catheters are the *Robinson* and *whistle-tip* types (Fig. 12-1), usually made of natural or latex rubber. Disposable plastic catheters of this type are available, but they have the disadvantage, especially for male patients, of greater stiffness and less pliability. These catheters are usually used for a single insertion such as the measurement of residual urine or to obtain a catheterized culture. They can be used as splinting catheters, as after plastic procedures on the ureter. The Robinson catheter has a solid rounded tip and may have two, four, or six eyes along its side. A large-diameter "multieyed" Robinson is often used in the presence of bloody urine, since there is less likelihood of catheter obstruction by clots. The whistle-tip catheter has two eyes, one on the side and one at the semirounded angle of the tip.

Another type of nonretentive urethral catheter is the *coudé* catheter, also known as the "elbow" or "natural curve" catheter. The advantage of this curve is that it can follow the contour of the bulbar and prostatic urethra as it curves beneath the symphysis pubis. This catheter is particularly useful in older male patients with elevation of the bladder neck by prostatic hypertrophy which may prevent insertion of straight catheters. The tip of the catheter may taper to a point or have an olive-shaped enlargement (olivary tip). These catheters are usually made of red rubber and are somewhat stiffer than Robinson catheters. Frequently they are impregnated with lead in small amounts so that they will be radiopaque and identifiable radiographically. Most coudé catheters have a single eye, and if they are taped in place for drainage, they must be observed often, since the single eye may become easily obstructed by mucus or blood clots.

Glass and metal catheters are used only for insertion into the female urethra. They have the advantages of indestructibility and easy sterilization which, however, are far outweighed by the disadvantage that they are rigid and potentially traumatic. Worst of all, should a glass catheter break while in use, there can be serious damage to the patient and serious trouble for the physician. Metal catheters come in graduated sizes and are useful for concomitantly obtaining a bladder urine specimen, dilation of the urethra, and insertion of antiseptic solutions. These instruments are actually female sounds (see later).

The most frequently used self-retaining catheter is the *Foley balloon* type, which actually consists of two tubes rolled into one. The larger tube is for drainage, and the smaller is a connection to a rubber balloon which is inflated from the outside after the catheter has been positioned. The inflated balloon thus prevents the catheter from slipping out (Fig. 12-2).

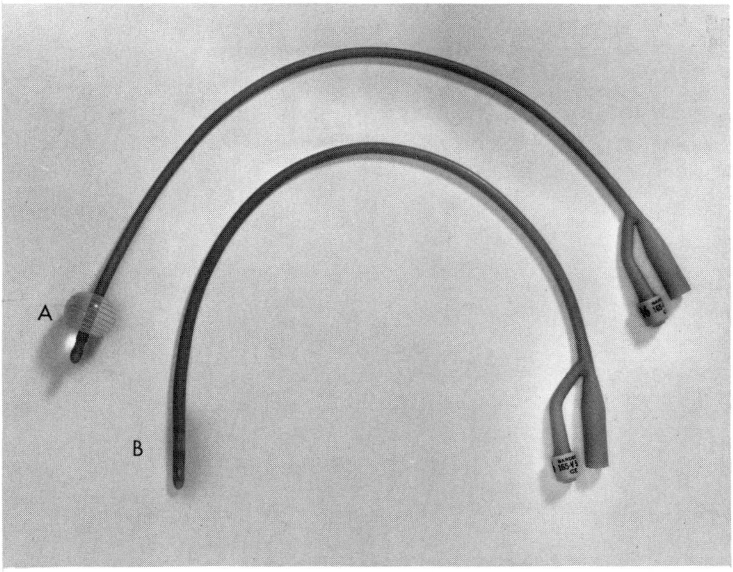

FIGURE 12-2. Foley catheters. *A*, balloon inflated; *B*, balloon decompressed. (Courtesy of Bard, Inc.)

Such catheters and their balloons are manufactured in a large variety of sizes. Commonly used balloon sizes are 5- and 30-ml capacity. The tip of the Foley catheter is of the Robinson type with one or two eyes on the side just past the balloon. Foley catheters with a coudé tip are available.

It is worth emphasizing some facets of the management of the balloon. The balloon is filled through the side arm with fluid, usually sterile saline or distilled water, by means of a syringe with an adapter. After the desired amount of fluid has been introduced, the side arm is bent back on itself and securely tied with stout string to prevent any leakage. Two new types of side arms are equipped with valvelike attachments that do not ordinarily require tying. One is composed of a rubber cork through which the fluid is injected with a small needle. The second version consists of a bicycle valve type of arrangement which can be opened by insertion of the hub of the syringe. Occasionally a dilemma arises when the valve is opened or the ligature cut, because the balloon will not decompress itself and the catheter cannot be removed. In such a situation, the insertion of 1 or 2 ml of ether or chloroform via the side arm will often break the balloon so that the catheter can be readily removed. It is good practice to check the integrity of the Foley balloon by distending and emptying it before the catheter is inserted into the patient. Foley catheters are usually used to drain the bladder either per urethram or through a cystotomy opening. They may not be advisable for use as nephrostomy drains, since the renal pelvis capacity is small and the presence of the balloon may of itself obstruct drainage of portions of the kidney. A new innovation is the self-inflating balloon. Once the catheter is in the bladder, a clamp is removed from the distal balloon arm, and fluid, presealed under pressure, automatically inflates the balloon.

Another group of retentive catheters includes the mushroom types (Fig. 12-3). The *Pezzar* catheter has one or two small holes in the side

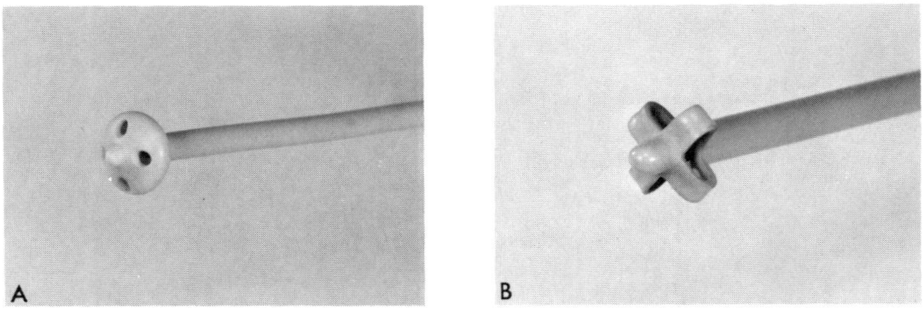

FIGURE 12-3. *A*, Pezzar catheter; *B*, Malecot catheter. (Courtesy of American Cystoscope Makers, Inc.)

and does not drain as well as the more commonly used *Malecot or batwing* catheter. The latter, while having a similar mushroom shape, has four large openings giving it a "winged" appearance.

A wire *stylet* (or mandarin) is needed to insert these catheters. The catheter is stretched over the wire to flatten the end (Fig. 12-4). A special loop on the handle of the stylet holds the catheter taut. Once the catheter is in position, the loop is released and the catheter resumes its original shape. The stylet must be used with great care, since serious injury can occur if the tip of the stylet should accidentally protrude through the

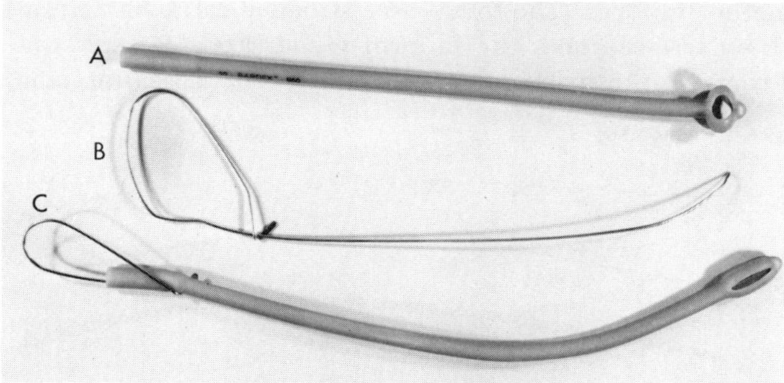

FIGURE 12-4. *A*, Malecot catheter; *B*, stylet; *C*, catheter with stylet inserted.

proximal end of the catheter. Since the catheter is now a rigid instrument, its insertion becomes the responsibility of the physician and not of the nurse. It is important that the stylet, as well as the outside of the catheter, be well lubricated. It is embarrassing to get such a catheter positioned in the patient and then be unable to remove the stylet. Though such catheters are self-retaining, it is wise to tape them to the skin for added security. Some of these catheters are available with a right-angle bend for cystostomy drainage. In general, we feel this offers no special advantage and may not drain as well from blockage at the bend.

Several other retentive catheters will be mentioned briefly. The three-way Foley catheter has three lumens—one is for the side arm and the other two are for the insertion and withdrawal of irrigating fluids. The disadvantage is that the lumina for irrigation and withdrawal must be small, and the likelihood of clogging with sediment and debris is high. The Oddi catheter is a variation of the Foley catheter with two balloons in tandem. One balloon is inflated inside the bladder and the second within the prostatic urethra to accomplish hemostasis following prostate surgery. There are numerous other variations in catheters, most of which seem to add little to the advantages of those more commonly used.

Filiforms and Followers

A filiform (also known as a "whip") is a small, somewhat stiff instrument used to traverse a strictured urethra. They are now made of plastic materials, but in the past were constructed of lacquered cloth or whalebone. They are available with various tips, such as an olivary tip, "rat-tail," and coudé curve, to negotiate the configuration of the stricture. In instances of false passages in the urethra, several filiforms may be necessary to occlude these passages until the stricture itself is traversed with another filiform. The follower, a stiffened catheter with a threaded tip, is then screwed onto the filiform guide (Fig. 12-5). It can then be guided through the strictured area. Followers of increasing diameter can

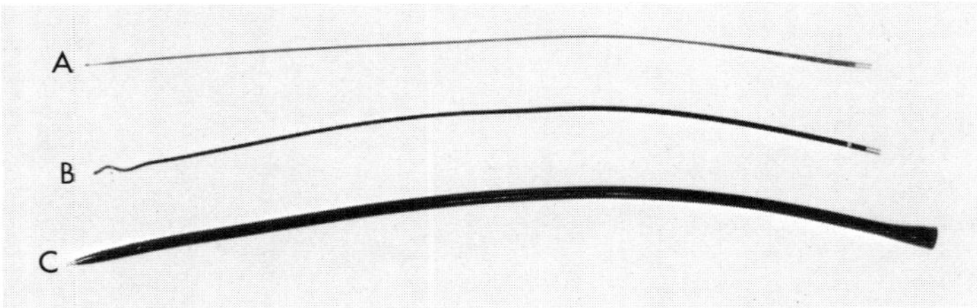

FIGURE 12-5. *A*, olivary-tipped filiform; *B*, rat-tail filiform; *C*, follower.

then be used to dilate the stricture. As the follower is introduced, the filiform portion merely coils on itself inside the bladder. The screw-on filiform guide may have either a male or female thread and, of course, the follower must have a corresponding thread to be of use. Frequently the follower must be left indwelling, particularly when it is desirable to dilate the urethra gradually over a course of several days. When this is done, the nurse must be careful not to dislodge the catheter and be certain that drainage is free, since the single eye of the follower can be occluded easily.

Bougies and Sounds

These are instruments used for dilation and calibration of the urethra. Bougies are semirigid instruments, commonly made of hard rubber, lacquered woven linen or nylon, or polyvinyl resins. Some bougies have permanently attached filiform guides. They are available with various tips. Bougies à boule are instruments with acorn and olivary tips used for calibration of strictures. The bougie is inserted gently and slowly withdrawn. The operator can then note the site and size of any constricting "hang" that is felt (Fig. 12-6).

Sounds are rigid dilating instruments, usually made of metal. Often the tip of the sound is tapered so that it is less than its maximum diameter.

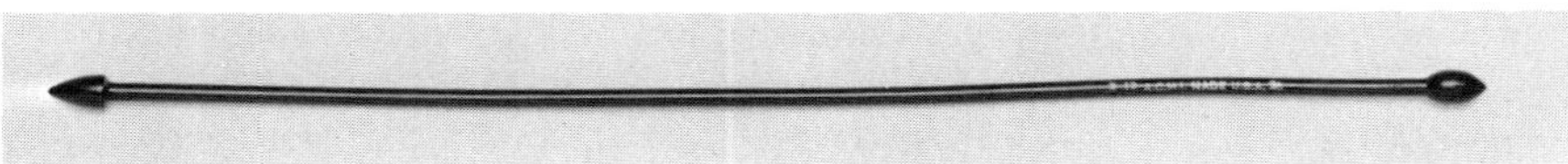

FIGURE 12-6. Bougie à boule. (Courtesy of American Cystoscope Makers, Inc.)

The proximal end of the sound is available with various curves to accommodate the male urethra. Some of these curves are illustrated in Figure 12-7. The most commonly used sizes vary from 18 to 24 F.

The illustrated urethral sounds are for use in the male patient. They must be inserted only by an experienced operator since, being rigid and curved, their injudicious use can result in severe damage to the tissues of the urethra. The curve of a sound is designed for a specific reason—namely, to negotiate the curvature of the bulbar and prostatic urethra beneath the symphysis pubis. Another type of urethral sound is for use in the female patient (Fig. 12-7*C*). These sounds are graduated and hollow

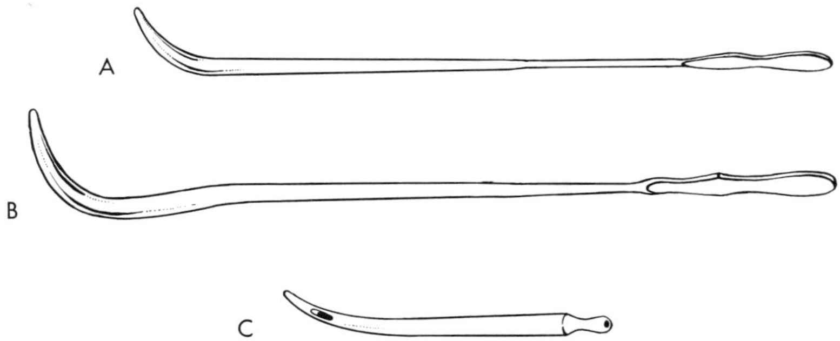

FIGURE 12-7. Varieties of urethral sounds. *A*, Van Buren curve; *B*, Guyon curve; *C*, combination female metal sound and catheter.

so that along with dilatation of the urethra, one can obtain a urine specimen from the bladder directly or insert medications. A curved stylet (mandarin) is sometimes used to insert a urethral catheter under difficult circumstances by the physician. It is inserted into the catheter as previously described in this chapter. Using great care and the technique for insertion of the male urethral sound, the catheter is positioned in the bladder and the stylet withdrawn.

Ureteral Catheters

Ureteral catheters are made in various shapes and sizes for insertion into or occlusion of the ureters. Again, for the many variations, the reader should refer to the catalogues of the various manufacturers. The commoner materials used in their manufacture are varnished woven nylon, silk, or solid polyethylene. The catheters may be x-ray opaque or non-opaque, depending on impregnation with radiopaque substances, and finally may or may nor be marked in centimeters. Graduation of catheters allows the cystoscopist to determine how far a catheter has been inserted up a ureter. Circular bands are placed at centimeter intervals. A single wide band identifies the 5-cm mark. Two wide bands identify 10 cm, and another wide band is added at each 5 cm until the five-band, 25-cm mark is reached.

Nonocclusive catheters are used for passage up the ureters in order to collect renal urine and for direct retrograde pyelography. Commonly used types are the whistle-tip, olivary-tip, and round-tip catheters. Other types include the *Garceau tapered whistle tip* which is useful mostly to occlude a ureter, particularly when selective urine specimens are being collected and one wishes to obtain an accurate volume measurement. At times it is difficult to introduce a ureteral catheter, particularly past the ureterovesical junction and especially when there has been some hooking of the lower ureters secondary to prostatic hypertrophy or cystocele formation. In such a situation, a *Blassucci flexiform spiral-tipped* ureteral catheter is often useful. These catheter tips are illustrated in Figure 12-8.

Another type of ureteral catheter that has a special use is the *wax-tipped* catheter. This kind of catheter is custom-made by the nurse when needed. To construct such a catheter, a whistle-tipped or round-tipped catheter is dipped into molten beeswax so that a drop gathers near the tip. After the wax has hardened and is noted to be smooth, the catheter is passed up the ureter with a twisting motion beyond a possible ureteral calculus. If a calculus is present, it will often imprint a spiral scratch on the wax. A neoplasm, on the other hand, will not scratch the wax. This technique, often forgotten, is particularly useful in the differentiation of persistent radiolucent ureteral defects.

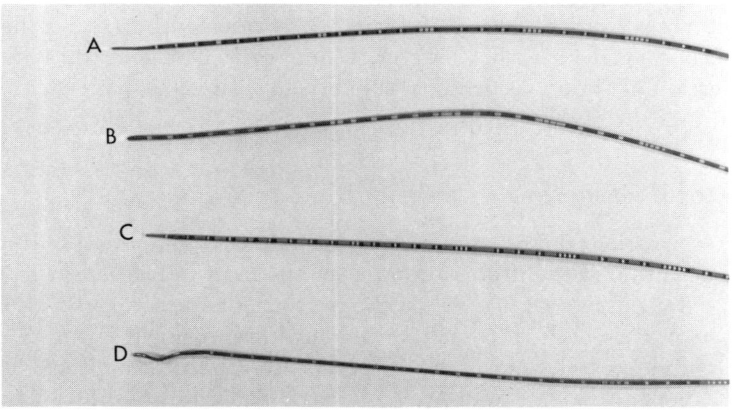

FIGURE 12-8. Various tipped ureteral catheters. *A*, tapered whistle tip; *B*, whistle tip; *C*, olive tip; *D*, spiral-tipped Blassucci.

There are three main types of occlusive ureteral catheters. Such occlusive catheters fit into the ureteral orifice much like a cork and allow the operator to fill the entire upper urinary tract (renal pelvis and ureter) for retrograde pyelography. The Braasch bulb is an onion-shaped tip that fills the ureteral orifice. The Foley tip is cone-shaped with the eye of the catheter in its center. Woodruff tips are metallic balls which screw onto a catheter. These balls come in sets of increasing size, so that with a single catheter the operator can tailor his size appropriately to the ureteral orifice (Fig. 12-9).

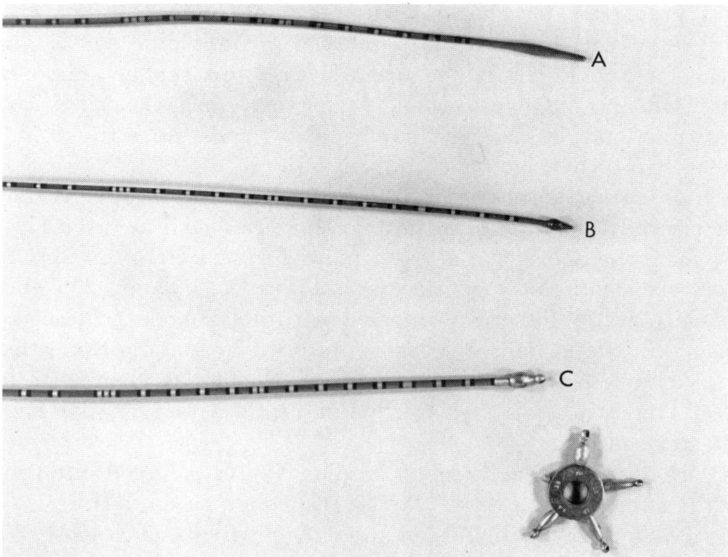

FIGURE 12-9. Catheters for occlusive retrograde pyelography. *A*, Braasch bulb tip; *B*, Foley tip; *C*, Woodruff catheter with various-sized tips.

Stone dislodgers are specially modified catheters sometimes used to grasp small calculi inside the ureter via the cystoscope. Many types have been devised and are in varying favor, depending on the skill and experience of the operator. The three main types include the Ellik loop, Johnson basket, and the corkscrew. The Ellik loop is a catheter with a nylon string attached to the eye. Tension on the string causes the tip of the catheter to loop on itself, at which time the calculus has hopefully been included in the loop. The loop and calculus must then be drawn down the ureter. Baskets, of which the Johnson basket is a prototype, consist of several wires exposed for a few centimeters along the catheter.

By external manipulation the wires are spread apart, and if the calculus falls between wires, they are placed on tension and the entrapped stone is removed with the catheter. The corkscrew, as its name implies, is screwed into the lowermost ureter to grasp a calculus in this location.

Sterilization and Care of Catheters

The sterilization and care of catheters vary enough from the routine of surgical instruments to warrant special emphasis. In view of the time and care required for maintenance, disposable catheters are becoming more popular. In addition, catheters that are left indwelling in the patient are best used only for that patient and then discarded. For example, urethral Foley catheters can be purchased in individual sterile packages from the factory. Polyethylene ureteral catheters can be similarly purchased, used once, and discarded. At present, however, such catheters will not completely replace the nondisposable type, since they tend to be either too stiff or too soft for certain situations.

The most important consideration in the care of catheters is that they be mechanically cleansed of all foreign material such as dried blood and mucus, since the debris can act as a nidus for bacterial growth. Urethral catheters are cleansed by gentle brushing on the outside. The lumen is cleared with water forcefully injected with a syringe. If there is much dried blood in the lumen, this can be softened by soaking the catheter in either hydrogen peroxide or special solutions such as Haemo-sol for ten minutes. The catheter is then washed in a mild detergent soap and dried prior to sterilization.

The care of ureteral catheters is similar. Water is forced into the distal end of the catheter, and debris can be pushed out through the eye. A wire stylet is passed through the lumen and out the other end to assure patency and to further remove foreign material. The eye of the catheter is then placed into a flask containing 10 per cent formaldehyde solution, and the other end of the catheter is allowed to hang over into the sink. By siphon action, the formaldehyde solution is dripped through the catheter for one hour. The catheter is then transferred to a flask containing distilled water for 15 minutes which, by siphon action, will wash out the formaldehyde. The lumen of the catheter can easily be dried by gently slapping the catheter. Well-cared-for woven ureteral catheters can on an average be used eight or ten times. It is good practice to test ureteral catheters once monthly by gently bending them near the eye to about 45°. If the catheter bends smoothly, it can be used again. On the other hand, if the varnish shows signs of cracking, the catheter is too brittle and should be discarded. It is certainly better to throw away catheters unnecessarily at times than to have the tip break inside the patient.

Catheters constructed of rubber or latex can be sterilized by boiling, autoclaving with steam or gas, and the use of chemical disinfectant solutions. Boiling the totally submerged catheter for 15 minutes is the simplest and most available method for destroying vegetative pathogens and their spore forms. However, repeated boiling will most rapidly shorten the life of the catheter. A less destructive method is the steam autoclave. The catheter should be soaked in water and wrapped while still wet immediately prior to autoclaving. This ensures more effective sterilization and prevents superheating. The latter more rapidly deteriorates rubber and latex. Two autoclave settings are either 270°F at 27 pounds per square inch (PSI) or 250°F and 15 PSI. The former combination is used for 3 minutes and the latter 15. Autoclaves for both combinations are available for nonhospital use.

Ethylene oxide gas sterilization techniques are becoming more popular in recent years. The main advantage of this method is that delicate articles such as cystoscopes, electrical cords, and plastics can be reliably sterilized at relatively low temperatures. Furthermore, a preliminary rinse in distilled water is unnecessary to remove potentially harmful chemicals before use in the patient. The ethylene oxide is mixed with an inert gas such as freon. The gas mixture determines the exposure time, which can range from five to eight hours. The specific settings are available in tables provided by the various manufacturers. However, the temperature and pressures are relatively low (110°F, 8 to 10 PSI). Special wrapping paper and low-temperature autoclave tape are used with this method.

Formalin gas is commonly used in a technique that will kill many but not all vegetative bacteria and is relatively ineffectual against spores. The dried instruments are placed on trays in a specially designed cabinet. Catheters must be scrupulously dry; otherwise, rubber and latex will be destroyed. One gram of formaldehyde pastilles is placed on a heat generator inside the cabinet. The generator is turned on and the cabinet locked. The pastilles vaporize in 1 hour and the gas is circulated for 12 hours, after which the cabinet can be opened. This time-honored method can be considered bacteriostatic rather than bactericidal and is therefore mainly valuable as a storage medium for sterilized instruments. Formaldehyde is extremely irritating to mucous membranes, and all instruments and catheters thus disinfected need careful rinsing before use.

Numerous chemical solutions are available for cold sterilization. Most of these solutions will kill most vegetative bacteria but have varying effects on tubercle bacilli, spores, and fungi. Certain of them are corrosive to instruments and others quite irritating to mucous membranes. Chemicals used in the past include oxycyanide of mercury, formaldehyde, alcohol, and aqueous benzalkonium chloride (Zephiran). The most effective presently available disinfectant is glutaraldehyde solution (Cidex). Ten-minute exposure to this solution will kill all vegetative bacteria and the tubercle bacillus. However, a three-hour exposure is necessary to kill spores. The instruments should be rinsed in distilled water prior to use in the patient. Such a solution is particularly suited for the doctor's office where sounds and catheters may be used several times during the day. At the conclusion of office hours, the catheters can be removed from the tray, cleansed mechanically, and dried, and thus be ready for soaking the following day. Catheters that have been sterilized in chemical solutions such as benzalkonium should not be autoclaved subsequently, since some of these solutions under heat and pressure will attack rubber. Once a catheter becomes discolored, loses elasticity, or develops cracks in its surface, it should obviously be discarded.

A useful time-saving technique for catheters that are less frequently employed is to individually package and sterilize the catheter, so that it will be available at a moment's notice. Flexible Sierra nylon plastic tubing is one such packaging material. The clean, dried catheter is inserted into the tubing, and a suitable length is cut. The ends are sealed over with striped tape which changes color after adequate sterilization. Such packages should be dated and can be considered sterile for at least one month. If muslin is used for wrapping, the article will be sterile for one week, and if wrapped in special kraft paper, for two weeks.

Woven nylon and plastic catheters can be boiled according to the manufacturer, but fare much better with gas or chemical sterilization. Endoscopic equipment can be sterilized only by gas or chemical solutions. The use of heat will melt the cement holding the lenses in place. To put it emphatically, *cystoscopic equipment should never be boiled or steam autoclaved.*

REVIEW QUESTIONS

1. Define the French scale for the measurement of instruments. How are these numerical values converted to millimeters?
2. Describe the following catheters and discuss their advantages: Robinson, "multieyed" Robinson, coudé, Foley, Malecot.
3. Describe the following instruments and how they are used: filiform and follower, bougie à boule, urethral sound.
4. Identify the following ureteral catheters and discuss their individual advantages: whistle tip, Garceau tip, Blassucci tip, wax tip, Foley tip, Braasch bulb, Woodruff tip.
5. Discuss the methods for cleaning ureteral catheters.
6. Discuss the methods of sterilization most appropriate for each of the following: rubber, polyethylene, metal, varnished woven material.
7. What methods are inappropriate for these materials and why?

CHAPTER 13
Endoscopic Instruments

ENDOSCOPIC instruments are important tools in the urologist's diagnostic and therapeutic armamentarium. They are used for visual inspection of the lower urinary tract, for investigation of the upper tracts, and for the treatment of many lower tract disorders. The development of these instruments by the specialty of urology has laid the groundwork for the design of the numerous other endoscopic tools now used in all branches of modern medicine.

As with other urologic instruments, there are numerous varieties. However, the principles of operation and construction are similar and a discussion of a commonly used type, the *Brown-Buerger cystoscope*, can be used as a baseline for study by the nurse. A detailed description is important so that the nurse can appreciate the delicate and complicated construction of this equipment and accordingly maintain it properly.

The Cystoscope

Briefly, a cystoscope is an instrument that is inserted into the bladder for examination. The instrument is basically an optical one with a complicated lens system. In order for the urologist to see into the bladder, its interior must be illuminated. Consequently, a light source consisting of an electric lamp is located on the interior end of the cystoscope. This lamp requires wiring within the equipment connecting with an external source of electric power. Furthermore, provisions must be made for the introduction of an aqueous irrigating medium to distend the bladder so that its wall can be pushed away from the objective lens in order to see the lining of the organ. Finally, space must be provided within the confines of the instrument for the introduction of ureteral catheters, biopsy forceps, and the like.

The main components of the cystoscope are the *sheath*, the *obturator*, and the *telescope* (Fig. 13-1). The sheath is the tubular structure that defines the outer limits of the instrument. The external surface of the sheath is in intimate contact with the mucous membrane of the urethra. Its diameter is commonly measured by the French scale. Because the outer surface comes into contact with delicate tissues, it must be free of any irregularities and scratches. The sheath must not be dented or bent; otherwise, the internal components, manufactured to a very close

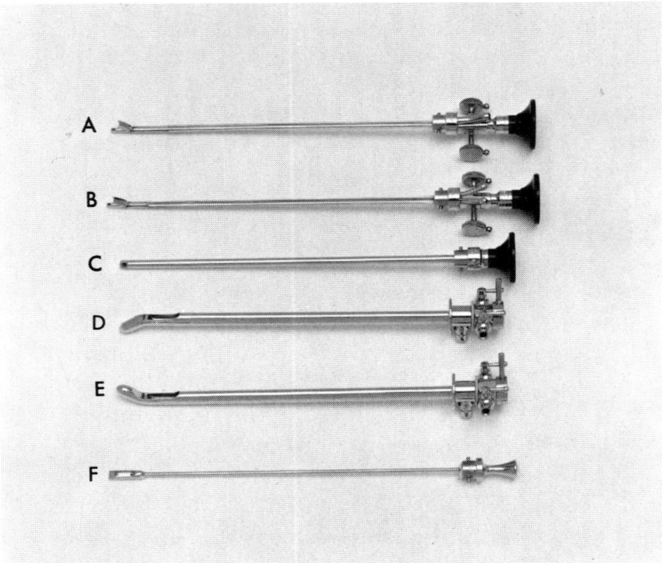

FIGURE 13-1. Components of a Brown-Buerger cystoscope. *A*, single catheterizing telescope; *B*, double catheterizing telescope; *C*, observation telescope; *D*, convex sheath; *E*, concave sheath; *F*, obturator. (Courtesy of American Cystoscope Makers, Inc.)

tolerance, will not fit or function properly. Obviously, no part of these instruments should ever be handled roughly. They will not tolerate dropping and handling with potentially damaging instruments. They should be picked up and placed down gently. An appropriate dressing forceps should be used to remove them from trays, formalin cabinets, etc.

The Brown-Buerger sheath is made with a curved beak, which allows for easier introduction into the bladder through the prostatic urethra. The sheath may be concave or convex, depending on the relationship of the internal opening (fenestra) to the curve of the beak. If the fenestra is on the same side as the curvature of the beak, it is known as a concave beak, and vice versa for the convex instrument. The light bulb is within the beak of the Brown-Buerger cystoscope. Other instruments may have the bulb incorporated into the removable lens system. Two wires in the wall of the sheath carry electricity from an external source on the outside end of the sheath. Also on the outer end are a pair of stopcocks used to control the introduction of irrigating medium into the bladder. A rotating lock mechanism is also placed here. Once a telescope has been inserted, it is locked into place not only to provide a watertight connection but also to prevent any movement within the sheath.

The obturator is used to occlude the fenestra of the sheath for introduction of the cystoscope. When it is inserted properly, it serves to make the sheath smooth so as not to damage the urethra.

The telescope is the optical portion of the cystoscope. The lens system consists of an ocular externally, an objective lens on the inside which peers through the fenestra of the sheath, and multiple achromatic lenses and prisms set in the shaft of the telescope (Fig. 13-2). The latter lenses are carefully inserted in place and sealed watertight during manufacture in a completely dehumidified room. If the seal is ever broken to allow moisture to enter or if the telescope is dropped, the chances are great that the unit will not function properly and will require repair.

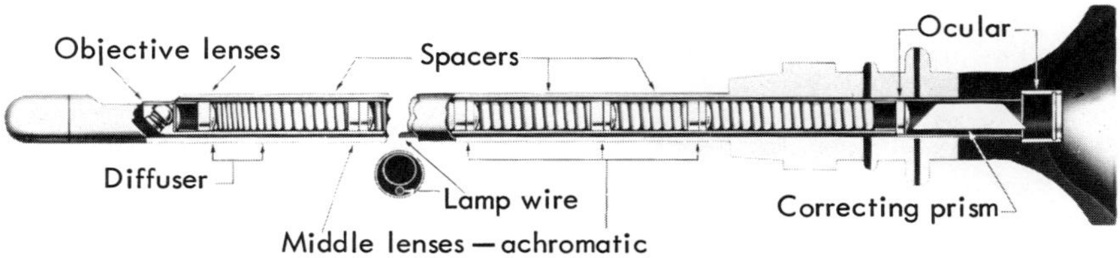

FIGURE 13-2. The internal components of an observation telescope.

Optical systems are available with different fields of vision. The most commonly used is the Foroblique system which has an angle from straight ahead to about 55° to the side. Other types include the direct forward, right angle, and retrograde system, wherein the operator can look almost directly backward, as in examination of the bladder neck (somewhat like a rearview mirror in an automobile). The various angles of vision are shown in Figure 13-3.

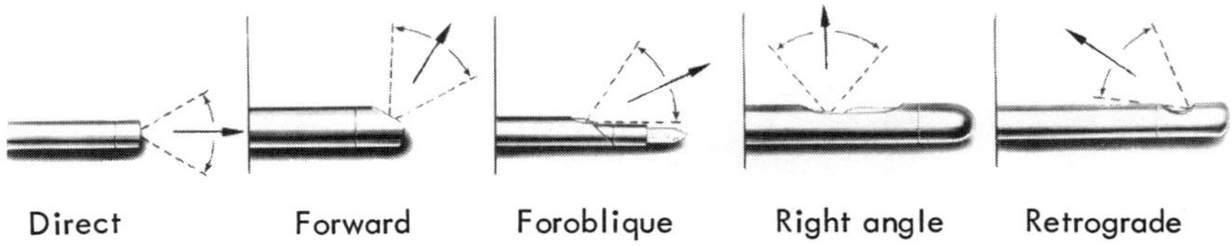

FIGURE 13-3. Angles of vision of various lens systems.

A "working unit" is a telescope which has a narrower stem (and thus a smaller field of vision) than the observation telescope, thus allowing catheters, biopsy forceps, and other instruments to be introduced through the cystoscope alongside the telescope into the bladder. An example of a working unit is shown in Figure 13-1*A* and *B*. A ureteral catheter can be introduced via the catheter tunnel through the sheath into the bladder. The catheter can then be deflected by means of a little lever (deflector) which operates through the fenestra of the sheath. The operator manipulates the lever by means of a control knob from the outside. Should it be necessary to insert two ureteral catheters simultaneously, crossover and snagging of catheters can be prevented by insertion of a longitudinal fin along the telescope stem, thus creating two separate catheter tunnels. Rubber nipples are placed on the tip of the catheter guides to make a watertight connection. When the catheter guide is not in use, the hole can best be plugged by insertion of a rounded sterile toothpick into the opening. Working units are available with larger guide openings for insertion of large instruments such as biopsy forceps.

Electricity to light the lamp must be obtained from an external source supplying about two volts. Two commonly used sources are the Wappler safety battery box (Fig. 13-4) and a stepdown transformer connected to

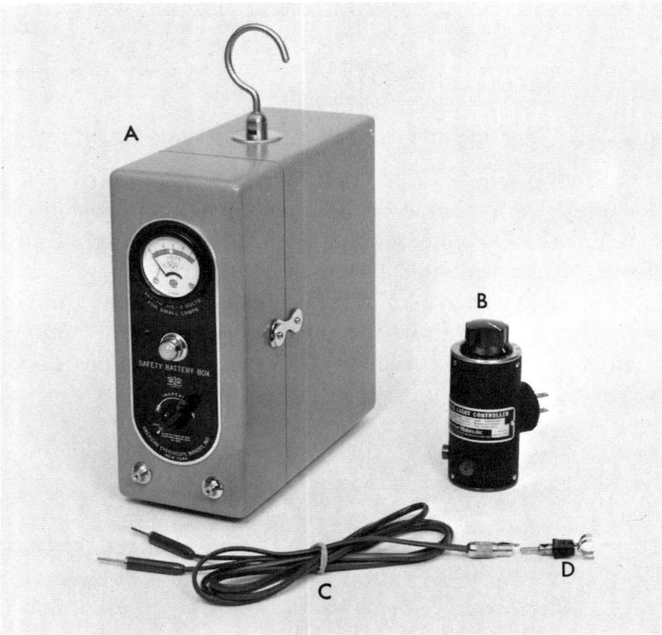

FIGURE 13-4. Electrical connections for cystoscopy. *A*, Wappler safety battery box; *B*, stepdown transformer; *C*, light cord; *D*, rotating contact. (Courtesy of American Cystoscope Makers, Inc.)

house current which has a variable rheostat. For pediatric instruments with more delicate bulbs, an additional resistor must be used to further reduce the voltage. The battery box has a rheostat incorporated into it and a voltmeter on the outside. After electrical connections have been made, the control is gradually turned clockwise until the needle is in the narrow white area of the meter wherein optimum illumination can be obtained. Below this level (the green area), the intensity of light will be too weak. Above it (the red area) there is danger that the bulb will burn out. If a shortcircuit is present, a buzzer in the box will sound a warning. The battery box is connected to a light cord. Two plugs in the cord will fit into corresponding sockets on the box. The other end of the cord has a connector which snaps onto the rotating contact on the cystoscope (Fig. 13-4).

The contact, also known as the lightpost, has a circumferential groove around which the connector can be rotated. In this groove, on opposite sides, are two black circles. When the connector is on these circles, the current is disconnected. Rotation of the connector 90° will turn the current on again. The rotating contact snaps onto the corresponding areas on the end of the cystoscope. As the cystoscope is turned to various positions, the contact can also be turned to prevent the light cord from winding around the instrument. Commonly used sizes of the Brown-Buerger instrument are 16, 21, and 24 French.

The Panendoscope

The Brown-Buerger cystoscope is probably the most widely used examining instrument in the United States, but its nearly right-angle view, while excellent for the inside of a sphere such as the bladder, is deficient for viewing down a cylinder such as the urethra. Numerous other instruments are available. One other will be described in detail, since it typifies those permitting a view along a tube. The *McCarthy Foroblique panendoscope* is a straight instrument which is often used in sequence with the Brown-Buerger instrument. It is particularly useful in examination of the urethra, and especially for evaluation of prostatic urethral intrusion. The field of vision is identical with that seen with the various resectoscopes used for transurethral surgery, which will be mentioned subsequently. The instrument consists of a telescope, sheath, and bridge assembly (Fig. 13-5).

The sheath is straight with a beveled blunt end. A lock and stopcock are attached to its outer end. In contrast to the Brown-Buerger instrument, the lamp of the panendoscope is part of the telescope, and the rotating electrical contact is attached to the outer end of the lens system. The telescope fits onto the bridge assembly, which in turn secures and positions the telescope in the sheath of the instrument. The plate on the bridge may be solid and watertight or may be perforated. The former assembly is used for examination alone and the latter when one wishes to insert ureteral catheters. However, this instrument is not as adaptable for manipulative work as the cystoscope. Various-sized perforated plates are available for the bridge. Although the panendoscope has no directing lever,

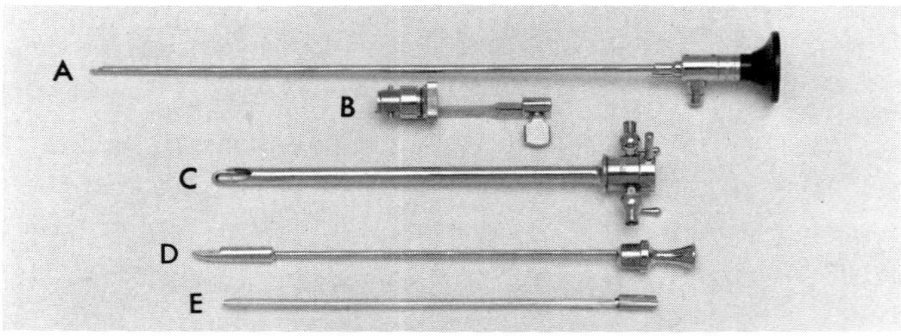

FIGURE 13-5. Components of the McCarthy panendoscope. *A*, foroblique fiberoptic telescope; *B*, bridge assembly; *C*, sheath; *D*, obturator; *E*, detachable fin. (Courtesy of American Cystoscope Makers, Inc.)

some guidance can be obtained by use of a fin which is snapped onto the telescope itself. An obturator is available, but this instrument may be introduced under direct vision.

Fiberoptic Instruments

The application of fiberoptics has opened a new era in urologic instrumentation. Fiberoptics utilizes the principle that light which enters the end of a glass fiber is trapped within the fiber and is transmitted to its opposite end by internal reflections. If many such fibers are placed side by side in an orderly fashion, a coherent image can be transmitted as well as light alone.

Fiberoptics has a number of advantages. The fiber bundle, being flexible, can be bent. One can therefore transmit light or an image around varying corners. The transmitted light intensity can be very high so that extraordinary illumination can be obtained. The amount of heat generated at the opposite end of the cord is usually not great enough to cause tissue damage.

The source of light is a parabolic lamp which can be housed in a small box which has appropriate condenser and cooling attachments. One end of the fiberoptic cord is connected to the light source. The other end can then be connected to various endoscopic instruments which contain light-carrying glass fibers either in the sheath or in the telescopic system. The free end of the bundle can be used directly at the operating table in those situations where intense illumination may be needed in a restricted area. This intense beam can be used clinically for transillumination, as in the evaluation of scrotal masses. These are presently the greatest clinical advantages of this new development.

There are some drawbacks to be considered at the present stage of knowledge. The fiberoptic cord is relatively heavy and, albeit flexible, it is not as mobile as the usual electrical cord used with standard light sources.

This somewhat hampers the maneuverability of the operator during endoscopic surgery. In addition, the glass fibers naturally take up more space than the fine wires in the sheath of standard instruments. Consequently, the internal caliber of cystoscopes containing the fibers in the sheath is slightly less than that of older-style instruments. When the fibers are incorporated into the telescopic system, the field of vision seems somewhat diminished. Regardless, as time goes by, further refinements in manufacture are to be expected. Fiberscopes, or instruments which transmit an image directly through the glass fibers, have yet to be perfected to a degree where they are really useful in urologic practice. Instruments of larger caliber, however, are now being used extensively in other branches of medicine, such as gastroenterology. Figure 13-6

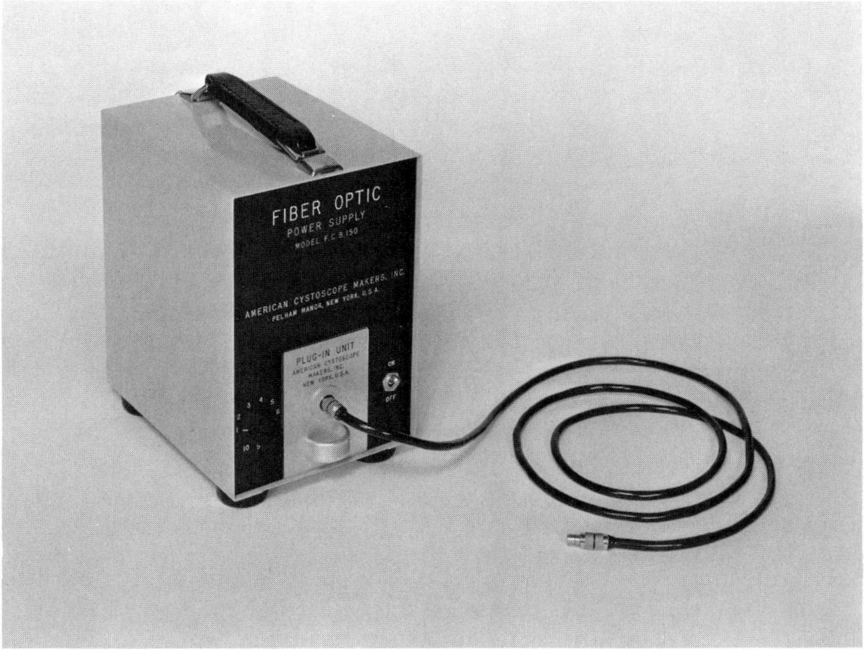

FIGURE 13-6. Fiberoptic light source with attached light-carrying bundle. (Courtesy of American Cystoscope Makers, Inc.)

illustrates a fiberoptic light source with the light-carrying bundle attached. Note that the bundle is coiled several times, yet the light appears at its end.

Fiberoptic cords must be sterilized without the use of heat. Cold antiseptic sterilization is preferred. An important point is that the solutions used must be colorless, since any pigments present may coat the ends and interfere with the quality and intensity of the transmitted light.

Cystoscopic Forceps

Many kinds of instruments are available for use through the cystoscope, and several common ones will be described. These include *cup biopsy* forceps, *alligator* forceps, *meatotomy scissors*, and *coagulating electrodes*. These instruments are introduced through the center channel of the cystoscope and are manipulated from the outside. The commonly used cup biopsy forceps can be obtained with a flexible or rigid stem. The former is preferred since it can be manipulated with greater ease within the bladder. The inner end of the forceps has a small hollow cup which can be opened by spreading the outside scissors type handle (Fig. 13-7).

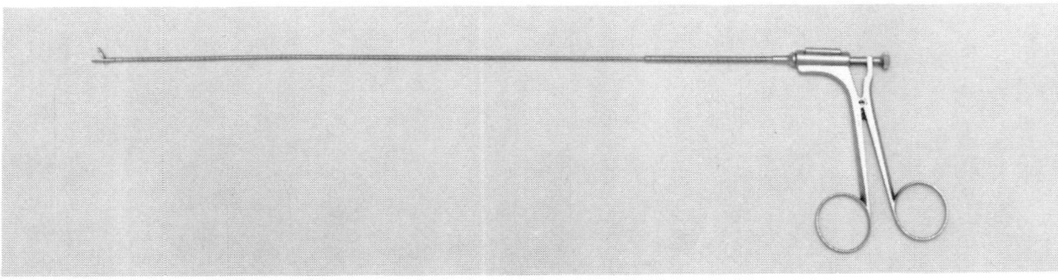

FIGURE 13-7. Cystoscopic biopsy forceps. (Courtesy of American Cystoscope Makers, Inc.)

The edges are sharp. The opened cup is directed against a lesion of the bladder, the cup is closed, and a biopsy is thus obtained. The alligator forceps and other instruments similar in construction have a serrated jaw which is used to grasp small stones or foreign bodies in the bladder. The meatotomy scissors consist of a small scissor tip used to cut within the bladder, usually a ureteral orifice. Its mechanical action is similar to that of the other forceps described.

Fulgurating or coagulating electrodes have tips of varying shapes which convey a high-frequency electrical current. The wiring connecting the tip to the outer end of the electrode is covered with appropriate insulation to the outer end which is connected by an adapter to an electrosurgical generator. The electrode is flexible so that the tip can be directed with the cystoscopic deflector against the lesion. After the electrode is properly placed, the current is then applied as necessary under control of a foot switch to the generator.

Maintenance of Cystoscopic Equipment

The maintenance of cystoscopic equipment is covered in large part in the section on sterilization. However, several points are worthy of re-emphasis. The various parts of the instrument should be checked to ascertain that they fit properly before the instruments are handed to the operator and after they have been cleaned at the end of the day. The obturator and the telescopic lens system should slide easily in and out of the sheath. If these need to be forced into place, something has been bent and the instrument will require return to the factory for repair. These instruments are delicate, should be handled gently, and will usually require repairs if dropped. Except for some experimental models, they should be thoroughly cleaned with soap and water. An appropriate soft-bristled brush is run through the sheath of the instrument to mechanically wipe out debris. Mechanical cleansing is as important as sterilization to maintain good performance. The lens system should be wiped clean. A toothpick is useful for small particles. At the end of the day, the ocular and objective of the lens system are wiped firmly with a gauze pad lubricated with a water-soluble jelly and washed. The bulbs are checked to see that they are in working order. Blackened bulbs should be replaced, since they are on the verge of burning out. When a bulb is changed, the socket must be perfectly dry and the filament at the base of the bulb kept straight so that adequate contact is made inside the socket. Any water in the socket will shortcircuit the system. Worn electrical connectors are replaced. The nurse should look through the telescopic system herself to make sure that vision is clear. If the lenses are at all fogged after mechanical cleansing, one must assume that moisture has been introduced inside the optical system, and this will require factory repair. The utmost gentleness in the handling of these instruments will result in a long life despite their delicate construction.

REVIEW QUESTIONS

1. Describe the cystoscope and its component parts. Describe the way this instrument is used by the urologist.
2. List the fields of vision of the various telescopes.
3. Describe the panendoscope, its component parts, and the use of this instrument.
4. What are fiberoptic instruments? How are they presently used in urologic practice?
5. Name three types of cystoscopic forceps.
6. Discuss the maintenance and care of endoscopic instruments.

CHAPTER 14
The Cystoscopic Examination

THE basic material prerequisites for the performance of a cystoscopic examination are as follows: (1) an appropriate table with stirrups, so that the patient may be placed in the lithotomy position; (2) an apparatus for delivery of irrigating solution to fill the bladder; (3) a source of electricity to illuminate the interior of the bladder; and (4) the cystoscopic instruments, sterile drapes, gloves, and gown.

Meticulous cleanliness should be observed in the cystoscopic suite just as it is in the operating room. Often the walls and floors are tiled to permit frequent scrubbing, and only the necessary equipment is kept in the room. The light in the room should be subdued, and the windows are usually covered with black shades to prevent excessive glare. Sink facilities should be available either in the room or close at hand so that the operator can go through a surgical scrub. It is advantageous, but not necessary, to have a central drain in the floor, which is slightly slanted to drain off any fluid that is spilled during the examination.

Examining Table

The examining table may be of the Hugh Young type. A movable pan at the lower end of the table is available to catch urine and irrigating solution from the bladder. The table may or may not be provided with a cassette holder and x-ray equipment so that intravenous pyelograms, cystourethrograms, and retrograde pyelograms may also be performed, thus combining the features of a cystoscopic and x-ray examining table. Newer models are motorized so that the height and horizontal plane of the table can be adjusted by means of a foot switch (Fig. 14-1). The table usually has two breaks—at the head and foot. It is important for the nurse to know how to adjust the table into various positions since, during a procedure, various adjustments may be necessary which the doctor will not be able to perform himself. It is also important for the nurse to know how to disassemble removable parts so that the table can be thoroughly cleaned after each use. In practice, the surface of the table is washed off between patients with an antiseptic solution. It is also important to place the patient directly on the table and to remove any cushions beneath him, since these may interfere with x-ray examinations.

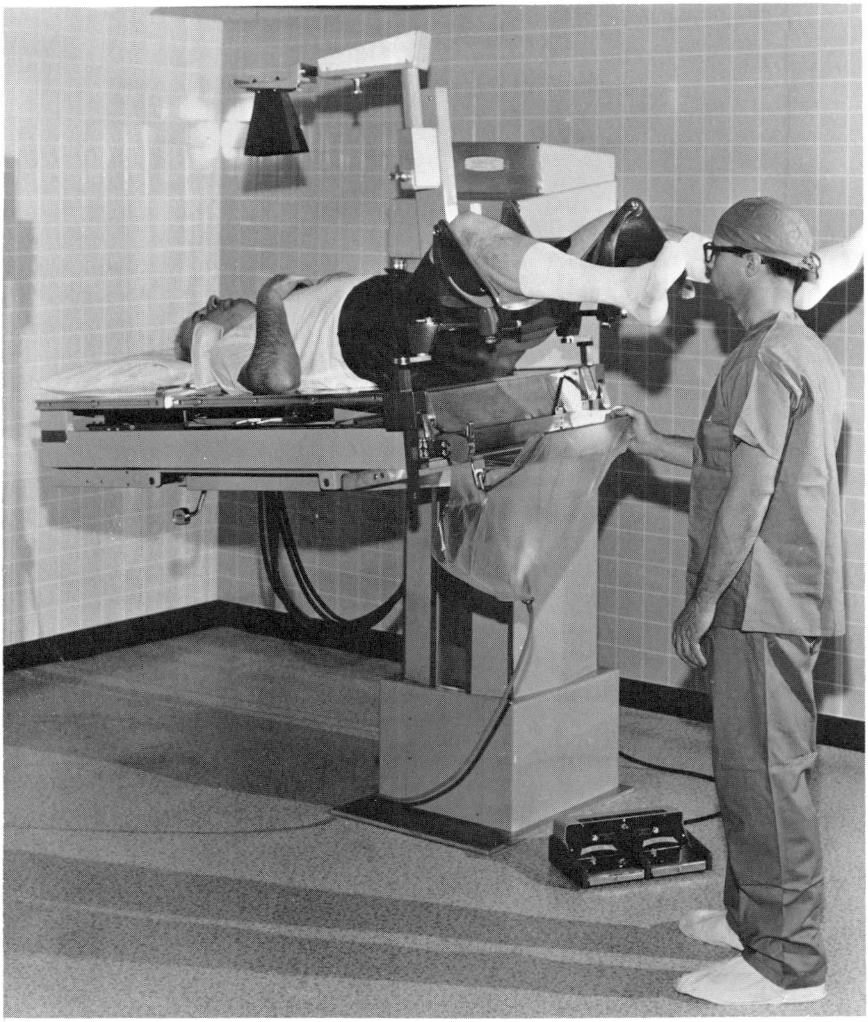

FIGURE 14-1. Modern cystoscopic table with x-ray attachments. (Courtesy of Liebel-Flarsheim Co.)

Irrigating Solutions

An irrigating solution must be available to fill the bladder. This can be placed in either wall tanks connected to the lower end of the table by means of sterile tubing, a sterile Valentine flask which is set up at the beginning of the day and periodically filled with irrigating solution, or in recent times disposable plastic irrigating flasks. Irrigating solutions commonly used are water, 5 per cent dextrose, isotonic glycine (1.5 per cent), and sorbitol-mannitol solution. The best visualization of the bladder interior is obtained with water. The danger of hemolytic reactions with the use of water (which can be absorbed through open veins) is minimal for purely cystoscopic examination. An electrolyte solution such as isotonic saline cannot be used since it can transmit current, and electrical equipment is used in such procedures.

The irrigating solution should be sterile and at a temperature between that of the room and the patient. Especially in cold weather, the irrigating solution should be heated to body temperature. Cold solutions may induce significant hypothermia, particularly in infants and children, thus leading to untoward reactions. The height of the supply bottle should be approximately thirty inches above the level of the bladder. Sterile tubing, either rubber or plastic, is then connected from the supply source to a stopcock on the cystoscope. By manipulation of the stopcock, the examiner is able to control the flow of solution. The solution may be taken from the sterilizer in a sterile pitcher and then delivered to the jar, or the fluid may be added directly from sterile bottles obtained from the manufacturer, or from a tank that sterilizes the solution and replenishes the supply by means of an automatic float mechanism. Regardless of the delivery system employed, the nurse must be certain that there is an adequate amount in the jar throughout the entire examination. Between examinations only that section of tubing adjacent to the patient (which is sterile) is replaced with fresh sterile tubing, but the technique would be somewhat better if the whole were changed each time.

Following completion of the day's examinations, the bell jar and tubing may be sterilized by boiling, autoclaving, or as is frequently done, being filled with an appropriate antiseptic solution and allowed to soak until the following day. If the jar is boiled or autoclaved, it is either wrapped in sterile wrappers or placed in a formalin cabinet until it is used again. Antiseptic solutions must be drained and discarded and the jar and tubing rinsed with sterile water before use to avoid introduction of irritative substances into the bladder. In an emergency situation where solutions are not readily available, an alternate method is to connect a bottle of 5 per cent dextrose and water intended for parenteral use with sterile intravenous tubing, which can then be connected to the stopcock on the cystoscope. One must be careful to read the label on the bottle of fluids used for cystoscopic examination. Although such fluids are sterile and chemically clean of extraneous substances, they are still not suitable for intravenous use, whereas fluids suitable for intravenous use can be safely used on an emergency basis for cystoscopic examination.

A standard cystoscopic setup is shown in Figure 14-2. Ideally the nurse should be in the room, particularly with female patients, not only for the

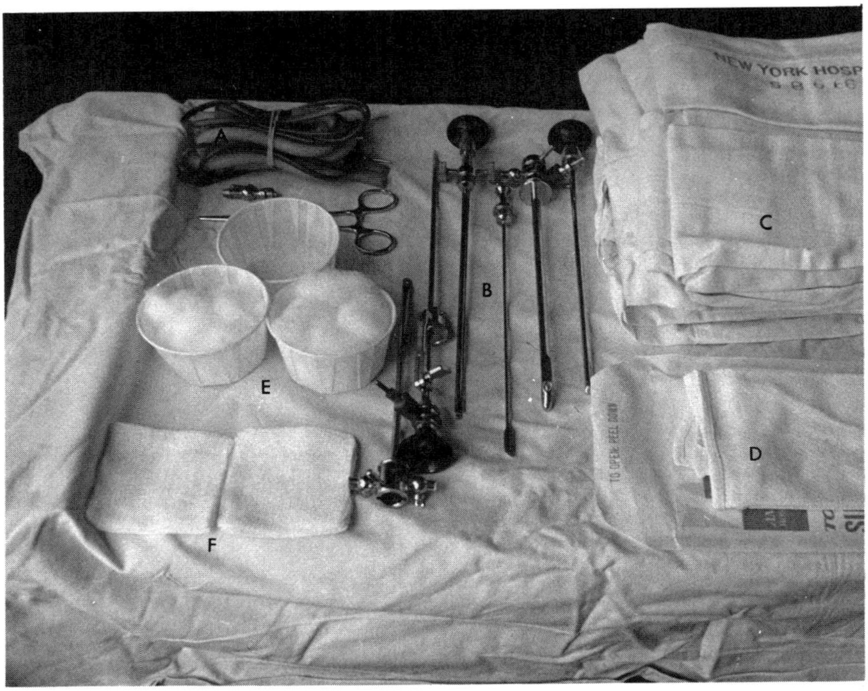

FIGURE 14-2. Standard cystoscopic setup. *A*, light cord and sterile tubing; *B*, sterile examining instruments; *C*, sterile drapes; *D*, sterile gloves and towel; *E*, hemostats and sterile cotton balls for preparation of genitalia; *F*, sterile gauze squares for lubricating jelly.

purpose of proper chaperoning but also to obtain any additional equipment the doctor may require at the last minute. The basic setup includes a panendoscope with its examining parts, a cystoscope with similar parts, several dry sponges to clean off lenses, toothpicks, the sterile electrical cord, and irrigation tubing. If retrograde pyelograms are to be performed or biopsies obtained, or a small lesion requires fulguration, appropriate equipment is then supplied as necessary. If the equipment has been sterilized with formalin gas or cold antiseptic solution, it must be rinsed in sterile water beforehand to avoid irritation of the operator's eyes and the mucous membranes of the patient.

Preparation of the Patient for Cystoscopy

Basic Preparation

Cystoscopic examination can be performed using no anesthesia, local, general, or spinal anesthesia. The preparation of the patient for this examination is determined by what the operator intends to do and the type of anesthesia to be used. If the examination is to include retrograde pyelography, the patient may be given enemas or cathartics on the night prior to examination. No anesthesia may be needed or a local anesthetic will frequently suffice, particularly if the examiner is gentle. General anesthesia is usually required for infants and children and may be necessary for the tense, fearful adult. Retrograde pyelograms can also be obtained without anesthesia, especially in adult female patients. If difficulty is anticipated—such as the presence of a tight urethral stricture which may require dilation, the presence of a small papillary lesion which may need fulguration, or extensive manipulation—then some form of anesthesia may be required. Under all circumstances, an operative permit should be obtained from the patient. If the patient is under the legal age or is mentally incompetent, permission is necessary from the parents or legal guardian. In rare instances when an emergency procedure is necessary and the legal guardians are not available, clearance should be obtained from the hospital administrator.

If he is an inpatient and no anesthesia is to be used, premedication with adequate amounts of a narcotic, a barbiturate, and frequently an oral tranquilizer should be used to provide relaxation, but the patient should be observed for the effects of these medications after the examination has been completed. If local anesthesia is to be used, it is advisable to prepare the patient beforehand with a barbiturate since this will diminish the severity of any allergic reaction to the local anesthetic. The patient should be asked if local anesthesia has been administered in any form previously and if untoward reactions occurred. Most patients have previously had some dental work with local anesthesia, and the doctor or nurse can usually find out if there were untoward reactions. Should general anesthesia be required, the patient is allowed nothing by mouth for at least eight hours prior to the examination. Approximately one hour previously, premedications are given intramuscularly. The nurse should routinely make certain that the patient's chart is complete, that the operative permit has been properly signed and witnessed, and that premedications are recorded and signed. Often adult patients will not be given a general anesthetic until an electrocardiogram, chest x-ray, urinalysis, and complete blood count have been obtained and recorded on the chart. Where this is the policy, the nurse must be certain that this information is properly recorded.

Local Anesthesia

Local anesthesia is accomplished by instillation of appropriate materials into the bladder and urethra and the use of ointments containing these compounds on the sheath of the examining instruments. One must remember that such anesthetic compounds can be absorbed from the patient's mucous membranes into the bloodstream. There is always some danger in their use. Of course, they should not be used when the urinary tract is acutely inflamed or while there is active bleeding, since the likelihood of resorption is greater.

Adequate local anesthesia of the male lower urinary tract can be accomplished by gentle instillation of 20 ml of a dilute local anesthetic such as 1 per cent lidocaine in aqueous form into the urethral meatus using a syringe with a short catheter tip. The injection should not be forceful, to avoid trauma and possible absorption. A penile clamp (Fig. 14-3) is then applied just below the glans penis and kept in place for five

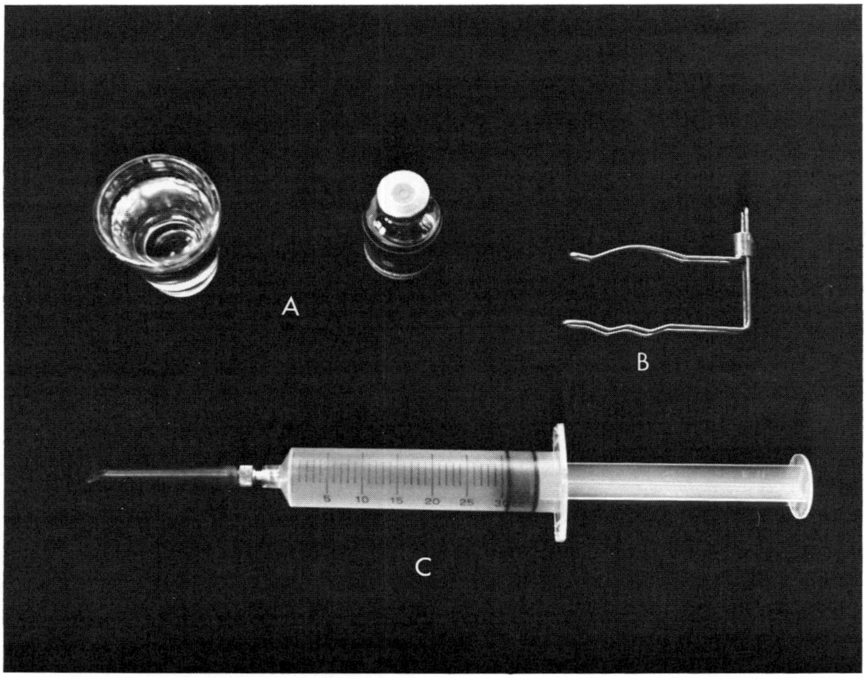

FIGURE 14-3. Equipment for local anesthesia of the male urethra. *A*, local anesthetic solution; *B*, penile clamp; *C*, syringe with short catheter.

minutes, during which time adequate anesthesia of the urethra should be obtained. One may then insert a small catheter into the bladder and introduce an additional 15 to 20 ml of dilute solution after the bladder has been emptied. After another five-minute wait, an examination can then be performed with minimal discomfort.

Experience shows that routine cystoscopic examinations can be performed in female patients without anesthesia, and indeed in many male patients as well. Many patients will come to the doctor either having had a stressful experience elsewhere or having had warnings by well-meaning friends of the extreme discomfort of this examination. If some time is spent with the patient describing exactly what is to be done, much of this apprehension can be allayed. If the patient is going to be examined on an ambulatory basis, he is told beforehand that if the examination becomes uncomfortable, the procedure will be discontinued immediately and that no attempt will be made to put him through a regrettable experience. With most patients who have been properly prepared, there is usually little difficulty.

Positioning the Patient

Cystoscopic examination is usually performed with the patient in the lithotomy position. The nurse should see that the patient is positioned so that there is optimal relaxation of the muscles of the legs and perineum. On placing the legs in stirrups it is important that the nurse be certain that circulation is not interfered with and that pressure points are padded to avoid possible damage to the popliteal nerve. This is particularly important in the patient who is to be examined under general anesthesia and can therefore not call attention to any discomfort. The common peroneal nerve travels over the outer edge of the fibula just below the knee joint, and lateral pressure at this level can temporarily damage the nerve and cause a foot drop. The popliteal arteries travel beneath the knee in the midline, and no sharp points should contact this area. Should a physical condition such as arthritis of the hips prevent positioning of the patient in the lithotomy position, some other position, usually the supine, is used. Sometimes a midposition between the full lithotomy and strictly supine position may be required, and the ingenuity of the doctor and nurse come into play. The legs can be separated and supported at the knees using adequate pillow and sandbag support.

Once the patient is in position for examination, the external genitalia are thoroughly cleansed with a soap scrub and an antiseptic solution (such as 1:1000 benzalkonium chloride) and dried with a sterile towel. The patient is then covered from the lower chest down to and including the feet with a sterile drape. The genitalia are exposed through a hole properly placed in the drape. Sterile disposable paper sheets are labor savers and convenient. The drawer of the cystoscopy table should also be covered by a sheet. Meanwhile, the operator scrubs in the accepted fashion for any surgical procedure and is gowned and gloved. The examining equipment, which has been thoroughly checked beforehand, is brought alongside the foot of the table and the examination is performed.

The Examination

One end of the sterile tubing is handed to the nurse, who connects it to the irrigating supply. The operator opens his end to wash air out of the system. The light cord is also handed to the nurse, who connects it to the electrical source so that the light can be adjusted to its proper intensity before the instrument is inserted into the patient.

Usually the urethra is examined first with the panendoscope. The endoscope may be inserted into the bladder with obturator in place, but it is better practice inserting the instrument under direct vision with continuous flow of irrigating solution, which will distend the urethra ahead of the instrument as it is guided through the urethra into the bladder. The anterior urethra and prostatic urethra are examined for evidences of disease, particularly any element of intraurethral prostatic intrusion.

The endoscope is then removed and the cystoscope is inserted with obturator in place. The obturator is removed and the examining telescope inserted. The operator will examine the interior of the bladder as irrigating solution is being introduced to note the evenness of bladder expansion. For example, a mass on one side of the bladder may expand at a slower rate and this can be noted. An idea of the bladder capacity is obtained with the bladder full, and the operator can note whether the media of the bladder are perfectly clear, bloody, or snowflaked, as seen with severe infection. The interior of the bladder is examined in a routine fashion for evidence of disease such as abnormalities of the bladder wall, inflammation of the mucosa, the presence of neoplasia, foreign bodies, and calculi. The ureteral orifices are examined for size, shape, position, and the appearance of urinary efflux from the upper tract on either side. Any further manipulation or examination depends on the findings at that time. The bladder is usually emptied before the instrument is removed at the end of the examination. The cystoscope should be removed with the obturator in place to prevent abrasion or irritation of the urethral mucosa from the sharp edge of the sheath alone.

Failure of Illumination

Failure of illumination can be tracked down in the following order. First, one must be sure the light bulb is secure in its socket. If the bulb appears blackened, it has probably burned out. Next, the light cord is examined for any signs of fraying. If questionable, it should be replaced. The tightness of the connections at either end of the cord should be checked, particularly with the lamppost on the cystoscope. Finally, if no other source of difficulty has been located, the battery box should be changed. If the lighting system is working properly and yet the operator can see nothing on peering into the telescope, he must be sure that the telescope has not been introduced into the sheath upside down. The optical system is properly inserted when the cystoscope lock and a pin near the ocular of the telescope are on the same side.

Postcystoscopic Care

Unless there is a significant contributing abnormality, the discomfort experienced by the patient following cystoscopic examination is usually not severe. There may be some burning and frequent urination. It is not uncommon for the urine to be slightly bloody for a short time. Meperidine (Demerol) or other narcotics in small doses, an increased fluid intake, and warm sitz baths will often take care of these problems promptly. Symptoms of abnormalities, however, may be exacerbated. For example, a patient who has significant prostatic difficulty which is barely compensated may go into retention following the examination. If the urinary tract is already infected, there is some danger of a febrile response, which should be adequately covered with appropriate antibiotics started prior to the examination. The nurse should reassure the patients that these minor problems are not uncommon and that they will pass. The passage of grossly bloody urine with clots, shaking chills and fever, and an almost total inability to void constitute a different story, however, which should be reported to the doctor promptly. Following examination, the patient's temperature should be checked every 4 hours for a period of 24 hours. The vital signs should be checked at frequent intervals, not less than twenty minutes apart, until they are stable, and a record should be kept of the frequency and volume of urination.

Following general anesthesia, the patient should be observed closely until conscious and fully reactive. Diet and ambulation are progressed as tolerated and as requested by the physician. Following retrograde pyelography, the patient should be watched more closely, particularly if the examination involves insertion of a catheter up a ureter and especially if a bilateral examination has been done. After ureteral catheterization an occasional patient will experience flank pain on the affected side similar to that noted with renal colic. This is due to the formation of small clots which can cause pain as they pass down the ureter.

Occasionally following renal function studies wherein a catheter has been indwelling for longer periods, there can be enough edema of the ureter to cause a temporary anuria. More often than not this will subside spontaneously. However, such obstructive anuria, erroneously known as "reflex anuria," may last as long as 48 to 72 hours. Rarely recatheterization may be necessary to start the flow of urine again. Patients who have divided renal function studies are told that their urine may be bloody for up to 24 hours. In such examinations, large ureteral catheters are used to totally occlude the ureters in an effort to obtain the complete volume output of each kidney during the examination. The likelihood of anuria when such divided function studies are done using an osmotic diuretic such as urea becomes less, since the diuretic effect continues for several hours after the catheters have been removed. Regardless, severe flank pain, chills, fever, and decreased urinary output should be promptly called to the attention of the physician so that appropriate management can be prescribed.

Studies for Neurogenic Dysfunction of the Bladder

Neurogenic dysfunction of the bladder is corroborated by cystometric studies. The clinician will be well aware of such dysfunction, since signs of neurogenic deficit involving other than the urinary tract will be present in the patient on careful examination. An "isolated" neurogenic bladder is a rarity, particularly since the nerve supply to the bladder and the rectal-perineal area are of common origin. A purely isolated neurogenic bladder can conceivably be obtained when the bladder is stripped clean, as might occur with pelvic surgery of adjacent organs, particularly in radical hysterectomy. Except for these iatrogenic situations, a neurologic defect is usually demonstrable.

Cystometric Studies

During the performance of a cystometric study, the patient must necessarily be awake in order to cooperate with the doctor. The intravesical pressure is measured with different amounts of solution in the bladder instilled through a urethral catheter. Certain points are noted, such as whether the patient does or does not feel the sensation of bladder filling. The volume and pressure at which the initial desire to void occurs are noted and recorded, and subsequently recognition of warm and cool solutions in the bladder. One also notes the maximum capacity, the maximum voluntary intravesical pressure, and the presence or absence of involuntary bladder contractions.

In the normal patient, the bladder capacity varies considerably anywhere between 250 and 600 ml. The first desire to void usually occurs when a minimum of 150 ml are in the bladder but may occur sooner if the lower urinary tract is irritated and inflamed. With 200 or 300 ml of fluid in the bladder, the patient is told to attempt micturition and normally should be able to raise the pressure of the water column in the manometer to more than 45 cm of water. The type of neurogenic abnormalities are legion, and so a pure form of deficit is not commonly seen. These may vary from the totally flaccid neurogenic bladder as seen in tabes dorsalis (wherein the bladder acts simply as a passive bag that can be distended to over a liter) down to the automatic uninhibited neurogenic bladder which has little capacity and contracts involuntarily with only a very small amount of fluid in the cavity.

A standard cystometric form sheet, as used at The New York Hospital–Cornell Medical Center, is illustrated in Figure 14-4 with a superimposed normal curve. Various instruments have been devised for cystometric study. The simplest and probably the most adequate equipment is shown in Figure 14-5. Fluid is introduced into the delivery jar which enters into a Y tube. One limb of the tube is connected to the catheter and the other limb to a simple water manometer. Air bubbles must be removed from the system before the connections are made. The manometer is adjusted to zero, which is approximated to the level of the neck of the patient's bladder. The tubing to the manometer is then clamped and water is allowed to drip into the bladder at a slow rate, no greater than 20 to 30 ml per minute. If a faster rate is used, the bladder may contract involuntarily in the normal patient. After a small aliquot, usually 50 ml, is instilled, the supply tube is clamped off and a manometric reading is obtained and recorded. The manometer is then clamped and additional fluid is introduced into the catheter in increasing amounts. During this time the various questions are answered—namely, does the patient feel the solution enter the bladder, at what point is an initial desire to void experienced, and at what volume has the bladder reached its maximum capacity? The maximum voluntary pressure is recorded, and during the manometric observation one looks for involuntary contraction, which will be manifested when the patient, lying comfortably, will suddenly raise the column of water quite high in the manometer. To obtain the maximum voluntary pressure, the patient is instructed to strain down as if voiding, but caution should be observed that the patient does not manually compress the bladder, since this will falsify the reading. It is important to realize that the normal bladder will contract involuntarily when its maximum capacity is approached and also when the rate of introduction of fluid is too rapid.

Usually the examination is well tolerated and is painless. When warm and cool solutions are introduced into the bladder to evaluate the patient's temperature sensation, the shrewd examiner does not ask the patient if the water feels cold or hot—he simply asks the patient if anything abnormal is felt. In the normal situation, the patient will spontaneously tell the examiner whether the solution is cold or warm. When the hot and cold solutions are requested from the nurse, the examiner should not forewarn the patient. Before these solutions are introduced into the bladder, it is best to feel them on the back of one's hand, since abnormally hot or cold solutions may be quite uncomfortable and possibly damaging.

Fancier cystometers have been invented, consisting of equipment that can record pressure changes continuously and directly by means of a direct writer on graph paper. These instruments are expensive, and

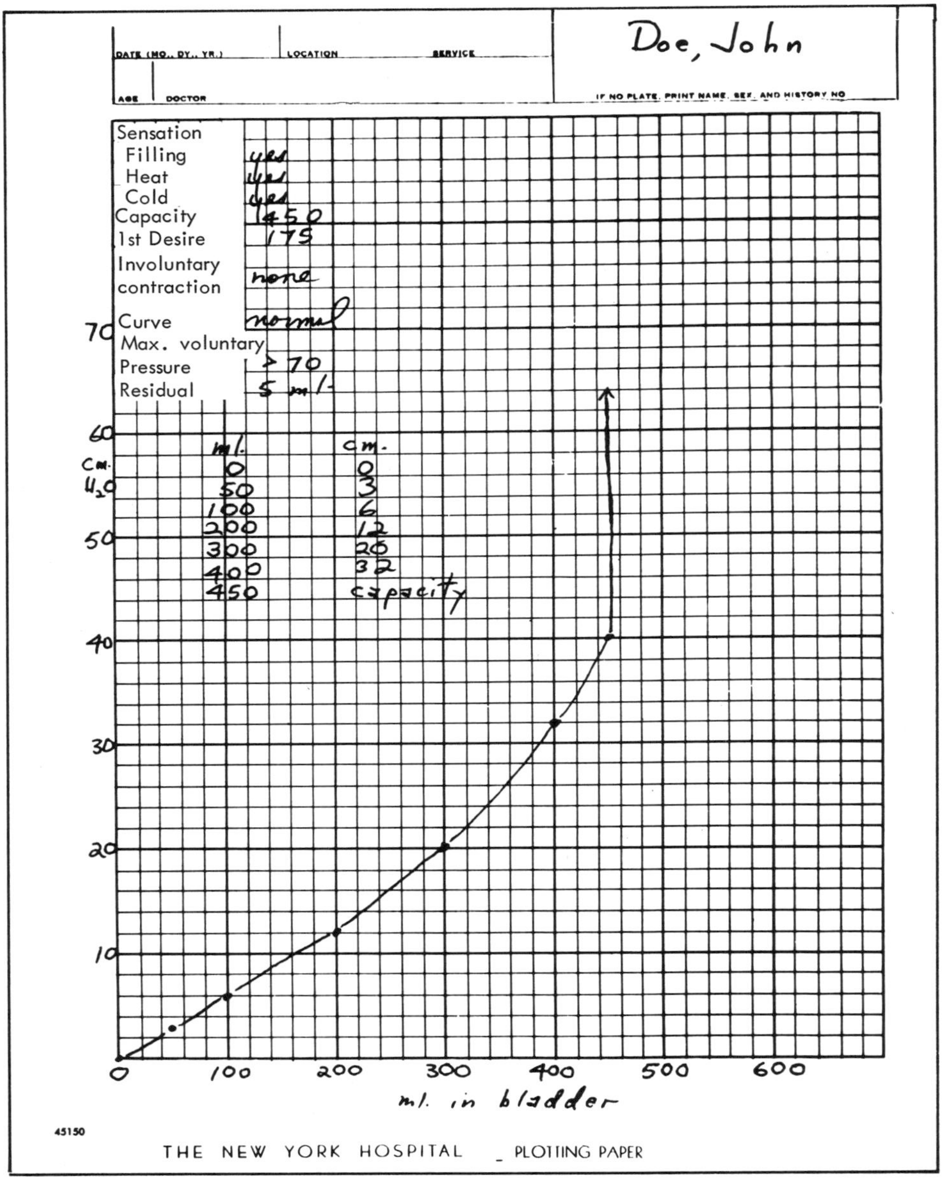

FIGURE 14-4. A normal cystometrogram.

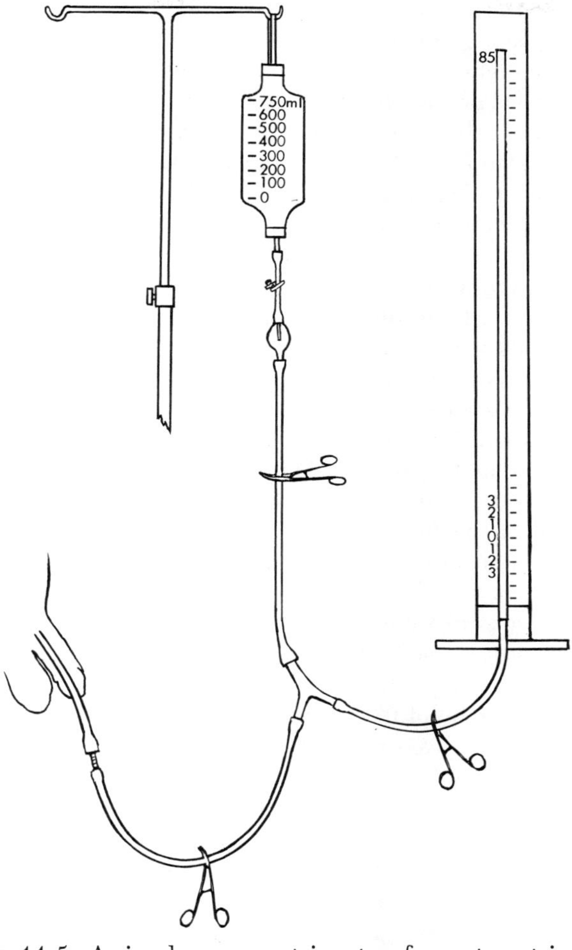

FIGURE 14-5. A simple manometric setup for cystometric studies.

usually all the information that is necessary can be obtained with simpler equipment.

Needle Biopsy of the Prostate

Needle biopsy of the prostate is usually performed to establish the diagnosis of carcinoma. It is our practice to do such a biopsy more often in patients in whom a radical prostatectomy is not contemplated, but the clinical diagnosis needs confirmation before embarking on specific treatment such as castration or estrogen therapy. There is a theoretical disadvantage in sampling a solitary nodule of cancer, in that tumor cells may be seeded along the path of the needle. Furthermore, should the biopsy be negative for cancer, one cannot always be certain whether the nodule was reached or the prostatic tissue was truly negative for neoplastic changes. Consequently, unless other circumstances dictate to the contrary, an open surgical biopsy by the perineal route is usually recommended for a solitary nodule, particularly if the plan calls for radical prostatectomy.

The biopsy is obtained using one of several available varieties of prostatic biopsy instruments. The Franklin modification of the Vim-Silverman needle probably enjoys the greatest popularity. With the patient in the lithotomy position, the needle is introduced into the perineum, which has been prepared under sterile conditions and suitably draped. With a guiding finger in the rectum, the operator directs the needle with its stylet toward the suspicious area of prostate using the opposite hand. The stylet is withdrawn. The biopsy blades are inserted through the lumen of the needle into the biopsy area. While holding the biopsy blades steady, the needle is advanced into the prostate using a rotatory motion to cut out the core of tissue between the blades. The blades and needle are removed together, containing the biopsy which is promptly placed in a fixative solution to avoid dehydration of the specimen. The procedure can be done under local anesthesia. Often it is helpful to make a small nick in the perineal skin to facilitate introduction of the needle. An operative permit is required, and mild sedation such as a small dose of a narcotic and a barbiturate is helpful. An alternate approach to needle biopsy of the prostate is a direct transrectal insertion of the needle into the prostate through the overlying rectal mucosa. Although many urologists favor this route, it is not used at our hospital.

In most instances, there is relatively little risk to the procedure. The main consideration is to rule out any bleeding tendency. As mentioned previously, certain patients with extensive prostatic carcinoma may have markedly elevated levels of circulating fibrinolysins. All patients in whom needle biopsy of the prostate is considered should be tested for this condition beforehand. Following biopsy there may be slight oozing in the perineum which can be controlled by simple pressure. On rare occasions there may be transient urinary retention, hematuria, or fever which is easily controlled by appropriate measures.

Renal Biopsy

A renal biopsy is often useful to identify an underlying renal parenchymal disorder. This may be achieved by an open operation, wherein a biopsy is obtained under direct vision, or by closed percutaneous needle biopsy.

Renal biopsy is usually performed on one of several indications, which includes renal disorders of indeterminate cause wherein all other diagnostic methods have failed to elucidate a definitive diagnosis. Such disorders include the nephrotic syndrome, unexplained albuminuria, hypertension in which a renal factor may be present, and unexplained hematuria; another aim is to identify an undiagnosed systemic disease which may involve the kidneys. However, the procedure of closed renal biopsy should not be taken lightly, since complications, when they occur, may be serious. The most common ones are lacerations and gross hematuria of a severe enough nature to require transfusion, operation, and possible nephrectomy. Other complications are the laceration of organs other than the kidney, particularly the liver and spleen, and an increasingly recognized incidence of iatrogenically produced renal arteriovenous fistula. Consequently, biopsy should not be performed when the patient is severely uremic, since hemorrhage is more likely and a possible nephrectomy could be most detrimental. Other contraindications include a solitary kidney, blood dyscrasia, abnormal position of the kidney, infection, potentially curable cancer, and marked hypertension.

Prior to renal biopsy, as much information as possible should be gleaned regarding the urinary tract by other means. The size and location of the kidneys must be defined. Blood dyscrasias are ruled out and blood should be available for the patient if transfusion is necessary. The needle biopsy is done with the patient awake, and thorough explanation of the procedure to him beforehand is necessary to obtain adequate cooperation and a good biopsy.

The patient is given nothing by mouth, beginning the night before, and a signed permission is obtained. Appropriate sedation is administered prior to the procedure. The patient is placed in the prone position on an x-ray table with a sandbag or rolled sheet beneath the upper abdomen to help immobilize the kidney to the back. The back is prepared and draped under sterile conditions. A preliminary ink mark correlating with previous x-rays is made over the lower pole of the kidney, usually the right one. The use of an image intensifier may help to direct the needle under direct visual control.

After adequate local anesthesia of the skin and subcutaneous tissues, a long spinal needle is inserted toward the lower pole of the kidney. A definite change in the consistency of tissue encountered will usually confirm that the kidney has been reached. This will be further confirmed by a to-and-fro swing of the needle as the kidneys move with respiration. The depth of insertion of this needle is noted. It is withdrawn and replaced with the Franklin modification of the Vim-Silverman biopsy needle. The needle is advanced as the patient holds his breath in deep inspiration. When the renal capsule is reached, the patient is asked to breathe, and the needle should go through the characteristic respiratory excursion.

The patient is again instructed to hold his breath in inspiration and the biopsy is taken by inserting the cutting prongs into the kidney and twisting out the plug of renal tissue. The specimen must be placed promptly in the appropriate fixative before it has an opportunity to dry out, particularly since the volume of tissue is not great.

Following the procedure the patient's blood pressure and pulse are checked hourly for the first four hours and every four hours for at least the next two days. All voided urine is examined for gross bleeding, with an eye to the presence of clots. Also, careful attention is paid to the possible presence of colicky flank pain. Should gross hematuria appear, the frequency of observations is increased and the physician notified. The ambulatory medical treatment of the uremic syndrome is strictly palliative.

REVIEW QUESTIONS

1. What are the basic material prerequisites for the performance of a cystoscopic examination?
2. Describe the irrigating solutions available for use during cystoscopy.
3. What factors will determine how the patient is prepared for cystoscopic examination?
4. Discuss the role of the nurse during cystoscopy.
5. Mention several common causes for instrument failure during cystoscopy and how they can be remedied.
6. What should the nurse look for in the care of a patient following a cystoscopic examination?
7. What is a cystometrogram? What information can be provided by such a study?

REFERENCES—UNIT II

Barnhill, Sue E., and Elizabeth E. Chenoweth: "Cleansing of the Perineum," *Amer J Nurs*, **66**: 566, 1966.

Bonnell, G. E.: "Urological Investigative Procedures," *Canad Nurse*, **59**: 825–28, 1963.

Craig, Ilsa: "Collecting Specimens of Urine: The Nurse Holds the Key to Diagnosis of Infections," *Nurs Times*, **62**: 531–32, 1966.

Cravitz, Leo, and Virginia Tyler: "Sterilization of Cystoscopy Instruments and Accessories," *Hosp Top*, **38**: 103–106, 1960.

Dineen, Peter: "The 'Sterilization' of Endoscopic Instruments," *JAMA*, **176**: 772–75, 1961.

Dison, Norma Greenler: *An Atlas of Nursing Techniques.* C. V. Mosby Co., St. Louis, 1967.

Emmett, John L.: *Clinical Urography*, 2 vols. W. B. Saunders Co., Philadelphia, 1964.

French, Ruth M.: *Nurse's Guide to Diagnostic Procedures*, 2nd ed. McGraw-Hill, New York, 1967.

Geist, Dorothy I.: "Round-the-Clock Specimens," *Amer J Nurs*, **60**: 1300–1302, 1960.

Glenn, James F., ed.: *Diagnostic Urology*. Hoeber Medical Division, Harper & Row, New York, 1964.

Guze, Lucien B., and Paul B. Beeson: "Observations on the Reliability and Safety of Bladder Catheterization for Bacteriological Study of the Urine," *New Eng J Med*, **255**: 474–75, 1956.

Harrow, Benedict R., Jack A. Sloane, and Louis Salhanick: "Clinical Evaluation of Renal Function Tests," *J Urol*, **87**: 527–34, 1962.

Hart, Elizabeth L., and Margaret J. Magee: "Collecting Urine Specimens," *Amer J Nurs*, **57**: 1323–24, 1957.

Kark, Robert M.: "Office and Bedside Examination of Patients Suspected of Having a Renal Disorder," *Med Clin N Amer*, **46**: 785–94, 1962.

Kelly, Ann, and Goffredo Gensini: "Renal Arteriography," *Amer J Nurs*, **64**: 97–99, 1964.

Kennelly, John M., Jr.: "Bacteremic Shock: Sequel to Genitourinary Tract Instrumentation," *J Urol*, **79**: 549–53, 1958.

Lapides, Jack, and John M. Bobbitt: "Preoperative Estimation of Renal Function," *JAMA*, **166**: 866–69, 1958.

Lenkowski, Michael F.: "Catheterization of the Male Patient," *Amer J Nurs*, **51**: 401–403, 1951.

Mainwaring, Cathryn: "Clean Voided Specimens for Mass Screening," *Amer J Nurs*, **63**: 96–97, 1963.

Marshall, Victor F.: "Fiber Optics in Urology," *J Urol*, **91**: 110–14, 1964.

Merritt, Donald, and Joy Sanford: "Sterile Voided Urine Culture," *J Lab Clin Med*, **52**: 463–70, 1958.

Milberg, Max, and Harold Hermann: "Pyrexia Following Cystoscopy," *J Urol*, **86**: 823–28, 1961.

Mohammed, Mary R. B.: "Urinalysis," *Amer J Nurs*, **64**: 87–89, 1964.

Page, Lot B., and Perry J. Culver, eds.: *Syllabus of Laboratory Examinations.* Harvard University Press, Cambridge, Mass., 1960.

Reagan, James W.: "Cytological Studies," *Amer J Nurs*, **58**: 1693–95, 1958.

Roland, Samuel I., and Victor F. Marshall: "The Reliability of the Papanicolaou Technique When Cancer Cells Are Found in the Urine," *Surg Gynec Obstet*, **104**: 41–44, 1957.

Silvis, Virginia, "Continuous Urine Specimens from Infants," *RN*, **22**: 37–39, 1959.

Smith, Alice L, *Carter's Principles of Microbiology*, 4th ed. C. V. Mosby Co., St. Louis, 1961.

Stewart, Bruce, Richard A. Schacht, Robert C. Bishop, and James Conway: "Differential Function Studies in Renal Hypertension: Indications and Techniques," *J Urol*, **94**: 7–14, 1965.

Tyler, Virginia R.: "Gas Sterilization," *Amer J Nurs*, **60**: 1596–99, 1960.

UNIT III

Surgical Treatment of Urologic Disorders: General Principles and Nursing Considerations

CHAPTER 15
Preoperative and Postoperative Care

A SURGICAL procedure is an integral part of the treatment of many urologic disorders. Except in emergency situations, most patients do not undergo operation until a complete evaluation not only of the urinary tract but of the patient's general state of health has been performed. During the preoperative period the necessary steps are taken to help the patient attain an optimal state of physical and psychologic preparedness for the anticipated surgery. The total care of the patient requires the active cooperation of all members of the health team.

Nurse's Role

The nurse plays an important role during every stage of the preoperative period. Information that the nurse obtains by observation and conversation with the patient may be invaluable. Although the physician tries to make the initial history and physical examination as complete as possible, the nurse, by more frequent contact with the patient, may glean additional useful data. Often a patient may neglect to give information because he feels it is unimportant or because he is unaware that his established way of life, normal in his eyes, is really quite abnormal.

There are innumerable examples illustrating how the nurse can discern these abnormalities. A patient may claim that he has no problems with urination, yet the nurse may observe that he goes to the bathroom or asks for a urinal at unusually frequent intervals. The patient may say that he is in "good shape," yet the nurse may notice he becomes short of breath just walking. The patient's reaction to such simple procedures as venipuncture or catheterization is often a good indication of his level of anxiety and pain tolerance. When the patient's response is extreme, whether very bland and nonchalant or overreactive, the nurse and doctor will need to more carefully explore the patient's perception of the situation in order to enable him to cope effectively with the imposed stresses.

Pertinent and concise nurse's notes are important to make certain that information is conveyed to the physician and others involved in the patient's care. By intelligent observation, the nurse can assist the doctor in the accumulation of the necessary data to evaluate and treat the patient. During this period, she will also be actively involved in assisting with the diagnostic work-up as well as administering the prescribed medical regimen. How well she assumes her responsibilities in these areas may well determine how quickly and adequately the patient will be prepared for his operation.

Physical Preparation for Surgery

Age is an important consideration in the preoperative preparation of the urologic patient. Urologic disease may affect patients of all ages, from young children with congenital abnormalities to elderly men with prostatic obstruction. Although nonurologic congenital anomalies may be associated in the patients of the pediatric age group, the general state of health of these children is usually good and operations are well tolerated.

The picture changes in the geriatric group wherein many of the disorders associated with aging may be present. These conditions will require evaluation and treatment as part of the overall management of the patient. Cardiovascular disorders may necessitate the use of digitalis, diuretic medications, oxygen, and ancillary treatment. The patient with chronic pulmonary disease such as emphysema may benefit from preoperative regimens utilizing intermittent positive-pressure breathing apparatus, mucolytic agents, and appropriate antibiotics for pulmonary toilet. Should the patient have diabetes mellitus, his disease will need to be regulated preoperatively and carefully monitored in the postoperative period to prevent complications. If a hypertensive patient has been receiving any medications for the lowering of blood pressure prior to admission, this fact should be noted and the medications identified. On rare occasions, patients who have ingested rauwolfia compounds such as reserpine during the ten days prior to anesthesia may become severely hypotensive during operation. Such ingestion does not negate anesthesia and surgery in emergency situations, but having this information the anesthetist is better equipped to handle such hypotension should it occur.

Many elderly patients, either because of lack of motivation, poor eating habits, or simply lack of funds, may suffer from malnutrition. This may not be severe under ordinary circumstances but may be sufficiently inadequate to lower the patient's resistance and tolerance of an operative procedure. The nurse, working closely with the dietitian may need to revise the dietary regimen to include the patient's preferences yet be nutritionally adequate. Vitamin and mineral supplements such as ascorbic acid and iron may also be prescribed. At times, in the markedly anemic patient, blood volume determinations and preoperative transfusions may be indicated.

In planning nursing care, the nurse needs to consider the physical and sensory limitations of the elderly patient. Those with impaired hearing or a language barrier may not understand instructions or explanations clearly. Special safety precautions must be taken with the patient with limited vision. Obstacles that may cause the patient to fall should be removed from harm's way. The feeble individual may need assistance in ambulation. Edentulous patients will need a diet free of tough, fibrous foods which are difficult to chew. Often the elderly patient has a very set way of life and may find adjustment to the hospital setting quite difficult. The nurse will need to be flexible and imaginative in manipulating hospital routines to meet the patient's needs.

Many elderly patients have a limited tolerance to medications. An exaggerated physiologic response is particularly common to the usual dosage of sedatives and narcotics. Barbiturates, for example, may cause agitation and mental confusion. In her planning, the nurse should establish goals for nursing care that are consistent with the physician's medical regimen but are also consistent with good nursing practice.

Psychologic Preparation for Surgery

It is the doctor's responsibility to explain the intended surgical procedure in sufficient detail so that the patient can understand what is planned and what to expect in the postoperative period. At times, particularly in the presence of a possibly incurable cancer or with a necessary but highly risky operation, the physician may prefer that discreet details be given to a responsible member of the family to spare the patient unnecessary emotional stress. It is wise for the nurse to know what has been told to the patient and what has been told to the family. She can do this by either being present at the discussion or speaking to the physician shortly thereafter. In particularly difficult situations, it is good practice for the physician to outline the details of these conversations in the progress notes of the patient's chart.

Several examples can be given to illustrate the kind of information that can be mentioned to both the patient and his family for various urologic procedures. In the case of a transthoracic nephrectomy, where the chest cavity is entered, the patient will often return to the unit with a chest drainage tube connected to underwater suction and may receive oxygen either by a nasal catheter or oxygen tent. If informed of this ahead of time, the patient and family will realize that this is part of the routine postoperative care and does not represent a "heart attack" or other major complication. Prior to any open operation, the patient should be advised that the incision will be painful for several days but that adequate pain medication will be provided. He should also be advised that soon after surgery the nurse will assist him in getting out of bed and walking. He will be asked to turn from side to side every few hours and to cough. Intravenous fluid therapy will be used for at least 24 hours following operation, and food and fluids by mouth are frequently withheld.

The patient who is to undergo bladder or prostatic surgery is advised that postoperatively he may have a strong desire to urinate due to the location of the surgery and the usually present indwelling catheter. Although a certain amount of discomfort of this nature is unavoidable, he should be instructed to inform the nurse of the duration and intensity of the pain in order for her to determine whether or not pain medication is needed. It is also important to tell the patient and his family that the urine after prostatic surgery is often bloody for several days. It is helpful to explain that as little as a teaspoon of blood can make a quart of urine appear quite red. Such simple explanations may prevent unnecessary fear and apprehension.

A philosophic question that frequently arises and about which there is considerable debate is, "How much detail of any contemplated procedure or possible complications should be discussed with the patient and his family prior to the operation?" Even the simplest surgical procedure involves some risk. Under an extreme circumstance, for example, a patient can die from a circumcision; on the other hand, the statistical chance is very remote, so ordinarily the possibility is not mentioned. Certainly the patient or his family must be forewarned of those complications that occur frequently—for example, total impotence is virtually guaranteed following a radical prostatectomy for cancer, and urethral fistulas after hypospadias operations are common. A 50-year-old sexually active man may choose to live a few years with his cancer and his potency rather than pay this price for a possible cure. Permanent urinary incontinence is a possible but rare complication following operation for benign prostatic enlargement. If this complication is discussed with undue emphasis prior to operation, many patients who would need such surgery may refuse to have it.

It is not possible or reasonable to discuss every potential complication before operation, but those that occur often and those seriously affecting the patient's future existence are worthy of note. Nevertheless, all questions raised by the patient and his family must be answered by the doctor as thoroughly and as frankly as reasonable. Failure to do so is an injustice to the patient and will greatly undermine his confidence in those responsible for his care. Physicians vary about telling a patient he has cancer. Assuming that the diagnosis is established, the author nearly always tells the patient. Not to tell the patient deprives him, as well as his family, of the right to openly and honestly work through the emotional crisis that such a diagnosis brings. Withholding the diagnosis may also jeopardize how realistically the patient plans his own future as well as that of his family.

What is the nurse's role in these discussions? In the first place, it is helpful if she knows what the doctor has told the patient so that she may clarify points already discussed by him. It is generally preferable that ambiguous questions or those with several different interpretations be referred directly to the physician in charge. Slightly different answers to the same question by several people may leave the patient confused and mistrusting. It is important, therefore, that both the doctor and nurse frequently share pertinent information so that the patient's trust in the health team be encouraged and sustained.

The nurse can and should discuss the routine details of the immediate preoperative and postoperative management with the patient. She can point out that a consent for operation must be signed by the patient and appropriately witnessed. She will want to discuss the necessity for preanesthetic fasting, and the administration of medication for the purposes of sedating the patient and reducing the amount of anesthesia necessary. She will explain to him that he will awaken in the recovery room, if one is available, and that he will stay there until he has adequately recovered from the immediate effects of the anesthesia. During his stay in the recovery room, blood pressure, pulse, and temperature will be taken frequently along with observation of drainage on dressings and from catheters. Morbid details need not be included. The patient who knows what to expect is the one who is better equipped to cope with the psychologic stresses of surgery.

Catheter Drainage Systems

Catheters are used to ensure adequate drainage of urine both preoperatively and postoperatively. Prior to surgery, the urinary tract is optimally prepared. Infections, so often present, may be treated with appropriate antibacterial agents. For this reason, it is particularly important to know whether the patient has had any untoward reactions to such medication in the past. The treatment of urinary infections with antibacterial agents is usually ineffective as long as an underlying urinary obstruction is present. However, obstructions that contribute to infection or impairment of renal function may be temporarily ameliorated by catheter drainage until such time as infection subsides and function improves. The catheter may also be used to relieve urinary retention caused by prostatic enlargement. The presence of the catheter, a foreign body, will of itself cause and promote infection, but the rewards of unobstructed urine flow are usually greater than the potential impairment caused by such an infection. Again, it must be emphasized that infection may be present in the first place.

Postoperatively, the catheter has several functions. When considering clamping a catheter, even temporarily, remember that it has nearly always been put in for drainage—not to be obstructed for some trivial reason! Of primary importance is the maintenance of free urinary drainage, since bleeding and edema may obstruct the lumen of the urinary tract at the operative site. The catheter also makes it possible to accurately monitor the volume of urine flow as well as estimate the amount of bleeding by observing the color and viscosity of the urine. In certain plastic procedures on the ureter and urethra, the catheter may secondarily serve to splint the operative site.

Types of Systems

The two most frequently used systems are *straight* and *decompression* drainage. The principles governing the use of each will be discussed. Also to be discussed, though used infrequently, are tidal and suction drainage.

STRAIGHT DRAINAGE. As its name implies, straight drainage is gravity-dependent drainage of a catheter directly to a collection device (Fig. 15-1*A*). It can be used anywhere in the urinary tract from the kidney level down to the bladder. The system consists of tubing attached to the end of the catheter with the collection container either at the bedside or

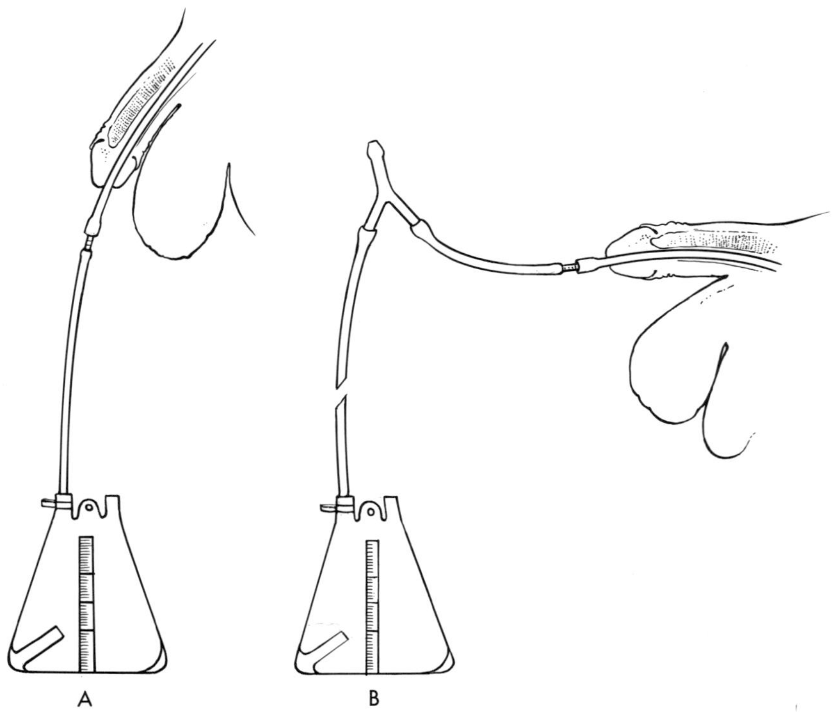

FIGURE 15-1. *A*, straight drainage; *B*, decompression drainage.

connected to a bag on the patient's leg. Since the purpose of a catheter is to drain urine, one must be constantly certain that drainage is free and unimpeded. The tubing should not be so flexible that it can become readily blocked by kinking or twisting. On the other hand, it should not be stiff or rigid. Ideally the flexibility should be such that it will naturally fall, or can be placed, in loose coils. The lumen should be adequate to accommodate a urine flow of up to a liter an hour. Most tubing used for urinary drainage has a diameter of one-fourth to three-sixteenths inch. The tubing should be long enough to allow the patient movement without undue tension on the catheter, but not so long that dependent loops allow urine to pool before emptying into the collection container. For patients on bed rest, 5 ft is the usual length if the container is at the side of the bed. Longer tubing may be necessary if the container is at the foot of the bed. The tubing must be connected in such a way that the distal end does not come into contact with the accumulated urine or the sides of the container. Since urine decomposes quickly at room temperature and bacteria flourish, this separation reduces retrograde ascent of organisms into the urinary tract. The collection container must always be lower than the level of the area being drained to ensure free gravity flow. It is equally important that the container be properly vented, since air must be displaced as urine flows into the container. If the air is unable to escape, pressure will gradually rise in the system, impeding the flow of urine. This can be partially obviated by the use of a distensible receptacle such as a plastic bag which can expand outwardly.

Drainage tubing is most commonly constructed from rubber or plastic materials. The former are being supplanted by the plastic materials, which have numerous advantages. These can be obtained prepackaged sterilely along with a collecting bag. Their cost makes it possible to discard these after a short period of use and replace them with a new sterile set. Furthermore, the plastics being clear, the nurse not only can see the color and consistency of the drainage but also can readily note if drainage stops. Lastly, the requirements of appropriate malleability are better met than with rubber.

Much has been written and discussed about the contribution of catheters and drainage systems to instigating or exacerbating urinary tract infections. There are those individuals who strongly advocate rigorous protocols to maintain the sterility of the drainage system. Others, a relative minority, pay little attention to sterile precautions. Among the procedures used in attempts to prevent infection are daily replacement of tubing and container with sterile equipment, frequent meticulous cleaning of all connections with antiseptic solutions when connecting or disconnecting any portion of the system, and the addition of an antiseptic solution to the collection container which is emptied every eight hours. Also advocated by some is the frequent cleaning of the catheter at the urethral meatus with an antiseptic. This is done by wrapping a sterile gauze pad, saturated with an antiseptic solution, around the catheter at the meatus and leaving it in place for a short period of time. Reason and practicality dictate a middle road in the care of drainage systems. A complete disregard of sterile technique cannot be condoned. On the other hand, while consideration of the patient's health and safety is paramount, whatever system is used needs to be workable in the particular patient setting. If the system is elaborate and complicated in its protocol and requires much personnel time and expense, this could mean sacrificing the patient for the system on a busy urology service.

A method that has been used on the urology service at The New York Hospital–Cornell Medical Center that has been safe for the patient as well as practical for the staff utilizes the following technique. Sterile disposable plastic drainage tubing and bags are used. Sterility is maintained until the package is opened at the patient's bedside and the tubing attached to the catheter. The bag hangs by a strap from the frame of the bed in a dependent fashion. The urinary drainage is measured and emptied every eight hours. The entire system is changed at least every three days. The proximal end of the drainage tube is covered with sterile gauze when disconnected from the catheter. An antiseptic solution is used to clean both the end of the catheter and that of the tubing when they are reconnected. However, disconnection of the drainage tubing from the catheter is kept to a minimum. Catheters are not irrigated routinely unless a specific request is made by the physician or when drainage becomes impeded by debris or clots. Patients can be ambulated with the intact system including the collection container. The excess tubing is coiled and the collecting bag attached by means of a safety pin at a dependent position on the patient's hospital gown. The patient should be warned not to let the tubing kink, and particular attention is paid to maintenance of a dependent position of the bag when the patient is sitting.

DECOMPRESSION DRAINAGE. As its name implies, decompression drainage prevents the organ to be decompressed from emptying rapidly. This organ is almost invariably the bladder. Most often it is used to slowly empty a bladder that has been chronically overdistended or as an attempt to control vesical bleeding. One of the complications from rapid emptying of a chronically overdistended bladder is the onset of bleeding from the sudden filling and rupture of mucosal blood vessels. A profound diuresis is common after an obstruction with hydronephrosis has been relieved and may perhaps be made less abrupt by judicious decompression. With such rapid diuresis, the urinary flow is so great that insufficient amounts of sodium are resorbed in the renal tubules. The patient may lose enough salt from his extracellular fluid via the urine to go into shock from electrolyte depletion. Consequently, when a catheter is inserted in such a situation, the patient's urinary output must be measured and recorded hourly during the first few hours to be sure that such an excessive diuresis is not occurring. Hourly blood pressure, pulse, and respirations are also important during this period to forewarn of possible cardiovascular complications.

Decompression is accomplished by having the urine draining from the catheter go uphill for a prescribed height before it drains down into the collection device. This is done by connecting the catheter tubing to a Y tube attached to a bedside pole which is raised the necessary distance above the level of the bladder (Fig. 15-1*B*). Since the urine will have to go uphill against gravity, a certain quantity will always be in the bladder. One end of the Y tube is left open to the air as a vent so that if the pressure in the system becomes too high, a safety exit is present. The vent also prevents a siphon from forming, thus draining all the urine from the bladder. Therefore, the equipment needed for decompression consists of a bedside collection container, two lengths of drainage tubing, of which one should be 5 ft and the other 3 ft long, a straight connector, a Y tube with at least an 8-mm bore, and a bedside standard such as an intravenous pole and adhesive tape. The standard is placed alongside the patient's bed and the Y is taped in an inverted position to the pole.

The height of the apex of the Y above the level of the bladder determines whether the decompression is "high" (5 to 8 inches), "medium" (3 to 5 inches), or "low" (3 inches). The long piece of drainage tubing is connected to the proximal arm of the Y and the remaining piece to the distal arm down to the collection container. Urine will not drain until the volume of urine in the bladder is sufficient to overcome the resistance created by the height of the Y tube above the bladder. Raising or lowering the height of the bed will change the degree of decompression. Consequently, the nurse needs to be alert to such changes so that the proper prescribed degree of decompression is maintained. Usually the patient is started on high decompression, and the height of the Y tube is lowered over a period of several hours until low decompression and finally straight drainage are achieved. If the fluid level in the tubing moves freely with respiration or with gentle suprapubic pressure, the system is patent and draining properly.

Decompression is sometimes used to control bleeding from the bladder. The height of the Y tube above the bladder raises the intravesical pressure and in effect acts as a mild tamponade against venous bleeding. The method is usually quite ineffective to control arterial bleeding. The effect of this tamponade is the same as when light pressure is applied to a cut on the finger. When the urine is very bloody, the nurse must not be fooled by what seems to be a satisfactorily patent system. The bladder can be full of blood clots yet the system may seem to be working freely. Consequently, under such circumstances, it is wise to palpate suprapubically at fairly frequent intervals, since a bladder full of clots is often easily palpable. The nurse can be especially suspicious of this possibility if the drainage seems to be adequate yet the patient complains bitterly of suprapubic discomfort.

TIDAL DRAINAGE. Although popular in the past, tidal drainage is seldom used today. This system may still be used, however, by some physicians when patients require prolonged catheter drainage. Tidal drainage provides for the automatic filling and emptying of the bladder, thus theoretically simulating normal bladder function. The system fills by gravity flow and empties by siphonage. Approximately 200 to 300 ml of solution is allowed to flow into the bladder over a two- to four-hour period. When the desired intravesical pressure is reached, the siphon action begins and empties the bladder. The cycle is repeated over and over. This system is not used if there is intravesical bleeding and must be checked frequently to make certain the catheter is patent. Another disadvantage to its use is that the patient must remain in bed.

SUCTION DRAINAGE. Occasionally following the removal of a cystostomy tube, the residual fistula does not close spontaneously and continues to drain urine. Another instance of fistula formation may occur following radical prostatectomy when the urethral-vesical anastomosis fails to heal. When such drainage persists, a low-grade suction (usually no greater than 2 to 3 cm of water pressure) is attached to a urethral catheter to keep the bladder empty. This promotes the closure of the fistula, usually in two to four days. Should this system be employed, the nurse must check to make certain the amount of suction does not exceed that desired by the doctor. Too much suction may cause injury to the bladder mucosa, which can be drawn into the holes of the catheter, indeed plugging the catheter and defeating drainage itself. The suction may be disconnected for short periods to ambulate the patient but should be reattached when the patient is in his bed or chair.

Irrigation of Catheters

Various solutions are available for catheter irrigation. Whatever the material used, it must be sterile. Sterile purified water can be used but isotonic saline is most commonly preferred. The use of commercially prepared amino acids for routine irrigation is usually unnecessary. Suby's solution, more often known as "G" or simply "urologic solution," is a useful one. The latter name implies, however, that this solution is ideally suited for routine irrigation of urinary drainage systems. This is hardly so. Suby's solution is prescribed by the urologist only for specific situations. It is strongly acid and irritating to the urothelium. It is used primarily in patients with long-term cystostomy drainage wherein the bladder lining has accommodated to the presence of the foreign body. Its purpose is to prevent calcific precipitation, most often phosphates, in the lumen of such catheters so as to make catheter change a less frequent occurrence. This solution is so irritating that in the freshly catheterized patient vigorous use may start bleeding from the bladder lining. "G" solution irrigation is sometimes prescribed for use in long-standing nephrostomy drainage or with permanent indwelling cutaneous ureterostomy catheters, but only at the physician's direction.

Another solution that is sometimes ordered is Renacidin, a commercially prepared 10 per cent mixture of organic acids. Whether Renacidin is more effective than solution G is debatable but the former does appear more irritating. Renacidin has also been used with long-term, continuous irrigation apparatus to successfully dissolve already formed calculi within the kidney. However, several published reports of severe kidney damage and even death have precluded its use under ordinary circumstances. If Renacidin is used, it must be kept refrigerated, since the component organic acids in the mixture decompose rapidly at room temperature.

Under rare circumstances, other solutions may be ordered for irrigation. These include 0.25 per cent acetic acid solution which may be instilled for severe *Pseudomonas* infection. Five-tenths per cent (0.5 per cent) neomycin sulfate solution may be used to cut down the number of bacteria. The prescribed amount is instilled into the bladder, the catheter clamped for 20 minutes, and then released. This may be repeated two or three times a day. Neomycin solution also needs to be kept in the refrigerator when not in use to prevent decomposition. Numerous other irrigating solutions have been used in the past for various purposes, mostly as local antiseptics. This include dilute 1:10,000 potassium permanganate, acriflavin, and 1:20,000 benzalkonium chloride. Finally an old but still very useful solution is silver nitrate in a dilution of 1:5000. It is best used following a single intermittent catheterization. The patient must be cautioned that his urine may appear cloudy following silver nitrate instillation, since urinary chlorides will precipitate in the form of silver chloride.

Catheters are irrigated with different-size syringes depending on the size of the cavity being irrigated and the volume of fluid to be used. The basic equipment necessary is sterile irrigating solution, sterile basin for solution, sterile bulb syringe, and clean basin for waste solution. Irrigation of the bladder is best performed using a 2-oz Asepto syringe (bulb). These syringes are now available in plastic, disposable, sterile irrigating sets. The syringe is filled with the irrigating solution about two thirds the length of the barrel. If the syringe and the bulb are filled completely, one cannot note whether the fluid can be irrigated freely. The bulb of the syringe is squeezed, thus introducing the intended amount of solution. On releasing the bulb, the fluid should flow back freely, thus indicating unobstructed flow and good manometrics. Another method is to introduce the fluid, disconnect the syringe, and note if the fluid flows back readily into a pan alongside the patient. When the catheter is severely obstructed as with clots, a Toomey syringe can be used. Under these conditions, such irrigation is the doctor's responsibility, but in an emergency situation the nurse may have to take care of the problem. A Toomey syringe is a 50-ml piston syringe with a large-bore hub. This large diameter can accommodate clots that need to be removed. The syringe is filled with irrigating solution, and the fluid is introduced gently and withdrawn strongly. This to-and-fro motion accompanied by the powerful suction on withdrawing the plunger can often suck out obstructing clots.

Irrigation of catheters draining smaller cavities, such as ureterostomy and nephrostomy catheters, depends on the specific situation. Commonly small amounts of solution are used, only a few milliliters. A small piston syringe with a Christmas tree adapter is useful. If the nurse is required to perform these irrigations, it is the doctor's responsibility to specify exactly the volume and nature of solution to be used and the method.

THROUGH-AND-THROUGH IRRIGATION. This type of bladder irrigation may be used preoperatively or postoperatively when there is vesical or postprostatectomy bleeding. Naturally both urethral and cystostomy catheters must be in place. If bleeding is sufficient to require this technique, it may be used in conjunction with decompression rather than straight drainage.

To set up through-and-through irrigation, the following equipment is necessary: bedside standard, sterile solution flask, tubing and Y connector, and tubing clamp. The sterile flask containing the prescribed irrigating solution (usually 1000 ml) is hung on the standard at the patient's bedside. Tubing from the flask delivers the solution through one arm of the Y tube connected to the catheter. The other arm of the Y tube is connected by tubing to either a straight or decompression collection system. For intermittent irrigation, the doctor will usually request that 75 to 100 ml of solution be run through the system each hour. This is accomplished by releasing the clamp connecting the flask and catheter and clamping the tubing between the catheter and bedside collection container. This allows solution to run into the bladder. When the appropriate amount has been delivered, the clamping process is reversed, thus stopping the inflow of irrigating solution and allowing the bladder to drain. If the doctor wishes the patient to have continuous rather than intermittent irrigation, the nurse will need to titrate the flow of solution to the prescribed hourly volume. Also, if the patient has only a urethral catheter and the doctor desires continuous irrigation, a special double-lumen catheter will be inserted. The solution is delivered through one lumen of the catheter and drains through the second.

Through-and-through irrigation should be checked hourly to see that it is functioning properly. One should check, for example, whether the solution flows easily in and out, suggesting a patent system. Also, particularly with through-and-through continuous irrigation, the nurse should frequently palpate the bladder to determine the presence of distention. It can happen that the irrigating solution channels a path through a bladder full of clots. If only the volume of inflow and outflow were observed, everything might seem normal. In the meantime, however, the patient's bladder could be filled with clots and distended, easily detected by palpation. To reduce the likelihood of this happening, the inflow of irrigating solution is usually through the urethral catheter and the outflow through the cystostomy tube.

It is quite important that careful records be kept of urinary drainage when through-and-through irrigation is used. The patient can absorb significant and even serious amounts of the fluid, and we rarely use the method for this reason. It is best to determine these totals every eight hours. A special sheet should be kept at the patient's bedside. Initially, when the system is started, the volume of irrigating solution is recorded and the urine receptacle emptied. At the end of eight hours, the amounts of irrigating solution and urine are each measured and recorded and the urine receptacle emptied. The eight-hour urine output can be determined by subtracting the volume of irrigating solution used during this time from the recorded volume of drainage in the receptacle for the same period. In this way, it is possible to determine if the patient's urinary output is adequate as well as to make certain that the irrigation is running at the desired rate.

Anchorage of Catheters

All urinary catheters must be anchored in place by one method or another, whether they are situated in the kidney, ureter, or bladder. This is done to maintain their position so that they drain properly. As discussed in Chapter 12, some catheters, such as the Foley balloon type, are self-retaining. With sufficient force, however, they can be pulled out with the balloon intact. A Malecot catheter, albeit "self-retentive" in nature, can be removed with minimal tension. Regardless of the organ drained by these catheters, they will need external anchorage to prevent too much play and movement and more importantly, inadvertent removal. Although catheters may be temporarily stabilized by sutures in the immediate postoperative period, this is not sufficient. Obviously, it is also essential that straight nonretentive catheters be stabilized by external anchorage.

A method to immobilize nephrostomy, cystostomy, and splinting tubes that has been found highly satisfactory is the application of a "tape sandwich" to the catheter close to the point of exit from the body. The first layer of adhesive tape is applied to the skin. The catheter is then laid down over this tape and a second slightly shorter piece applied over this with the catheter fitted in between. The catheter can be placed in a

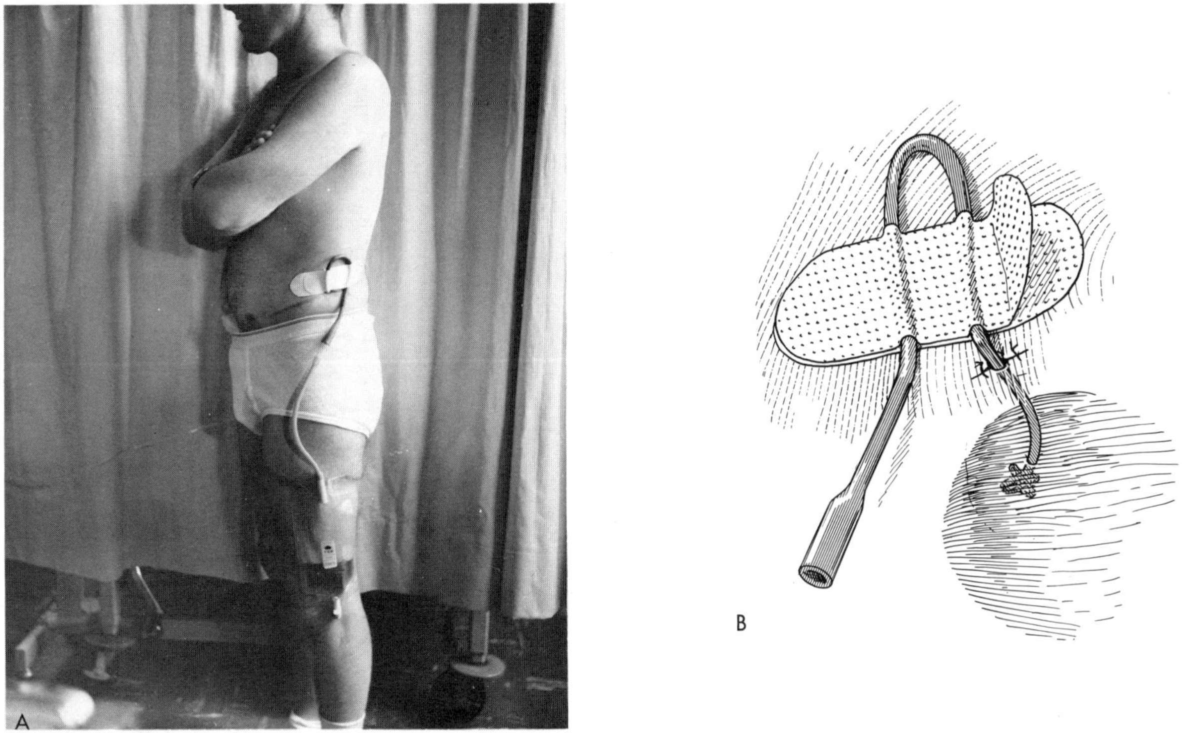

FIGURE 15-2. *A*, ambulatory patient on nephrostomy drainage, with leg urinal; *B*, details of method of anchoring a nephrostomy or cystostomy tube with adhesive tape.

straight line between the tape layers. If additional immobilization is necessary, it can be looped upon itself, so that a double length of tubing is incorporated (Fig. 15-2).

To remain adequately anchored, the tape should be at least 3 or 4 inches long and at least 1 inch wide. The first layer of adhesive is applied to clean skin to which has been applied a coating of compound tincture of benzoin which has been allowed to dry thoroughly. If the corners of the tape are rounded, there is less likelihood of the ends curling and the adhesive strips dislodging. If, after several days, the underlying skin becomes macerated, the sandwich can usually be reapplied to the opposite side of the incision. Indwelling urethral retention catheters can be anchored in the same manner by placing a sandwich on the inner thigh at the distal end of the catheter. Thus, there will be less tension and discomfort for the ambulatory patient from the weight of the collecting apparatus and a minimum of motion of the catheter in the urethra.

Indwelling urethral catheters are usually of the Foley balloon type. In certain situations, most often in the presence of a urethral stricture, a straight catheter or a filiform or follower may be left in place. In such instances, the catheter must be adequately secured with tape to the penis. Many techniques have been devised for this, of which Figure 15-3 is an

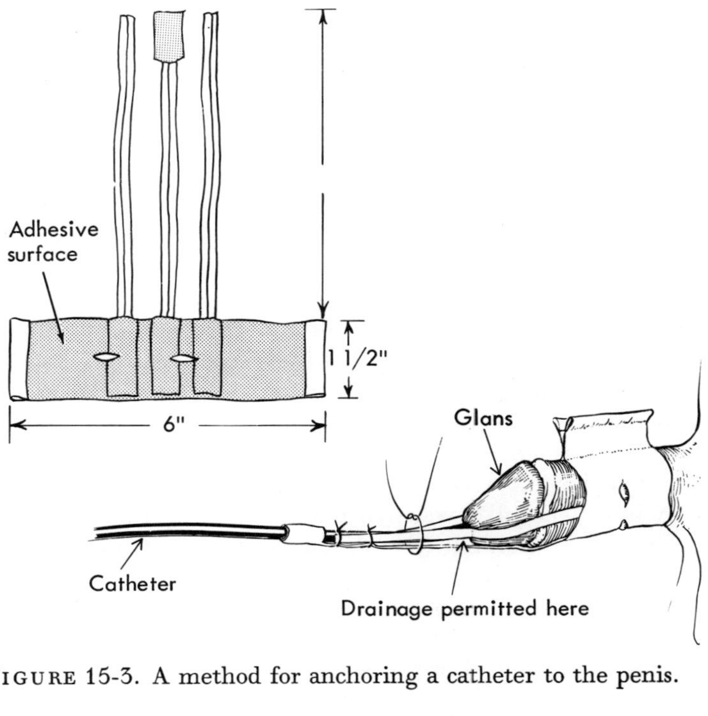

FIGURE 15-3. A method for anchoring a catheter to the penis.

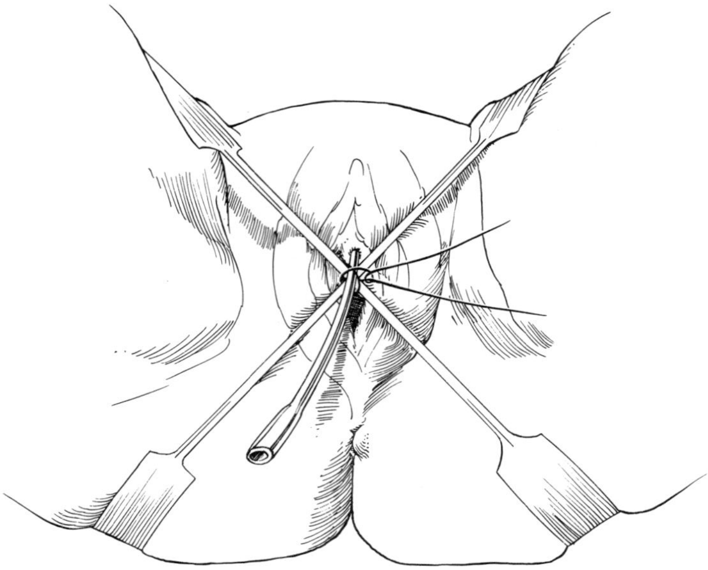

FIGURE 15-4. A method for anchoring a urethral catheter in the female patient.

example. The need to use an indwelling straight urethral catheter for the female patient rarely arises. A method of taping in such situations is illustrated in Figure 15-4.

Principles of Postoperative Care

In the first several hours following operation, the nurse will be concerned with the patient's recovery from anesthesia, measurement of blood pressure, pulse, and temperature, urine and wound drainage, and intravenous fluid administration. Most hospitals provide immediate postoperative care in a recovery room that is especially equipped and staffed so that, should any emergencies arise, treatment can be initiated quickly. Once the patient is awake and his condition is thought to be stable, he will be sent to his room on the patient unit.

If the patient has received a general anesthetic and is unconscious, it is vital that he be carefully watched for signs of respiratory obstruction. It is usually best to maintain the unconscious patient on his side until he is awake and responding. In this position, there is less apt to be pharyngeal obstruction by the tongue or aspiration should the patient vomit.

During this period, blood pressure and pulse are taken every 15 to 20 minutes and the temperature every hour. In order to establish a baseline on which to evaluate the significance of these findings, the nurse should check the patient's chart for those vital signs recorded before and during surgery. Certainly, a falling blood pressure and rising pulse are cause for alarm. Hypotension may result from the effects of the anesthetic agent, inadequate blood replacement at operation, or poor hemostasis with excessive bleeding. The surgeon's primary concern will be to determine, as quickly as possible, the cause of the hypotension and to initiate treatment. Hypotension is, in particular, poorly tolerated by the elderly patient and should be recognized and treated as early as possible. The nurse must be especially alert to the patient who is normally hypertensive, since his blood pressure at shock levels may fall within the normal range for the average person. It is equally important to identify as early as possible hypertension in the usually normotensive patient. Such an occurrence might suggest an overloading of the vascular system with fluids, and if the patient has had a transurethral resection of the prostate it may portend the presence of dilutional hyponatremia. Symptoms of hyponatremia include not only an elevated blood pressure but a slowed pulse, and the patient acquires an ashen appearance. Should the condition not be treated promptly, usually with 5 per cent saline, the patient can suddenly go into shock and die. (For a more detailed discussion, see page 279.)

For reasons of safety, the temperature should be taken by rectum in the immediate postoperative period, since the patient may be unconscious or groggy from heavy sedation. An exception to this rule is the patient who has had perineal or rectal surgery. In this instance, an axillary temperature is taken. Should the patient's temperature be below normal, extra blankets should be added to warm him. This may be particularly important following transurethral surgery, since the rapid exchange of fluids during the procedure may have allowed dissipation of some of the body heat. On the other hand, should the operated organ have been infected, which is not unusual in urologic surgery, the nurse should be alert to signs of bacteremia, such as fever, chills, and flushed appearance.

The patient's intake and output must be carefully monitored. Intravenous therapy is essential not only for the replacement of fluids and electrolytes but for blood and medication administration should this be necessary. The nurse will need to be particularly concerned with the position of the intravenous needle to make certain it is not inadvertently dislodged and that the solution is running in at the prescribed rate. If the patient is unconscious or restless, an arm board to stabilize the extremity as well as an appropriate restraint may be necessary. The nurse must make certain that the volume and kind of fluid received are accurately recorded. Should there be medications or electrolytes added to these fluids, these too must be recorded as well as the bottle accurately labeled.

Intravenous fluids are discontinued as soon as the patient has bowel sounds and can tolerate fluids in adequate amounts. Usually this is within 24 hours. Occasionally if the procedure has involved the upper ureter or kidney, the patient may develop a paralytic ileus. A nasogastric tube to suction may be necessary to remove gastric fluid and decompress the stomach. Nasogastric drainage is also necessary following ileal conduit construction and radical cystectomy. A record of intake is required until such time as intestinal function is adequate and allows the patient to eat and drink normally. Oral fluids, once tolerated, should be encouraged to a total of 3000 ml daily. Accurate measurement of intestinal drainage is important for accurate fluid and electrolyte replacement. Urinary output should be measured and recorded as long as catheters are in place and for several days after they are removed.

To prevent respiratory and vascular complications, it is important that the patient be turned and coughed every two to three hours and be ambulated as soon as the doctor allows. Patients with flank incisions are particularly loath to cough. A modified Fowler's or sitting position is the most conducive to adequate deep breathing. It also enables the nurse to more effectively support and splint the incision. Barring complications, patients are usually ambulated the night of, or first day after, surgery. Each day the patient's time up should be increased and activity to his level of tolerance encouraged.

The nurse must be particularly attentive to the elderly patient who may wish only to stay in bed and be left undisturbed. Because these patients are particularly subject to respiratory and vascular problems, the nurse may need to use all her persuasive powers, ingenuity, and added assistance of co-workers to get the patient up and moving. Elastic bandages on lower extremities are frequently used to prevent venous stasis and possible phlebothrombosis. The intermittent positive-pressure breathing apparatus, used in conjunction with mucolytic agents, may help to prevent respiratory congestion and pneumonia.

Wound dressings should be examined frequently to determine whether the drainage—in color, volume, and consistency—is within normal limits. Practically all wounds following urologic surgery will have rubber Penrose drains. Excessive bleeding, therefore, is usually apparent on the dressing. Bright red viscous drainage associated with clots and a fluctuating blood pressure suggests that the situation should be immediately reported to the doctor and the patient's condition watched closely. As a general rule, when excessive bleeding does occur, which is infrequently, it is most likely to be associated with procedures on the kidney or prostate.

It is well for the nurse to remember that when there is surgical entry into the urinary tract, the closure of the incised organ is never watertight. Following certain procedures—pyelotomy or ureterolithotomy, for example—urine frequently drains from the wound. It takes only a small amount of blood to make urine appear quite red. If bleeding is occurring in appreciable amounts, the drainage will be more viscous than normal urine and also contain blood clots. Unless specifically contraindicated, the dressing should be changed as frequently as necessary to keep the wound dry.

Initially, drains are tacked to the wound with a suture. The suture is cut when the drain is advanced, and once this is done, it is important not to inadvertently pull the drain out when removing the dressing. A sterile safety pin is then run through the drain to keep it from slipping into the wound. A dressing that is saturated through is a potential avenue for infection. Also, a constantly wet dressing may contribute to skin irritation and urine odor. Each time the dressing is changed, the skin should be washed with hexachlorophene and sterile normal saline or water, dried, and an appropriate antiseptic applied. A heat lamp to the area two or three times a day promotes healing and reduces inflammation. When urine drainage is copious, a temporary ostomy appliance attached to straight drainage will sometimes adhere over the drain. This is not always possible however, owing to the irregularities in the skin surface due to the sutures. On page 247 a special technique is described that is used to care for wounds with wire sutures. When changing dressings, one should adhere to the principles of sterile dressing technique.

The details of each dressing change—time, color, and quantity of drainage—should be recorded in the nurse's notes. If very accurate measurement of output is desired, a precise count of numbers of pads saturated with drainage should be recorded. In certain instances, the doctor may want the dressings weighed on a scale such as one used to weigh food for patients on special diets. For abdominal or flank dressings that need to be changed frequently, it is convenient to use Montgomery straps. Compound tincture of benzoin is first applied to protect the skin from irritation caused by the adhesive.

Care of perineal wounds consists of washing the area around the incision to remove any drainage, application of an antiseptic, and exposure of the area to a heat lamp. It is particularly important that the area be cleansed after the patient has a bowel movement and a sterile dressing reapplied. A T-binder is useful in securing a dressing in this area—a single T for the female patient and a double T for the male patient. As soon as the drains are removed and the wound has healed sufficiently, the patient begins sitz baths two or three times a day.

Care of wounds of the external genitalia is usually performed by the doctor. Usually the dressing is changed at least once a day. The nurse, however, should make certain that it is intact and that there is no unusual drainage or odor which might suggest complications, most particularly wound infection. When the wound is sufficiently healed, sitz baths may be ordered.

As with wound drainage, the color and amount of urine drainage from a catheter should be checked frequently. Red urine that is more viscous than normal urine and that contains clots is strong indication that bleeding is excessive. Bright red urine suggests arterial bleeding while dark red suggests a venous origin. The appearance of urine following prostatic surgery is particularly important, since abnormal bleeding will first be reflected in the urine.

It is important that the nurse know the placement and purpose of all catheters. Into what organ is the catheter inserted, and is its purpose to drain urine or splint and stabilize the operative area? All catheters should be labeled as to location and, where appropriate, right or left. Bedside urine collection containers should also be labeled accordingly. Dressings often make it difficult to identify catheters correctly, which can cause serious error in determining whether urine drainage is satisfactory.

It is imperative that the patency of the catheter be maintained. The catheter following urologic surgery is never clamped except on specific direction of the doctor. Catheters are usually not irrigated routinely. However, in the presence of heavy bleeding and blood clots, the doctor may wish to irrigate to ensure patency. He will use sterile water or normal saline. If the catheter is in the bladder, he may need large amounts, at least 2000 ml, of irrigating solution. A Toomey syringe should be available, since with this syringe it is possible to create the vacuum necessary to remove clots. Appropriately smaller syringes and volumes of solution will be used if the ureter or kidney is to be irrigated. Acid solutions such as Suby's G solution should not be used for irrigation in the early postoperative period; it is quite painful and irritating to a newly operated area and has anticoagulant properties.*

REVIEW QUESTIONS

1. Identify those additional considerations that may be necessary in planning preoperative and postoperative care of the elderly patient.
2. Outline the essential topics to be covered preoperatively in order to prepare the patient for surgery.
3. Why may catheter drainage be initiated prior to surgery?
4. Diagram and label a urinary straight drainage system. Identify those points in the system where contamination can occur and indicate those measures appropriate to prevent contamination.
5. Identify two situations where decompression drainage may be initiated and give the rationale for its use in each instance. How can the nurse determine whether the system is patent?

* References for Chapters 15–23 are listed at the end of Unit III (pages 293–95).

6. What are the relevant nursing considerations in caring for the patient with through-and-through irrigations?
7. Describe how you would anchor a nephrostomy catheter with adhesive tape.
8. Why is it particularly important to take the patient's temperature frequently in the early postoperative period following genitourinary surgery?
9. Identify major nursing considerations in the first 24 hours postoperatively for the following: intake and output, catheters and catheter drainage, wound dressing, vital signs, intake by mouth, pain medication, prevention of respiratory and circulatory complications.

CHAPTER **16**

The Urologic Operating Suite

THE urologic operating suite is basically organized in the same manner as any general surgical room, but with certain modifications in design to render it better suited to specialized urologic procedures. The lighting should be such that the room can be darkened adequately for transurethral surgery.

Operating Tables

It is convenient to have several types of operating tables available. However, the standard table with breaking points at the head, foot, and midportion can be adapted to *all* urologic procedures. Such tables have provisions for leg stirrups for the lithotomy position and a "kidney lift" for the flank approach. Although specialized tables for perineal surgery are available, the standard operating table is more than adequate. For transurethral surgery, a table with a drawer and tray to catch bladder irrigations that can be handled by the surgeon during the operation is a great timesaver, since the bladder will be filled and emptied many times. Otherwise, an assistant must constantly be on the alert to catch bladder contents in a basin during any transurethral operation. This method not only involves a lot of extra work for the assisting nurse but is also wasteful of operating time and, despite care, inevitably results in spillage and a generally messy situation. Transurethral tables can be obtained with a motorized unit allowing the operator to raise, lower, or tilt the table at will by operating a foot switch. Such motorized units are the ultimate in convenience but are also more expensive (Fig. 16-1).

Instruments

The instruments and setup used in the operating room are basically the same as those used for any major general surgical procedure. The equipment for transurethral surgery is quite different and will be described in a separate section. Specific additional instruments for various urologic procedures will be discussed in more detail.

Surgery of the Kidney and Upper Ureter

In addition to the usual major tray, rib instruments should be available, since the removal of a rib often facilitates operative exposure. These

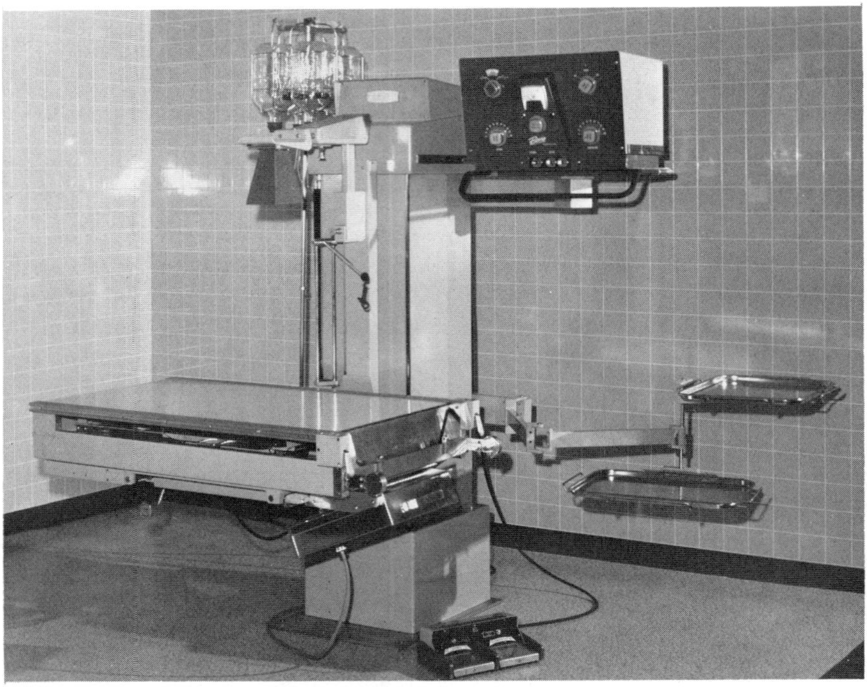

FIGURE 16-1. Motorized table for transurethral surgery. (Courtesy of Liebel-Flarsheim Co.)

include periosteal elevators, right- and left-handed Doyen rib raspatories, rib cutters, and bone rongeurs. Several sizes of self-retaining retractors of the Finichietto type will be useful, especially if the kidney is approached through the chest. Pedicle clamps (Fig. 16-2) are large clamps used to secure the renal pedicle. The preferred method of controlling the renal

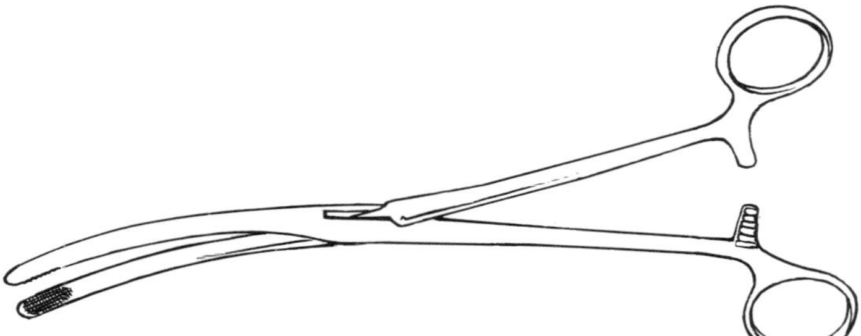

FIGURE 16-2. Pedicle clamp.

blood supply is to isolate and ligate the arteries and veins individually. Under certain conditions, however, mass ligation requiring these large clamps may be necessary. Randall kidney stone forceps are made in sets of increasing degree of curvature (Fig. 16-3). These forceps are inserted

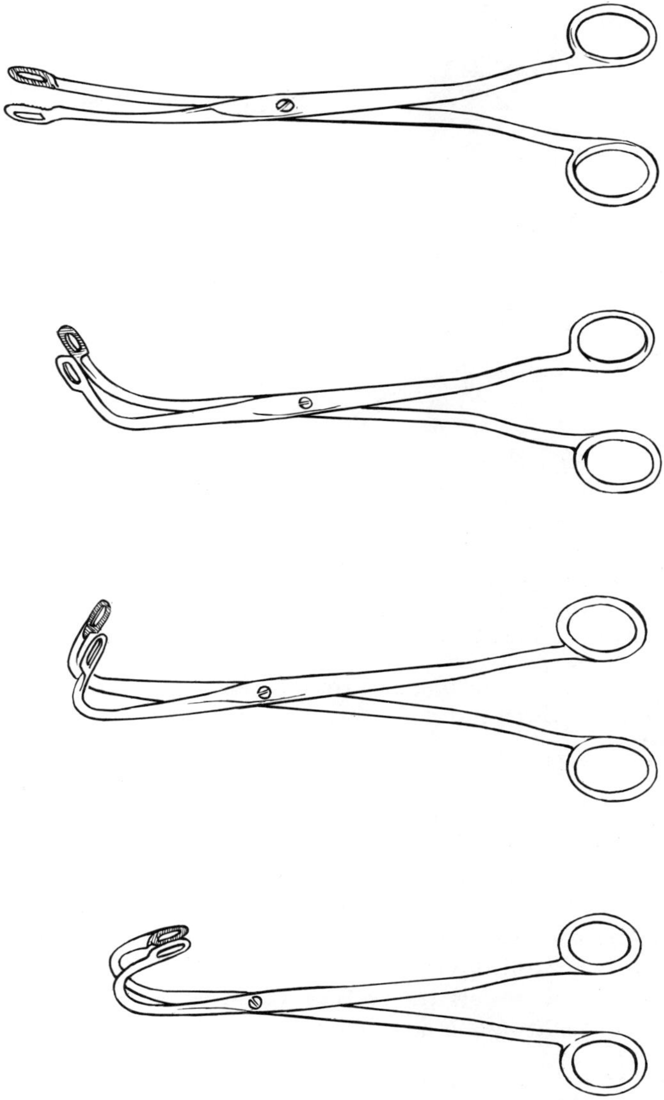

FIGURE 16-3. Randall kidney stone forceps of various curvatures.

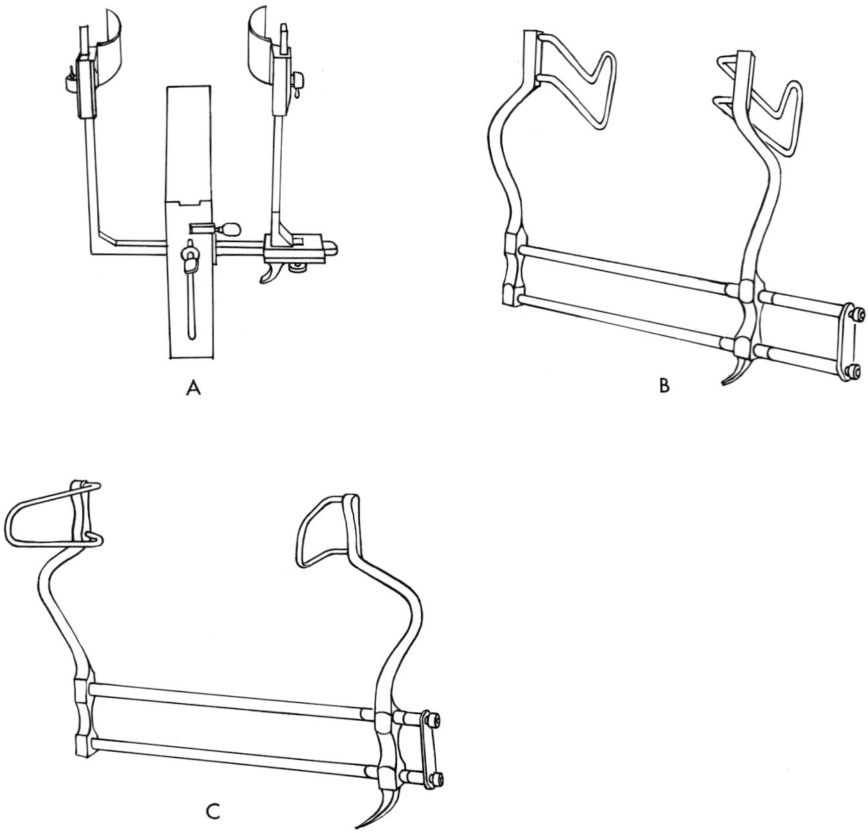

FIGURE 16-4. Self-retaining retractors for bladder and prostate surgery. *A*, Beneventi retractor; *B*, boot retractor; *C*, Balfour retractor.

through the opened renal pelvis and because of their different angulations can be used to explore the entire collecting system of the organ. The pressure to the jaws is controlled by the operator's fingers to prevent breakage of a calculus as it is removed. Other instruments particularly useful are the wide range of vascular instruments, especially those used to temporarily control the renal blood supply. They are used in surgery for diseases of the vessels themselves, during partial resections of the kidney, or in "splitting" procedures for removal of staghorn calculi.

Surgery of the Bladder and Prostate

For surgery of the urinary bladder and the anterior abdominal approaches to the prostate, the main additional instruments are various retractors particularly suited to visualize the interior of the bladder and the depths of the bony pelvis. These include self-retaining retractors such as the Balfour, Beneventi, and boot retractors (Fig. 16-4). For retraction inside the opened bladder, the Jackson and loop retractors are useful (Fig. 16-5) as are malleable retractors.

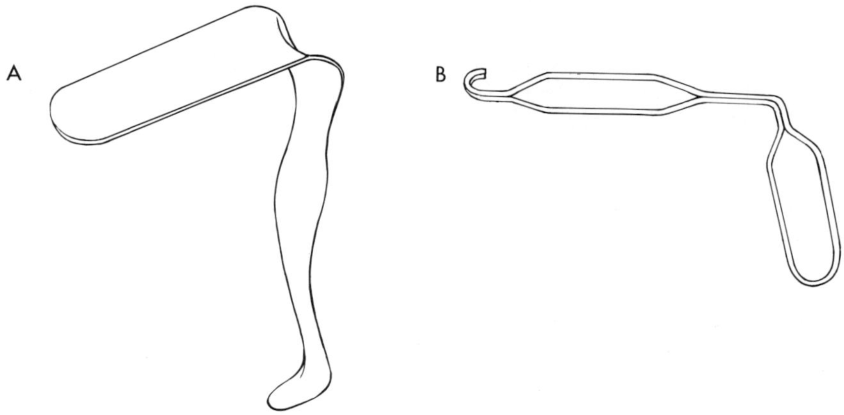

FIGURE 16-5. *A*, Jackson retractor; *B*, loop retractor.

Perineal Prostatic Surgery

A group of specialized retractors is designed for the perineal exposure of the prostate. These include the bifid, bulb, posterior (or rectal), and lateral perineal retractors (Fig. 16-6). The Lowsley curved seminal vesicle tractor and the long and short Young prostatic tractors are used to rotate and mobilize the prostate (Fig. 16-7). The standard instrument setups for several of the major types of procedures are listed in Appendix V.

Fulgurating Equipment

Fulgurating equipment should be available not only for transurethral work but also for open suprapubic fulguration of bladder papillomas and coagulation of bleeding points. This equipment will be discussed in the section on transurethral surgery.

Catheters

A varied selection of sterile catheters should be available in the operating room. These include many sizes of Malecot, latex, red rubber, whistle-tip, and coudé catheters. Foley catheters, particularly in the larger sizes, should be available with various capacity balloons. Five ml and 30 ml are standard sizes, but balloons of 75 ml are sometimes needed for hemostasis following prostatectomy.

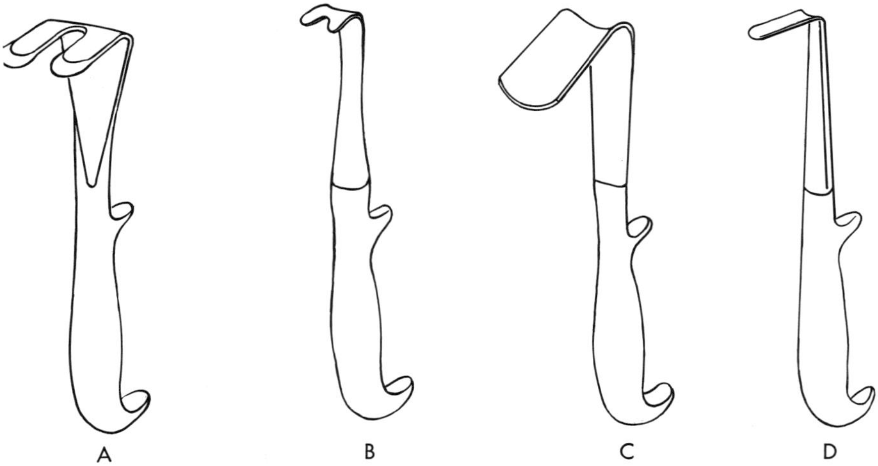

FIGURE 16-6. Retractors for perineal prostatic surgery. *A*, bifid; *B*, bulb; *C*, posterior (or rectal); *D*, lateral.

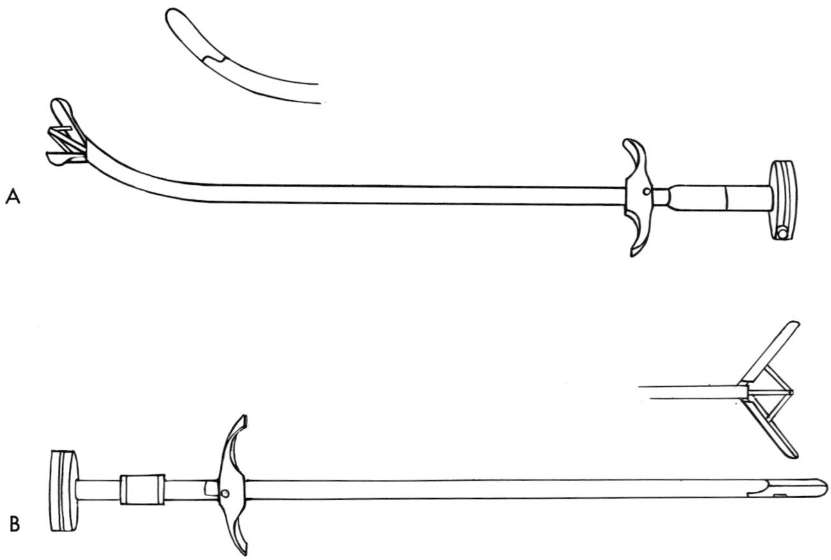

FIGURE 16-7. *A*, Lowsley curved seminal vesicle tractor (open and closed); *B*, Young prostatic tractor (open and closed).

Positioning the Patient for Surgery

Proper positioning of the patient on the operating table is important to accomplish good surgical exposure. Furthermore, good exposure may make the difference between a fairly simple and a difficult operation. Many different positions are used in urologic surgery, some of which can result in unusual strain and pressure on various parts of the body. The following are commonly used positions.

The *flank* (or exaggerated decubitus) position is used for the lumbar and transthoracic approach to the kidney and adrenal gland (Fig. 16-8*A*). The maximum benefit of the position is attained when the musculature between the lower ribs and iliac crest is taut. This will ensure wide exposure after the incision is made and the muscle layers divided. After the patient is anesthetized, he is turned on his side so that the operative side is uppermost. The iliac crest should be at the level of the mid "break"

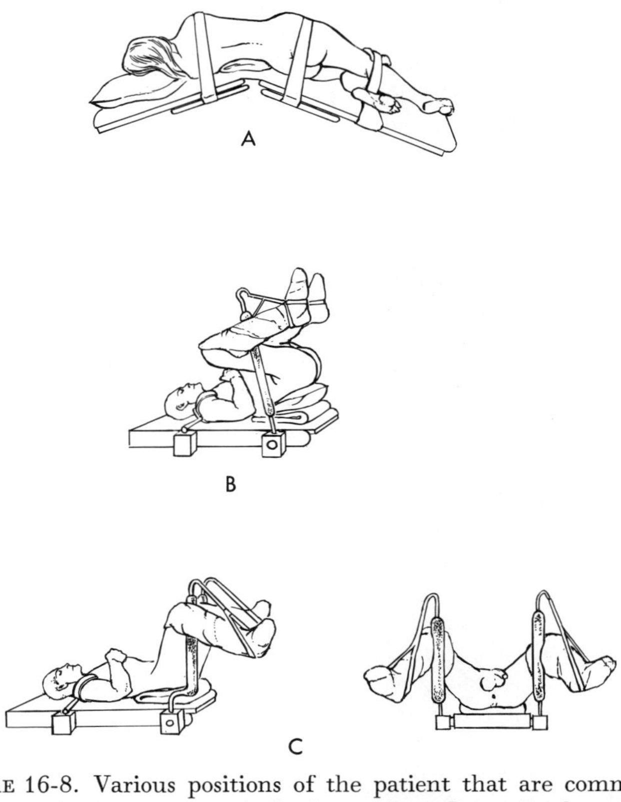

FIGURE 16-8. Various positions of the patient that are commonly used in urologic surgery. *A*, flank position; *B*, perineal position; *C*, lithotomy position.

in the table. The patient is stabilized by bending the knee of the lowermost leg. The uppermost leg is kept straight, and a pillow is inserted lengthwise between the legs. A wide strap is placed around the legs at the level of the knee. Pressure points should be protected with foam rubber pads, particularly at the outer aspect of the leg below the knee, since the common peroneal nerve runs around the fibula at this level. Pressure injury to this nerve may cause a foot drop. Needless to say, this is a distressing and avoidable complication.

The table is then "broken" by lowering the head and foot. The degree of flexion is increased until the flank is taut. This often requires elevation of the kidney rest. Once adequate position is obtained, the patient is further secured by a wide band of adhesive tape applied over the hip and attached on either end to the operating table. The shoulder girdle can be similarly secured by means of a narrow strip of tape across the point of the shoulder but not too tightly as to interfere with respiration.

The *supine* position is used for transabdominal surgery. When the upper abdomen is to be explored, as for nephrectomy, renal artery surgery, and so forth, the patient is placed perfectly flat. For surgery of the lower ureter, bladder, and prostate, somewhat better exposure can be obtained with the *modified Trendelenburg* position. Using the sacrum as a fulcrum, the head and feet are each lowered a few degrees. This simple maneuver tips the pelvis so that it becomes relatively more shallow.

The *lithotomy* position is used for cystoscopy and transurethral surgery. Depending on the type of table, its lower end is lowered or removed. The patient's legs are placed in stirrups and must be separated sufficiently so that the surgeon has adequate working room. Pressure points behind the knees and along the calves are padded (Fig. 16-8*C*). At the conclusion of any operation in the lithotomy position, the patient's legs are lowered gradually over a several-minute period while the blood pressure is monitored, particularly in the older patient and especially if there has been some blood loss. The lower extremities can hold 700 to 800 ml of blood. If the legs are lowered rapidly, this sudden decrease in central blood volume may be enough to drop the patient's blood pressure, possibly resulting in myocardial or cerebral ischemia.

The perineal (or exaggerated lithotomy) position is surprisingly well tolerated by most patients. When properly employed, the perineum will be parallel to the ceiling and floor (Fig. 16-8*B*). The patient is placed in this position gradually. He is first put into the standard lithotomy position except that the buttocks are brought down far enough to extend 6 to 8 inches beyond the lower end of the table. Each stirrup is turned inward 180° so that the patient's feet are pointed toward his head. The stirrups are then rotated downward as the patient's buttocks are elevated to place the perineum in the desired position. Once the proper position is reached, the patient's buttocks and lower back are supported by an adequate number of blankets or sheets which are secured in place with adhesive tape. A good part of the patient's weight is borne by the upper chest and scapulae in this position, and the patient is further stabilized by means of shoulder braces. These must be well padded and positioned carefully so that pressure is on the tips of the shoulders and not over the midclavicular area. Here injury to the brachial plexus can result in permanent disability to the hands. Even more so than with the standard lithotomy position, patients should be lowered very gradually out of the perineal position. The *prone* and *jackknife* positions are not used much by the urologist. A posterior approach to the adrenal gland is occasionally used, and rarely a transsacral approach to the prostate.

REVIEW QUESTIONS

1. Describe how the patient is prepared for the flank, supine, lithotomy, and exaggerated lithotomy positions. Indicate the specific precautions taken in each position to prevent pressure injuries.
2. Indicate those additional instruments that should be added to the general instrument setup for surgery on the following: kidney and upper ureter, bladder and prostate.
3. In taking the patient out of the lithotomy or perineal position, why are the legs lowered gradually over a period of several minutes?

CHAPTER 17
Surgery of the Kidney and Ureter

Incisions

THE kidney may be approached by one of three routes. The most commonly used is the classical *lumbar* or *flank* incision. The eleventh or twelfth rib may be removed to facilitate exposure. A second approach is directly through the pleural cavity, the *transthoracic* route, usually reserved for neoplastic lesions; and the third is the *transabdominal* approach.

In the transthoracic approach, the diaphragm is divided and the retroperitoneal space entered from above. An alternate "extrapleural" approach can be used by removing the eleventh rib, dividing the diaphragmatic attachments and reflecting the intact diaphragm upward. The abdominal approaches may be carried directly into the peritoneal cavity, which gives the surgeon the advantage of an exploratory laparotomy with the opportunity to examine the opposite kidney. The alternate anterior abdominal retroperitoneal approach is accomplished by dissecting off peritoneum and retracting it medially.

Surgical Procedures of the Kidney

Nephrectomy is the removal of a kidney. This may be accomplished in different ways, depending largely upon the disorder present. When operating on noncancerous conditions, the surgeon will open Gerota's fascia and dissect down to the renal capsule. The entire kidney is mobilized, the blood supply ligated, and after division of the ureter, the kidney removed.

A *radical nephrectomy* is removal of a kidney within its surrounding perirenal fat and intact Gerota's fascia. Such wide excision is the preferred method of removal for cancer and may also be used when nephrectomy is necessary following severe renal lacerations with organizing perirenal hematoma. The radical removal for cancer includes a local periaortic lymph node dissection. The transpleural or transperitoneal approach for renal cancer frequently is used, since the blood supply of the kidney can be reached and ligated before the tumor mass is mobilized, thereby reducing the possibility of tumor spillage into the bloodstream. Removal of the kidney with the entire ureter is *nephroureterectomy*. Common indications for this procedure are tumors of the renal pelvis and ureter.

A *partial nephrectomy* requires ligation of the blood supply to that portion of the kidney which is to be removed, following which the diseased area is resected. The numerous blood vessels on the cut surface of the kidney which is to remain must be individually ligated. Such operations are limited to localized disorders such as a hydronephrotic half of a double collecting system, a segmental infarction, or localized disease in a calyx. Renal cysts are treated by *decapsulation*. The dome of the cyst extending beyond the surface of the kidney is removed, leaving the base intact. The cut edges of the cyst wall are secured with a continuous hemostatic suture. Attempts to remove the cyst wall within the kidney are unnecessary and often result in excessive bleeding.

Renal calculi are handled surgically according to their size and location. Calculi that are movable may be removed through an incision in the renal pelvis (*pyelotomy*). The operation for removal of stones through this approach is called *pyelolithotomy*. The extraction of calyceal calculi by incision of the renal parenchyma directly over the stone is a *nephrolithotomy*. Staghorn or branched calculi frequently require *complete nephrolithotomy*, commonly known as the "kidney-splitting" operation. The kidney is opened down the middle from top to bottom like the pages of a book. Naturally the renal blood supply must be temporarily occluded at this time. The stone or stones are removed, and after meticulous suture ligature of the divided parenchymal vessels, the halves of the kidney are joined together.

A *nephrostomy* is an opening in the renal parenchyma through which a catheter is inserted for direct drainage of the kidney (Fig. 17-1). This can be performed by direct incision in the renal capsule and insertion of the catheter through the parenchyma into the pelvis. A safer technique, which better guarantees proper position of the tube, is to position the tube through a pyelotomy. A large clamp is inserted through the pelvis and out a thinned area of cortex. The tip of the catheter is grasped with the clamp and threaded into the pelvis, thus confirming its position under direct vision. Nephrostomy drainage is usually temporary and may be part of an associated operation such as a kidney split or pyeloplasty. It may be used as a "safety valve" in instances of marked hydronephrosis wherein the surgeon institutes drainage until renal function improves to the degree that a definitive procedure can be performed on the obstruction. At times, with marked obstruction and acute infection, a nephrostomy can be a lifesaving measure. The use of nephrostomy drainage permanently is to be avoided if possible, since it is fraught with complications when used on a long-term basis. These include persistent infection due to the foreign body effect, stone formation, as well as occasional bleeding or fever

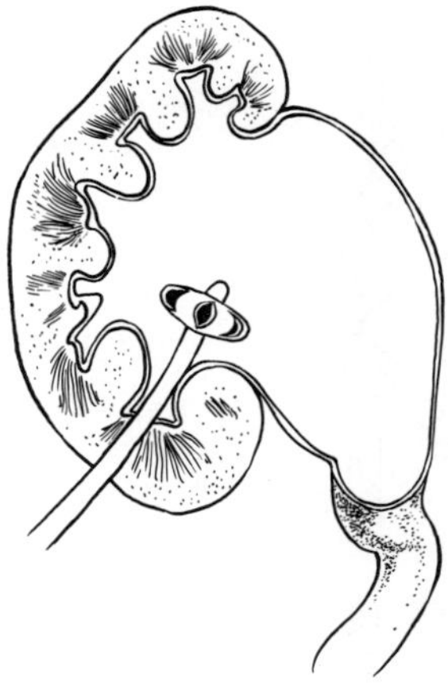

FIGURE 17-1. Nephrostomy tube positioned in renal pelvis.

following change of the catheter. Because of its large drainage holes, the Malecot catheter is a good nephrostomy tube. Foley catheters are less likely to come out inadvertently, but their balloons partially fill the renal pelvis and may of themselves internally obstruct a portion of the collecting system.

A *pyeloplasty* is a plastic operation to relieve an obstruction, usually congenital, at the ureteropelvic junction. One of the more commonly performed procedures is the Foley Y-V plasty (Fig. 17-2). The aim of such a repair is to relieve the obstruction and reconstruct the pelvic outlet so that it gracefully funnels widely in a dependent fashion into the ureter. The excess renal pelvis is excised to eliminate areas of stasis. Following such procedures, the kidney is usually drained by temporary nephrostomy drainage until operative edema subsides. Most surgeons will also splint the area of repair for two to three weeks by means of a catheter which is inserted through the area of repair, out the kidney, and onto the skin.

Specific Nursing Considerations

Hemorrhage is not common after kidney surgery, but it can be very serious. If a total nephrectomy has been performed, bleeding is not likely if the renal artery and vein have been individually divided and ligated. Postnephrectomy bleeding is more common when the entire renal pedicle has been grasped in large pedicle clamps and hemostasis accomplished by mass ligature. Serious bleeding may occur following nephrostomy from trauma to cortical blood vessels along the tract. With catheters of smaller caliber (10 to 18 F) than used in the past, such bleeding is less likely. Delayed bleeding may occur following partial nephrectomy or the

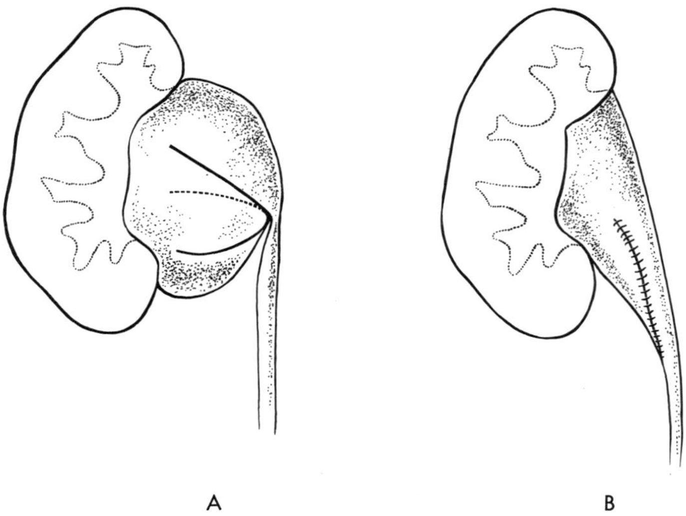

FIGURE 17-2. Correction of ureteropelvic junction obstruction (*A*) by pyeloplasty (*B*).

"splitting" operations where a large bare area of kidney has been exposed at surgery. Such bleeding, sometimes of alarming proportions, is most likely to occur 8 to 14 days after operation, since it is at this time that absorbable suture material begins to disintegrate and clots may break loose. Whenever surgery is performed on a kidney where the organ is not completely removed and the formation of urine is expected to continue, absorbable suture material is used. Otherwise, nonabsorbable material can remain as a nidus for encrustation, future stone formation, and persisting infection. Although hemorrhage is no longer a frequent complication after kidney surgery, its possible occurrence must be watched for carefully. After nephrectomy, partial nephrectomy, or "splitting" procedures, the patient will usually have his blood pressure and pulse taken and recorded hourly for the first 24 hours. After this period, the frequency of observations will be tapered, depending on how stable the vital signs have been and the amount of sanguineous drainage on dressings or in the urine.

Rubber tissue drains are almost always used to drain blood and fluid from the immediate operative site to the outside. Should this drainage not be provided for and instead allowed to accumulate, an infection with abscess formation could follow. The drains, usually two or three in number, will protrude approximately an inch from the skin. When drainage has decreased to an insignificant amount, the doctor will remove the drains completely.

During the first 24 hours after kidney surgery, the drainage may be quite red. The dressing may need frequent reinforcement or change. If bright clots appear on the dressing, a physician should be notified immediately. The number of dressing changes as well as the amount and character of drainage should be carefully recorded in the nurse's notes. The volume of drainage can be estimated by noting the number of gauze pads saturated with drainage. Sterile dressing techniques must be followed. After the first day, the drainage should be lighter in color. Serous drainage usually is minimal by the third day. Signs of excessive bleeding will be indicated by red, thick drainage, clots, or evidences of distention and tension at the suture line. While a massive hemorrhage would be reflected immediately in a falling blood pressure and rising pulse, a slow but excessive ooze might not be reflected in these signs for several hours. Consequently, checking the dressing, which may be the first indication of trouble, becomes extremely important. A key point when checking for bleeding is not only to examine the dressing but also to examine with one's hand the underside of the patient. Occasionally a patient has appeared to have a sparkling white, dry dressing but to the chagrin of the nurse was found to be lying in a pool of red drainage when turned.

If the renal pelvis has been opened as for a pyelolithotomy, there will nearly always be varying amounts of urine draining from the wound for at least several days and up to two weeks. Many surgeons do not attempt to achieve a watertight closure, not only since it may be impossible but because it may invite stricture formation. Finally, pyelotomy wounds seem to heal just as quickly when only a few approximating sutures are used. Any urinary drainage or leakage that occurs must have free access to the outside; otherwise, an accumulation (uroma) may cause fever and toxic symptoms, especially if infected. Dressings may need changing as often as every hour if urine flow is copious. If urine drainage is quite marked, it is sometimes feasible to apply a temporary ostomy bag around the drains attached to straight drainage. Such an arrangement may decrease the need for frequent dressing changes, conserving the energy of both the patient and the nurse.

The patient should be turned from back to operated side at least every two to three hours during the first 48 hours. By turning the patient to the operated side, the pressure of other organs helps to obliterate any dead space at the operative site and improves dependent drainage. Once drainage subsides, the patient can turn to either side. Should the patient have a nephrostomy or chest tube, one must make certain the tube is positioned properly, free of kinks, and draining well. A liberal use of pillows facilitates proper positioning and contributes to the patient's greater comfort.

Operations on the kidney may induce various degrees of paralytic ileus. Usually, however, when procedures are performed through a flank incision, a nasogastric tube is not necessary. The patient is often able to begin oral fluids in small amounts (30 ml per hour) the second postoperative day, and diet is progressed thereafter as tolerated. With the transthoracic or abdominal approach, the patient may need a nasogastric tube. Particularly with the abdominal approach, because of manipulation of abdominal organs, gastric drainage may be necessary from three to five days or until intestinal activity returns. As with gastric drainage following any type of surgery, it is important that the amount be measured at least once every 24 hours. A rectal tube, enemas, and medications may also be utilized to relieve gaseous distention.

Following the transthoracic approach, the patient will have a chest tube attached to underwater suction. While the tube will facilitate reexpansion of the lung, its main purpose is to drain fluid that may accumulate in the pleural space. The initial drainage is red and aqueous, and usually within 24 hours becomes pink or straw-colored. The total volume of drainage usually tends not to exceed 150 ml for the entire time the tube is in place, which is usually 48 to 72 hours. Red, thick drainage with blood clots is unusual and should be immediately reported to the doctor. With any chest tube, any accidents that would allow air to enter the pleural cavity must be avoided. All connections should be taped, the underwater-seal tube should always be below the level of fluid in the drainage collection bottle, and the catheter should never be disconnected from the water-seal bottle unless doubly clamped by the doctor. Should bubbles appear on the surface of the drainage collection bottle, this must be reported to the doctor, since this may signify an air leak in the pleural space. Occasionally, following this approach, the patient may be placed in an oxygen tent. In most instances, because of the cool, humidified atmosphere, the tent is used for the patient's greater comfort rather than his increased need for higher oxygen concentrations. Usually the tent is discontinued on the second or third postoperative day. A chest x-ray is usually taken after the removal of the chest tube to confirm that no air has entered the pleural space and that the lung is fully expanded.

Following kidney surgery, the patient will usually not have an indwelling urethral catheter. To ensure accuracy in collection of voided urine, a 24-hour collection container is convenient. This a is 3000- to 4000-ml plastic or glass bottle that is kept at the patient's bedside. Each voided urine is measured and recorded on a bedside intake and output sheet. The urine is then added to the total 24-hour specimen container. Once every 12 or 24 hours, the container's contents are measured, emptied, and replaced with a fresh, clean receptacle. If the patient does not void within 8 or 10 hours after surgery, the doctor should be notified. He may order catheterization to determine the volume of urine in the bladder in addition to relieving discomfort. If the volume of urine is small, the doctor may want the catheter left in so that output can be measured and recorded frequently. An average hourly output of 30 ml or less is usually cause for concern. An hourly specific gravity reading may also be ordered to determine if the kidney is able to concentrate the urine. A fixed specific gravity of 1.010 or less may be a bad omen, since this suggests the kidney has lost its ability to concentrate at this time.

After complete nephrectomy, the voided urine should be clear at once. Following other operations on the kidney, however, it is not unusual to see bloody discoloration for several days, which will gradually subside. If the urine is very dark or contains numerous clots, the doctor in charge should be notified promptly. A useful technique to gauge severity of hematuria and its cause is the use of *rack urines*. A few milliliters of each voided specimen is poured into a test tube which is then placed in a test tube rack. The tube is labeled as to time and date of voiding. This gross technique can be used to estimate whether hematuria is decreasing.

With nephrostomy drainage, it is essential that the position and patency of the tube be maintained. The tube is anchored at the incision with a black silk suture. It is further stabilized by adhesive tape to the skin. If a "splinting" catheter is in place, it usually emerges from the wound next to the nephrostomy tube. It is usually a Robinson-type catheter and is also fixed to the wound and skin in the same manner. Since its purpose is to stabilize the operative repair and not to drain urine, it is usually clamped or tied off. In the early postoperative period, when bleeding may be present, the nephrostomy tube should be checked at least every hour to assess the volume and character of the drainage. During this period, frequent "milking" (squeezing the tube in the palm of the hand) will help to dislodge blood clots in the lumen which may prevent free drainage. Should excessive bleeding occur, it will be readily apparent in the color and viscosity of the drainage.

Under no circumstances must the nurse clamp the nephrostomy tube unless specifically instructed to do so. Should one wish to disconnect the tube from the collection container temporarily—as, for example, when moving the patient from bed to stretcher—the end of the tube should be wrapped in sterile gauze and reattached as soon as the move is completed. Furthermore, a newly inserted nephrostomy tube should not be irrigated except by the physician. Although the nephrostomy tube has been inserted as a bypass, there are other available exits for urine, such as down the ureter or through the renal pelvis along tissue drains to the outside. Since a totally watertight closure of the renal pelvis is usually not accomplished or intended, it is common to have a fair amount of drainage through the drain sites in the immediate postoperative period until the pyelotomy begins to seal off.

A nephrostomy catheter is removed when it is no longer needed. In other words, complete relief of obstruction to the downward flow of urine must be demonstrated. This can be done in several ways. One is to insert contrast material into the pelvis, clamp the tube, and obtain x-rays at ten-minute intervals following the clamping to observe the rapidity of emptying. Another method is to clamp the nephrostomy tube on doctor's orders and observe the clinical course of the patient. Once the tube is clamped, the onset of flank pain or fever implies a significant degree of obstruction. When this occurs, the tube should be opened and reattached to straight drainage. The volume of urine that drains immediately on opening the catheter is measured and recorded as a "residual urine."

A more sophisticated and delicate measure for determining the patency of the urinary tract is the *burette test* which, when combined with the aforementioned x-ray studies, will give more complete information as to the necessity of continuing nephrostomy drainage. The burette test measures the pressure inside the renal pelvis over a period of time, at least 8 to 12 hours. If the pressure remains within certain normal limits, urine is draining freely into the bladder and the nephrostomy tube can be removed safely (Fig. 17-3).

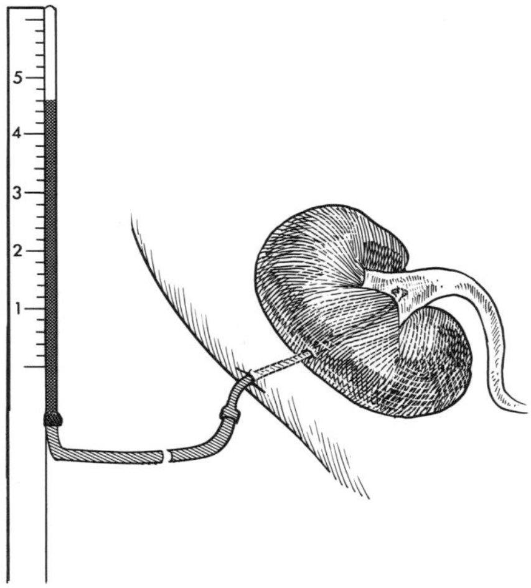

FIGURE 17-3. Schematic diagram of burette test.

The doctor initiates the study. A standard laboratory burette is taped to a stand at the patient's bedside. A centimeter scale is taped alongside the burette with the zero mark opposite the level of the renal pelvis. The lower end of the burette and the end of the nephrostomy are joined with sterile tubing. Sterile saline tinted with methylene blue dye is instilled into the burette up to the zero point, following which the height of the fluid column in the burette is recorded at hourly intervals. The addition of methylene blue facilitates these readings, and its first appearance in the voided urine can be noted, giving an indication of patency below.

Along with the hourly pressure readings, the temperature, activity, and position of the patient are noted at each reading. This information is placed on graph paper kept at the patient's bedside. Since the normal intrarenal pressure is 15 cm of water or less, the height of the burette column will not rise above this level as urine is produced if no lower obstruction is present. In the presence of complete obstruction, the fluid level in the burette may rise very rapidly; a partial obstruction will be manifested by a gradual rise in pressure above 15 cm. If there is flank pain, chills, or temperature elevation above 38.5°C, the test must be discontinued and the nephrostomy reconnected to straight drainage. Three or four consecutive readings of 25 cm or higher are also enough indication to discontinue the study.

Changes in position, movement, coughing, or sneezing will cause the pressure to rise. While the patient may sit up or have the head of the bed raised between readings, the nurse should make certain that he is quiet and flat for at least five minutes prior to a reading. For the period of the test (which is usually begun in the evening and carried through the night), the patient should be confined to his bed. Should he be in a high-low bed, it is important that the height of the bed not be changed once the test is started, since this would alter the zero point and give inaccurate figures. Breathing will cause a slight fluctuation in the water column of a centimeter or two. This small variation is negligible when the average is calculated at the end of the test.

If these studies demonstrate residual obstruction, the patient might be discharged from the hospital on nephrostomy drainage to be reevaluated at a later date. In such instances, the doctor may request that the nurse instruct the patient in nephrostomy care, anchorage of the catheter, whether or not irrigations should be performed, and what to do in case of an emergency.

Surgical Procedures of the Ureter

Positioning for surgery of the ureter depends on the level to be explored. The upper ureter is usually approached through the flank in the same position as for exposure of the kidney. The mid-ureter can also be exposed similarly. The lower ureter may be explored through a paramedian incision or a Gibson incision. The latter is a lateral oblique lower abdominal incision. Ordinarily, the peritoneum is not entered but is swept medially and the ureter identified in the retroperitoneal space. Rarely, the lowermost ureter may be reached through an anterior vaginal incision.

Ureterolithotomy is the most frequently performed operation on the ureter. Calculi larger than 1 cm in diameter will not readily pass spontaneously and often require surgical intervention. The three places most likely for a calculus to become lodged are at the narrowest points of the ureter—i.e., where it begins, where it ends, and where it crosses over the iliac vessels. At operation, the ureter is incised longitudinally and the calculus removed. The ureterotomy can then be left open or loosely approximated with fine chromic catgut sutures. The opening is drained to the outside with rubber tissue drains. All external urinary drainage should cease by the tenth to the fourteenth postoperative day if there is no obstruction to urine flow below the ureterotomy site.

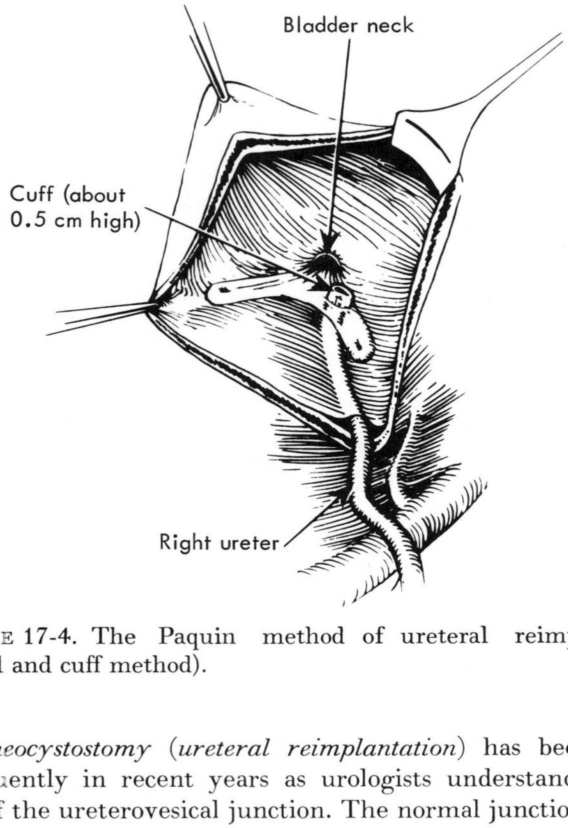

FIGURE 17-4. The Paquin method of ureteral reimplantation (tunnel and cuff method).

Ureteroneocystostomy (*ureteral reimplantation*) has been performed more frequently in recent years as urologists understand more about disorders of the ureterovesical junction. The normal junction functions as a passive valve which opens as urine flows down into the bladder. When the bladder contracts, the walls of the junction close so that there is no backflow or "reflux" of urine back into the kidney. There is convincing evidence that continued reflux eventually results in damage to the kidney by hydronephrosis and infection. Stenosis at this junction may also cause hydronephrosis and renal damage. There are many methods for re-implanting the ureter into the bladder and restoring this valve mechanism. The basic principles of all these procedures are the same. An adequately reconstructed valve mechanism that neither obstructs nor refluxes must have an obliquely inserted ureter, the walls of which must be pliable so that increased pressure in the bladder will firmly close this valve. The length of the ureteral tunnel must be about five times as long as the diameter of the ureteral orifice, and the tunnel should be placed in a location that will have adequate muscular backing, such as the bladder base.

The "tunnel and cuff" technique of Paquin is one that follows these principles. The ureter is divided at the ureterovesical junction. Through an opening in the back of the bladder, a submucosal tunnel is fashioned down to the trigone. The ureter is threaded through this tunnel to its new orifice. The end of the ureter is then turned on itself like a "French cuff" to yield a small-diameter orifice (Fig. 17-4). Other popular operations performed using the same principles are the Leadbetter-Politano, Hutch, and Lich procedures. Postoperatively many surgeons will splint these ureters by means of a catheter through the new orifice up into the renal pelvis, partly to ensure urinary drainage until inflammation subsides in the operative site.

Specific Nursing Considerations

The major nursing problem after ureterolithotomy is wound care because of the large amounts of external urinary drainage. As with pyelotomy wounds, frequent dressing changes may be necessary to keep the patient dry. Ureteral splinting catheters following reimplantation are usually small-diameter latex or red rubber catheters 8 to 12 F in diameter. The distal end of the catheter is often brought out through the bladder and abdominal wall alongside the cystostomy catheter (Fig. 17-5). The latter is usually of the Malecot or Foley type. Both catheters are anchored to the skin with suture and tape and connected with glass adapters to straight drainage. Occasionally the splint may be a smaller ureteral catheter of the type used for retrograde pyelography. In such an instance the catheter should be connected to the collector through the bulb of a medicine dropper (Fig. 17-6). The use of a needle as an adapter in such catheters will further compromise a small lumen, impeding urinary outflow, and should not be used.

The splinting catheter should be observed frequently to see if it is draining properly. If it is not, the cause may be poor position of the tube in the renal pelvis or occlusion by mucus. In the latter case, the doctor will attempt to irrigate it clear. If the catheter does not drain well, urine will usually drain around the splint into the bladder, although this is not the ideal situation. Attempts to reposition the tube for better drainage are strictly a physician's responsibility. If irrigation is necessary, the doctor will employ a small-piston syringe using 2 or 3 ml of solution at a time.

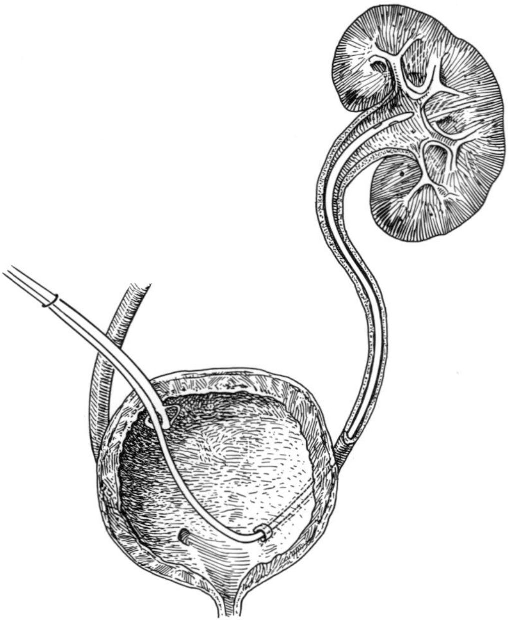

FIGURE 17-5. Splinting and cystostomy catheters, following reimplantation of ureter.

In view of these considerations, the measured drainage of each catheter is often meaningless, particularly with ureteral splints. More important is the combined total of measured output and reasonable assurance that all tubes are patent and unobstructed.

The splinting catheter is usually removed on the seventh to tenth postoperative day and the cystostomy tube a day or two later after suitable x-ray studies. These include withdrawal ureterograms to evaluate downward emptying and cystograms through the cystostomy tube to confirm the disappearance of reflux and an intact bladder closure. The abdominal fistula left after the cystostomy tube is removed will usually close spontaneously in a day or two as long as no distal obstruction is present. In the interim, gauze dressings are placed over the opening to absorb the urine.

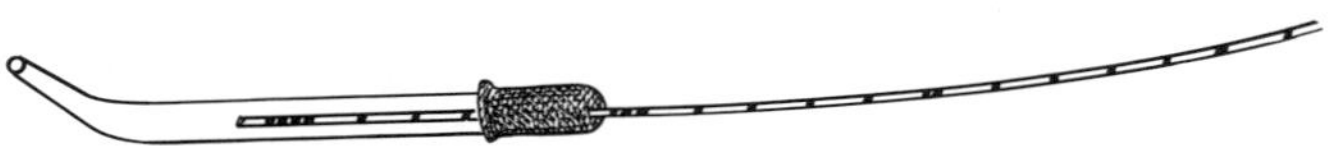

FIGURE 17-6. Attachment of ureteral catheter to medicine dropper for straight drainage.

REVIEW QUESTIONS

1. Describe three surgical approaches by which nephrectomy may be accomplished.
2. Define the following: radical nephrectomy, nephroureterectomy, kidney split, pyelotomy, nephrostomy.
3. Discuss postoperative hemorrhage following surgical procedures on the kidney, including relevant factors to be considered in giving nursing care.
4. Describe wound care following pyelotomy and ureterolithotomy.
5. Following nephrectomy, what specific observations should be made of urinary output? Indicate those conditions that would be cause for concern and should be reported to the doctor.
6. Discuss the several procedures that may be used prior to removal of the nephrostomy to determine patency of the upper urinary tract. What would be the nursing responsibilities in each?
7. Plan the nursing care for a 45-year-old female patient following radical nephrectomy (transthoracic approach) for the first 24 hours postoperatively. Identify the objectives of care for this period and the specific nurse-patient activities to achieve these objectives. By what means would you see that your plan was communicated to the other nursing personnel? At the end of 24 hours, how would you evaluate whether or not the objectives of the plan of care had been met?
8. Discuss the location and function of splinting catheters following Y-V plasty and ureteral reimplantation. How do these catheters differ, and what is the significance for nursing care?

CHAPTER 18
Permanent Urinary Diversion

MEASURES to permanently divert the flow of urine from the bladder may be necessary for a variety of reasons. Some of the more common indications include removal of the bladder for cancer, neurogenic bladder dysfunction with degenerating upper tracts, selected cases of incontinence, and other obstructions where kidney function is so poor that restorative procedures entail high risk or may not be possible. Permanent urinary diversion can be performed in many ways. The fact that the urologic literature is replete with many ingenious methods, however, implies that none have been entirely satisfactory. Presently the three most commonly used surgical methods are ureterosigmoidostomy, cutaneous ureterostomy, and the ileal conduit. Other less desirable methods involve the use of permanent catheter drainage in the form of either permanent nephrostomy, cystostomy, or an indwelling urethral catheter.

Permanent Catheter Drainage

A small group of patients with diseased urinary tracts will not be candidates for any corrective surgery. To ensure a free flow of urine, the urologist's only alternative may be to initiate permanent catheter drainage. Continual use of catheters is best avoided because, as a foreign body, the catheter predisposes to frequent infections and calculus formation. Permanent catheters may be in the kidney (nephrostomy), ureter (ureterostomy), or bladder (cystostomy). A cystostomy catheter is usually preferred over a urethral catheter when permanent bladder drainage is necessary.

If one is to reduce the risk inherent in permanent catheter drainage, it is imperative that the patient learn to care for himself at home according to the regimen established by his physician. The two primary areas of consideration will be irrigating and changing the catheter. Physicians differ in their philosophies of catheter irrigation. The primary purpose of the catheter is to drain urine. Some physicians feel, therefore, that so long as the catheter is draining, it need not be irrigated. Others feel that interval irrigation is necessary to ensure patency. All agree that the patient should know how to irrigate if drainage decreases or stops. Also, all agree that irrigation, if not done properly, can increase the likelihood of symptomatic infection.

The implication for the nurse is, therefore, that she must teach the patient to irrigate his catheter, using a safe technique. The physician will determine the circumstances under which he wishes the catheter irrigated and the type and volume of solution to be used. The physician may specify that he wants the catheter irrigated only if the free flow of urine is impeded. The patient can usually determine this by a noticeable decrease in volume of urinary ouput or a cessation of drainage. Both conditions are often accompanied by pain and an elevated temperature. The physician may, on the other hand, want the patient to irrigate routinely two or three times a week and additionally as may be necessary to ensure patency.

It is particularly important that the doctor specify the volume to be used because of the marked difference between capacities of the kidney pelvis and the bladder, and also because of the variations in these capacities that occur with age. The normal adult renal pelvis has a capacity of 4 to 6 ml. If the pelvis is hydronephrotic, the capacity may be 10 or even 100 times greater. The capacity of a child's renal pelvis may vary from 1 to 3 ml depending upon the age of the child; the younger the child, the smaller the capacity. Volume is not quite so significant when irrigating the bladder. For purposes of irrigation, the normal adult bladder will accommodate 75 to 90 ml, while children, again depending upon age, will tolerate approximately 25 to 75 ml. The nurse's principle of irrigation is not to lavage the organ but to maintain the patency of the catheter. (Irrigations to wash out the bladder are best done by the physician.)

For home irrigation, the solution commonly prescribed is sterile normal saline. This can be made by adding a teaspoon of common table salt to a pint of water, which is boiled for ten minutes. Occasionally, the physician may prefer a slightly acid solution which is prepared commercially. Such a solution may be obtained by the patient from the hospital pharmacy or his local druggist. Solution G (Suby's solution) is one of these (See Appendix VI, pages 380–81.)

Nephrostomy and cystostomy catheters are changed by the doctor. A urethral catheter is usually changed at the clinic, in the private office, or by the visiting nurse if the patient is female; it is changed by the doctor, a male nurse, or a specially trained orderly if the patient is male. How often the catheter is changed will be determined by the physician and his evaluation of the need for change. It may be once a month or as infrequently as every three months. Since changing external ureteral catheters is a relatively simple procedure, most patients with these are taught the technique. These are usually changed weekly.

A patient with a catheter needs a drainage bag. At night he can wear a leg bag or use bedside drainage, preferably the latter. The catheter must never be clamped. If two catheters must be worn—as, for example, with bilateral ureterostomies—a Y tube may be used to connect them to one bag. There are some physicians, however, who do not favor the Y tube because of the possibility of cross-infection; they prefer that each catheter be attached to a separate drainage receptacle. (See Appendix VI, page 381.)

Many physicians feel that when catheters are to be worn permanently, the incidence of calculus formation is reduced if the patient is placed on a low-calcium, low-phosphorus diet (Shorr diet) (see Appendix I, page 362) and aluminum hydroxide gel. The dietitian can be of great help in giving diet instructions. However, it will still be the nurse's responsibility to see that the patient understands the diet and the schedule for taking the accompanying medication.

It is extremely important that the nurse allot the necessary time in preparing the patient adequately for discharge. Too often teaching is left until the last minute, whereas, had there been a little forethought, she could have anticipated the need for homegoing preparation. At least three or four days should be allowed. The amount to be taught and the patient's ability to learn are essential factors to be considered. Most patients learn the irrigation procedure with little difficulty. The changing of a ureteral catheter, however, requires much greater time and effort. Nearly all patients are fearful of damaging the kidney and, initially, are timid and reluctant to perform the procedure. Their fears, together with their awkwardness in handling the catheter, make teaching more difficult, requiring patience, practice, and much reassurance. It is important that a responsible family member be included in the teaching. A visiting nurse should visit the patient at home to determine that he is handling the procedure correctly. (See Appendix VI, pages 378–82.)

Ureterosigmoidostomy

Ureterosigmoidostomy is a surgically formed opening between the ureter and sigmoid colon (Fig. 18-1). Over fifty methods of anastomosis have been devised, indicating the degree of difficulty involved in achieving success. The ideal result occurs when urine flows freely into the bowel without obstruction and there is no reflux of urine or fecal material into the kidney.

Ureterosigmoidostomy has two important advantages. The patient usually has urinary control per rectum and requires no external appliance. This seemingly ideal situation is marred by its complications. Despite the most meticulous surgical technique, there may be intermittent episodes of fecal regurgitation into the kidneys, causing insidious pyelonephritis. Intermittent or progressive obstruction at the anastomoses may cause hydronephrosis. Furthermore, the exposure of colonic mucosa to large volumes of urine over long periods of time results in resorption of urinary electrolytes, particularly chlorides. An unsuccessful attempt on the part of the body bicarbonate to adjust to this increased chloride results in a

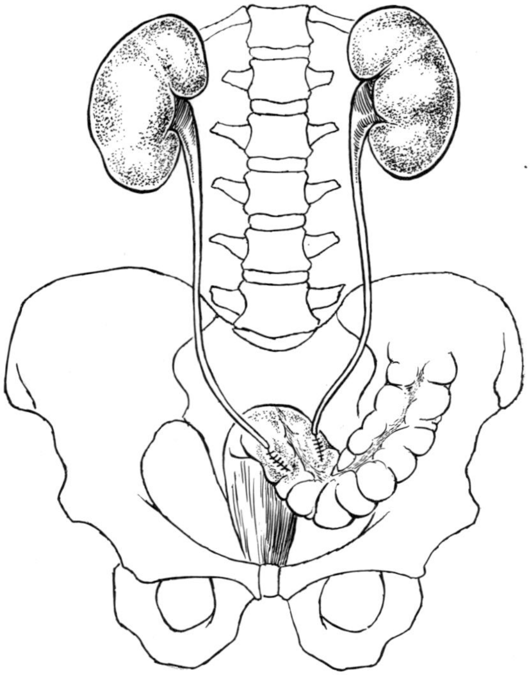

FIGURE 18-1. Ureterosigmoidostomy.

hyperchloremic acidosis. In addition, these patients tend to have a low serum potassium which, of itself, can cause renal tubular damage. This combination of events can gradually result in loss of kidney function. Patients are uncommon who have lived fifteen to twenty years following this type of diversion without evidence of some renal deterioration or clinical symptoms. Consequently, this procedure should seldom be performed if the patient is a child or young adult. Furthermore, such diversion is also contraindicated in situations where there is poor rectal sphincter control (neurogenic bladder or anal injury), radiation proctitis (as following treatment for carcinoma of the bladder), and diverticulitis, to name a few.

Special Nursing Considerations

Preoperatively the patient is placed on a regimen to prepare the bowel. The purposes of this regimen are twofold: to lower, as much as possible, the bacterial count of intestinal flora and to reduce the volume of formed feces.

Approximately three to five days prior to surgery, oral medications specifically effective against intestinal bacteria may be used. Medications commonly used for this purpose are neomycin and phthalylsulfathiazole (Sulfathalidine). Frequently a cathartic such as magnesium sulfate is given before the first dose. As the medication begins to take effect, the nurse will notice that the stool becomes more liquid and that there is a change in the characteristic odor. Decreasing the bacterial count may help to decrease the incidence of postoperative wound infections. During this period, the patient will be placed on a low-residue diet, which is usually changed to a clear liquid diet one or two days before surgery. The patient will also have either a daily cathartic or an enema, or both. Some surgeons use only mechanical bowel preparation consisting of cathartics, enemas, and a low-residue diet. On occasion, the use of oral antibiotics to change the intestinal flora has resulted in the complications of enterocolitis secondary to overgrowth with staphylococci or fungi. The nurse carries major responsibility for making certain that the prescribed regimen is followed. Most patients during this period are physically uncomfortable, which frequently only serves to heighten their anxiety. The nurse, therefore, should also be liberal in dispensing explanation, encouragement, and understanding.

Postoperatively, as with any intestinal surgery, the patient will have gastric drainage and intravenous therapy for three to five days. He will also have a large-lumen tube (28 to 34 F) inserted into the rectum and attached to straight drainage. Accurate measurement and recording of intake and output are important.

The rectal tube is held in position by adhesive strips attached to the buttocks. During the first several days, the position of the tube and amount of drainage should be checked every several hours. Should the tube become displaced or obstructed, back pressure may cause damage to the anastomoses. The doctor will reposition or irrigate the tube should either become necessary. The tube is left in place continuously for approximately the first eight to ten days. Thereafter, it will need to be inserted only at night. Should the patient have some leakage of urine after the use of the rectal tube is discontinued, frequent perineal exercises (tightening and relaxing the anal sphincter) usually strengthen the sphincter sufficiently to eliminate this problem.

There are certain facts of which both the patient and nurse must be aware. The patient should never take harsh laxatives or enemas, since these could produce abnormally high intrarectal pressures causing reflux of urine and feces. Postoperative constipation is virtually unheard of; if such symptoms occur, the likelihood is that the patient is developing a mechanical bowel obstruction. Most patients, however, return to their preoperative fecal evacuation schedule.

The patient should learn to empty his rectum every three to four hours whether he feels pressure or not. The rectum can, over a period of time, accommodate increasingly larger volumes of urine without causing discomfort. As mentioned previously, urinary electrolytes are resorbed through the intestinal mucosa. Keeping the intracolonic urine volume small by frequent emptying helps to reduce the rate of resorption. This, too, is the rationale behind the use of the rectal tube connected to straight drainage at night. At bedtime, the patient is instructed to lubricate a rectal tube, insert it approximately 4 inches, tape it to the skin, and attach it to bedside drainage. Some patients object strenuously to the use of the rectal tube and prefer instead to get up two or three times nightly to empty their rectum. While the patient is in the hospital, his blood chloride levels will be followed carefully. Should they become markedly elevated, the patient will be given oral sodium bicarbonate. Some patients may need to take bicarbonate permanently to avoid becoming too acidotic. Should this be necessary, the patient must understand the importance of the medication and why he must take it regularly.

The urine expelled from the rectum is usually cloudy with flecks of stool and has a strong, pungent odor. In the immediate postoperative period, the anal area must be kept as clean and dry as possible. Petrolatum provides a water-resistant coating for the skin. Abdominal pads cut to fit around the tube and between the buttocks help to absorb any leakage. A T binder holds the pads in place. A heat lamp to the area, twenty minutes three times a day, relieves irritation. Once discharged from the hospital, the patient will need perineal care with soap and water at least once a day. These patients are well advised to take tub baths instead of showers since the water is both cleansing as well as therapeutic. Should he use night drainage, he will need to wash all of the equipment thoroughly each morning.

Cutaneous Ureterostomy

Transplantation of the divided ureter to the abdominal wall is known as cutaneous ureterostomy (Fig. 18-2). In general, this method of diversion has more disadvantages than advantages. A major disadvantage is that the patient will usually have bilateral openings on the skin, each requiring appliances. Such appliances are more prone to leak than the ileostomy type of appliance. A second disadvantage is that urinary flow is continuous so that there is no voluntary control. Finally, a high percentage of cutaneous ureterostomies, particularly those involving a normal ureter with its delicate blood supply, will stricture particularly at the skin and fascial level. These ureterostomies, unless they can be revised successfully, will require drainage by permanent indwelling catheters. These catheters may leak on slight changes in position, need frequent irrigation and change, and also encourage infection and stone formation.

In their proper place, however, cutaneous ureterostomies have much to

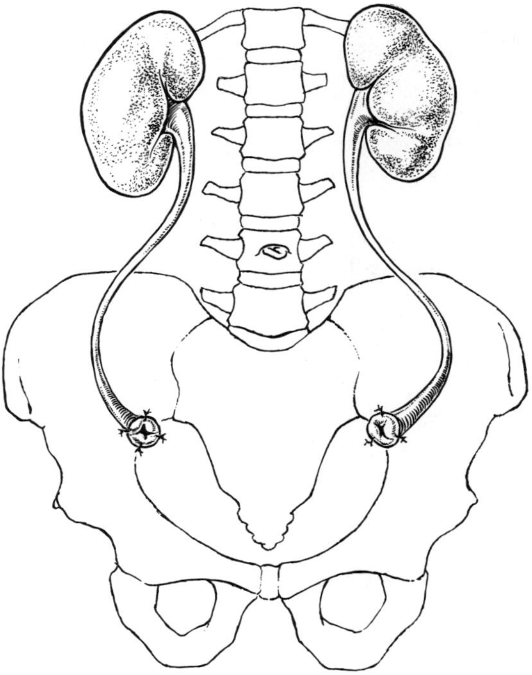

FIGURE 18-2. Cutaneous ureterostomy.

offer. When renal function is very poor as a result of long-standing obstruction, it may be the only type of drainage the patient can tolerate. Furthermore, a thick-walled, chronically dilated ureter as seen in such poor-risk patients tends to have a luxuriant blood supply and is more likely to yield a successful transplant not requiring a catheter.

Specific Nursing Considerations

In an effort to prevent slough and stricture, special care is given the ureteral stoma. In the operating room, the stoma is covered with a small gauze pad saturated with normal saline. For the next five to ten days, the stoma is kept constantly moist, using about 5 ml of solution. The nurse should moisten the pad hourly. The equipment for this procedure is most conveniently kept on a tray at the patient's bedside. It consists of a small glass bottle for the normal saline and a bulb syringe. A second bottle and syringe will be necessary if the ureterostomies are bilateral. If the equipment is covered with a sterile wrapper, it need be sterilized only once daily. Sterile cellophane or Saran Wrap over the wet pad keeps the outer dressing dry and prevents evaporation. If the dressing is applied carefully, the pad can be moistened merely by lifting the edge of the dressing. The pad and dressing are usually changed once a day by the doctor. Should the pad be adherent to the stoma, it is thoroughly saturated with normal saline and allowed to soak until it can be removed without resistance. Otherwise, frequent abrasion of the delicate ureteral mucosa may enhance stricture formation.

Since many patients who undergo this procedure have poor kidney function, fluids and electrolytes must be carefully monitored postoperatively. The patient will have a Robinson-type splinting catheter in each ureterostomy. It is usually tacked to the skin with a black silk suture and further stabilized with adhesive tape. The catheter is attached to straight drainage. Since the catheter goes directly to the kidney, it should be checked hourly during the first 48 hours to see that it is draining properly. Even when the catheter is patent, urine will occasionally leak around it. This may be caused by temporary obstruction because of position change. Persistent leakage, however, suggests that the catheter needs to be repositioned. Usually, a 1/4-inch adjustment of the catheter in or out until it irrigates freely is all that is necessary. In the early postoperative period, the doctor will adjust and irrigate the catheter as needed. If the ureteral stoma has healed satisfactorily, the catheter is removed on about the tenth day, and withdrawal ureterograms are obtained to demonstrate prompt emptying of the kidney.

Should the patient develop chills, fever, or flank pain, it is relatively certain that residual urine is present. The doctor will then catheterize the ureter to determine the amount of residual present. If it is excessive, the catheter may be left indwelling for a longer time until future studies demonstrate it can be removed safely. This process may be repeated several times before the doctor is able to determine whether the ureterostomy needs to be managed with an appliance or catheter. Because of this uncertainty, the permanent appliance is usually not ordered until it is established that an indwelling catheter is unnecessary.

Ileal Conduit

The ileal conduit is constructed by implanting the ureter into a short segment of isolated terminal ileum (the Bricker procedure). This segment, with its own blood supply, is separated from the remaining small intestine which is reanastomosed to restore the integrity of the intestinal tract. The divided ureters are anastomosed directly to the conduit with no attempt at obliquity. The proximal end of the conduit is closed, and the distal end is brought out as a stoma, usually in the right lower quadrant of the abdomen (Fig. 18-3).

A properly functioning conduit contains very little urine at any time, since the urine is constantly expelled by peristalsis and the conduit has no reservoir function. Consequently, since the ileum is virtually empty, reflux up the ureter is of little significance. For the same reason, absorption of urinary electrolytes is not a problem if the conduit is kept less than 20 cm in length. When compared with cutaneous ureterostomy, the conduit has the advantages of a single, healthy stoma of a size that can be fitted with an effective external collection device. On the other hand, with severely depressed renal function, direct drainage by cutaneous ureterostomy should be used. In general, it is unwise to use intestinal segments for diversion when the blood urea nitrogen is consistently over 40 mg

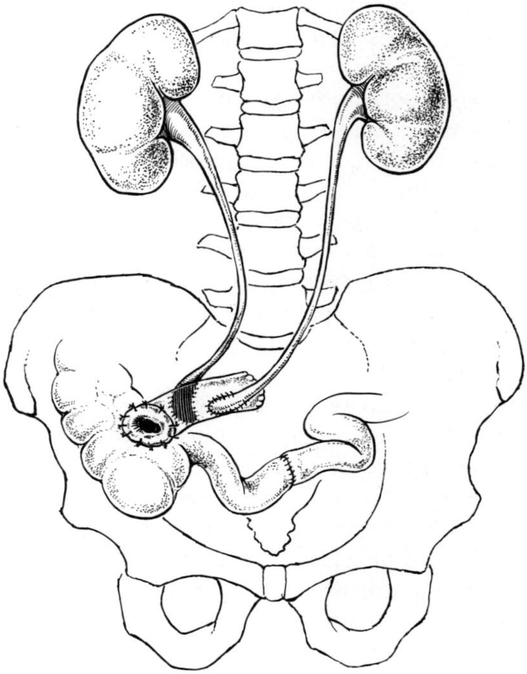

FIGURE 18-3. Ileal conduit.

per cent. In addition, the several anastomoses and rearrangements involved in construction of the conduit are accompanied by a moderate percentage of postoperative complications such as ureteral obstruction and intestinal obstruction.

Specific Nursing Considerations

Preoperatively, the patient's bowel is prepared for intestinal surgery (see page 211). The patient will usually have nasogastric drainage and intravenous therapy for approximately five days postoperatively, or until the intestinal tract has begun to function normally. Urine will be collected by either a temporary ostomy bag or a catheter attached to straight drainage. It is therefore necessary for the nurse to carefully measure intravenous fluids, gastric and urinary drainage so that the doctor is able to determine necessary fluid and electrolyte replacement.

Conduit construction is undertaken through a lower abdominal incision. The ileal stoma is usually within 2 to 3 inches of the incision with the result that wound and urine drainage, edema, and surface irregularities may interfere with the adhesion of the temporary appliance. A leaking appliance makes accurate measurement of urinary output difficult and may also contribute to skin irritation and wound infection. Consequently, care of the skin and incision is very important. Irritation around the stoma is usually minimal if the temporary appliance is used properly and changed not more than once in 24 hours. If the incision becomes wet with urine, dressings are changed as often as necessary. At the first signs of irritation or inflammation, the area should be exposed to a heat lamp at least three times a day. Fecal or urine drainage from the incision is rare and indicates that one of the anastomoses has broken down. Usually these fistulas will close spontaneously. In the interim, however, the nurse will need all of her ingenuity to devise methods to protect the skin. One of the most generally applicable and effective preventatives and treatments for skin problems is a paste made from karaya powder and water to coat the exposed areas.

Because of problems with temporary appliances and the failure of the conduit to drain adequately because of paralytic ileus, some urologists prefer catheter drainage of the conduit. The catheter is usually of the multieyed Robinson type. It is inserted several inches into the stoma and fixed to the skin with adhesive tape. The distal end of the catheter is attached to straight drainage. In the early postoperative period, large amounts of obstructing mucus are secreted by the ileal segment. The nurse should check the catheter hourly for such obstruction shown by a decrease in volume of drainage or urine leakage around the catheter. If she suspects obstruction, the doctor should be notified immediately, since back pressure in the ileal segment could damage the various suture lines. He will usually either irrigate the catheter with several milliliters of normal saline or replace it with another catheter. When the catheter is removed, a temporary bag is applied. Usually, peristalsis will return to the ileal conduit simultaneously with return of intestinal peristalsis. The following chapter discusses the selection and use of temporary and permanent appliances, skin care, and considerations necessary in teaching the patient to care for his ostomy.

REVIEW QUESTIONS

1. Explain why permanent urinary drainage by catheter is avoided if at all possible.
2. Describe the disadvantages of urinary diversion by ureterosigmoidostomy.
3. What is the purpose of the bowel regimen preoperatively? Describe this regimen.
4. What procedures, if followed by the patient, may help prevent long-term complications of ureterosigmoidostomy?
5. Describe the care of the anal region postoperatively.
6. Why is special care of the ureteral buds so important until healing is well advanced postoperatively? Describe the essential factors to be considered in planning this care.
7. Differentiate between the nurse's and the doctor's responsibilities in maintaining proper functioning of the indwelling ureteral catheter.
8. What are the advantages of urinary diversion by ileal conduit as compared to ureterosigmoidostomy or cutaneous ureterostomy?
9. Describe the care of the ileal conduit postoperatively.

CHAPTER 19
Appliances for External Urinary Diversion

AFTER urinary diversion to an external opening, such as ileal conduit or cutaneous ureterostomy, a collection device must be worn. Both temporary and permanent devices are available. Temporary devices, disposable and made of clear plastic, are usually used in the early postoperative period. Prior to discharge from the hospital, however, the patient is fitted with a permanent appliance and is instructed in its application and care. The permanent device is commonly made of latex rubber or durable plastic material, both of which last for months if cared for properly.

The selection and the application of both types of appliances are usually the responsibility of the nurse. She must be acquainted with the various temporary and permanent appliances available so that she can select the model most appropriate to the specific needs of the patient. She must also know how to use the appliance selected in order to teach the patient the necessary skills before he is discharged from the hospital. It is unfortunate that many nurses, charged with these responsibilities, do not have the knowledge required to provide adequate nursing care.

If in the early postoperative period the patient is allowed to experience frequent soiling, he soon becomes discouraged and may feel he will never be able to return to his former way of life. He will worry whether any device is leakproof and if he ever will be able to master its application. Skin breakdown from leaky, improperly fitted bags causes the patient not only physical discomfort but also severe emotional stress. The nurse who enters the patient's room, carrying his new appliance, and announces, "I've never used one of these before, but we'll read the instructions together," is hardly one to inspire confidence or elevate flagging spirits.

The following information is intended to highlight the essential factors in the selection, fitting, and use of appliances. Although the products of all manufacturers have the same basic components—namely, faceplate, pouch, outlet, and belt—the construction and design vary from product to product. A partial list of manufacturers producing ostomy equipment and supplies is given in Appendix VIII. The interested reader should contact these companies directly for brochures and other information describing their products. Local surgical supply houses also provide excellent counsel. Suffice it to say that the nurse who selects and fits an appliance should have a broad knowledge of the type of equipment available.

Temporary Appliances

After construction of an ileal conduit, the surgeon usually sends his patient from the operating room with a temporary postoperative pouch connected to straight, dependent drainage. Some surgeons, however, leave an indwelling catheter in the conduit for several days before introducing the temporary appliance. Diversion by means of cutaneous ureterostomy requires drainage through an indwelling catheter for ten days to two weeks before an appliance is substituted. Major considerations in selecting the temporary pouch include the type of adhesive used on the faceplate, the length and width of the pouch, and the outlet of the pouch. These considerations must be correlated with the configuration of the patient's abdomen, the location of the stoma relative to bony prominences and the surgical incision, and the patient's body build.

The faceplate design which generally has proved most satisfactory is one with adhesive material mounted on a thin, flexible paper, plastic, or cloth backing. Since the stoma is brought out of the abdomen through a skin wound and sutured in place, the surrounding skin area is convoluted and puckered. Adhesives with heavy or stiff backings and faceplates with cardboard rings for belt attachment often are not flexible enough to follow irregularities of the skin surface. Since urine is liquid, leakage occurs where there is the slightest crease or separation between the adhesive and the skin.

The faceplate may come with or without a precut center opening. If a precut opening is desired, the one-half- or the three-quarter-inch openings are most practical. In some cases, these may be too small but can be enlarged and shaped to specific stomal requirements. A blank faceplate is preferable when the opening must be cut eccentrically, as when the stoma is close to the surgical incision.

Temporary bag pouches are usually available in both a large and a small size. The large pouch is approximately 4 inches wide by 16 inches long with a 4-inch-diameter faceplate. The small pouch is usually 3 by 12 inches with a correspondingly smaller faceplate. The small bag is appropriate for children, and either size may be used for an adult. Even smaller temporary devices are becoming available for infants and toddlers.

The upper end of the temporary pouch is always sealed. The lower end may be sealed, open, or sealed with an adapter outlet. Since a sealed pouch cannot be emptied unless completely removed, it is unsatisfactory for urinary drainage and is more appropriately used for fecal drainage after gastrointestinal surgery. Pouches with adapter outlets are much more convenient but are significantly more expensive. The open-ended pouch (ileostomy-colostomy) can be easily adapted for urinary drainage using a glass or plastic adapter and an elastic band. Figure 19-1 illustrates several types of temporary bags.

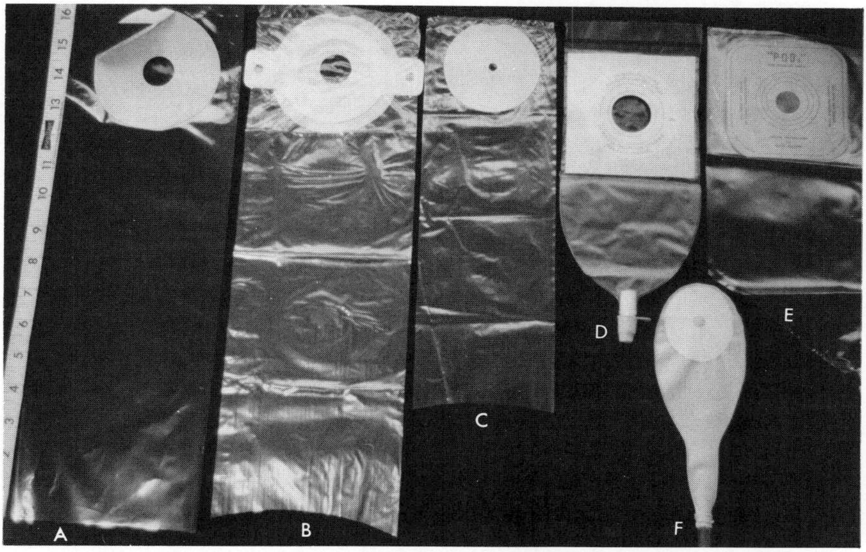

FIGURE 19-1. Temporary appliances. *A*, adult open-ended bag with backing folded to show clear, thin, adhesive backing; *B*, bag demonstrating cardboard ring for belt attachment; *C*, child-size bag; *D* and *E*, bags showing variation of shapes and built-in outlets for easy emptying of attachment to straight drainage; *F*, child or infant bag, tapered for insertion and snug fit for connector.

Preparation of the Temporary Appliance for Application

The nurse who changes the temporary bag for the first time postoperatively should make a paper pattern of the size and shape of the stoma. This pattern is left at the patient's bedside so that it is readily available when a new bag is applied. The pattern not only serves as a timesaver but also ensures greater accuracy in refitting the faceplate, thus reducing the likelihood of leakage and the need for frequent bag changes. As a general rule, the faceplate opening should be just large enough to expose the stoma and a thin rim of surrounding skin. When the skin around the stoma is puckered from suturing the stoma to the skin edge, however, the faceplate opening must be large enough to clear the irregularities; urine pooling in these indentations would undermine the adhesive bond. During the early postoperative period the pattern may need revision as stomal edema subsides. The opening is placed in the center of the faceplate unless proximity to the surgical incision or bony prominences dictates otherwise.

The length of the bag is a factor in its preparation. If a 16-inch open-ended bag is used, more efficient drainage results when 4 to 6 inches are cut off the end of the bag before the glass drainage connector is attached. A longer bag tends to kink and obstruct the outflow of urine. When the bag does not empty properly, the weight of accumulated urine may pull the faceplate away from the skin. The following method of joining the glass connector to the dependent portion of the bag ensures a watertight connection:

1. After the faceplate opening has been cut according to the pattern and the bag shortened, the open end of the bag is inverted and pulled through the faceplate opening for a length of two inches.
2. A medium-size glass connector is placed in the folds of the open end of the bag. The tip of the connector is placed even with the cut ends.
3. An elastic band is wrapped several times around the bag and connector. Without releasing the band, the ends of the bag are cuffed back and the band wrapped tightly around the cuff.
4. The glass connector is pulled back through the faceplate opening (Fig. 19-2).

The final step in the preparation of the bag is removal of the protective backing overlying the faceplate. If desired, a solvent thinly applied to the adhesive suface and allowed to dry seems to increase its tenacity. The bag is set aside until the skin surrounding the stoma is prepared.

Preparation of the Skin for the Temporary Appliance

It is of paramount importance to be gentle when removing the temporary pouch and adhesive residue from the skin. A solvent should be used, preferably one manufactured specifically for this purpose. These are characteristically nonflammable, quick, and less irritating to the skin. Solvents such as ether, benzene, and acetone not only are irritating and drying but are highly flammable and unpleasant smelling; they should be avoided. Carbon tetrachloride is another potentially dangerous solvent because of its hepatic and renal toxicity if absorbed. Although some adhesive residue may remain after cleansing, the skin should never be vigorously scrubbed.

The pouch is removed by applying solvent to the adhering surface between the faceplate and the skin. A medicine dropper is useful in this situation. After using the solvent, the skin is washed with soap and water and is thoroughly dried. Under no circumstances should the bag be ripped off.

The skin around the stoma must be perfectly dry if a watertight seal is to be achieved. Consequently, the stoma must be covered with an absorbent material to keep the surrounding skin dry until the pouch is applied. Several materials can be used to construct "wicks" for this purpose, such as fluffed cotton, gauze, or facial tissues. This absorbent material can be held more easily if placed in the open end of a test tube or a small bottle to serve as a "handle."

Whether or not the patient is ambulatory determines the best position for the pouch outlet. Dependent urinary drainage is the important consideration. Consequently, for the ambulatory patient the pouch should be oriented in an up-and-down axis; for the patient on bed rest the pouch should be directed transversely. To apply the pouch to the patient, hold the faceplate directly above the stoma with the pouch outlet appropriately aligned, remove the "wick," and promptly press the faceplate onto the skin surface. Once the faceplate is in place, secure the seal by using the fingers to press out wrinkles and crevices around the stoma opening and faceplate surface. Many people also apply compound tincture of benzoin

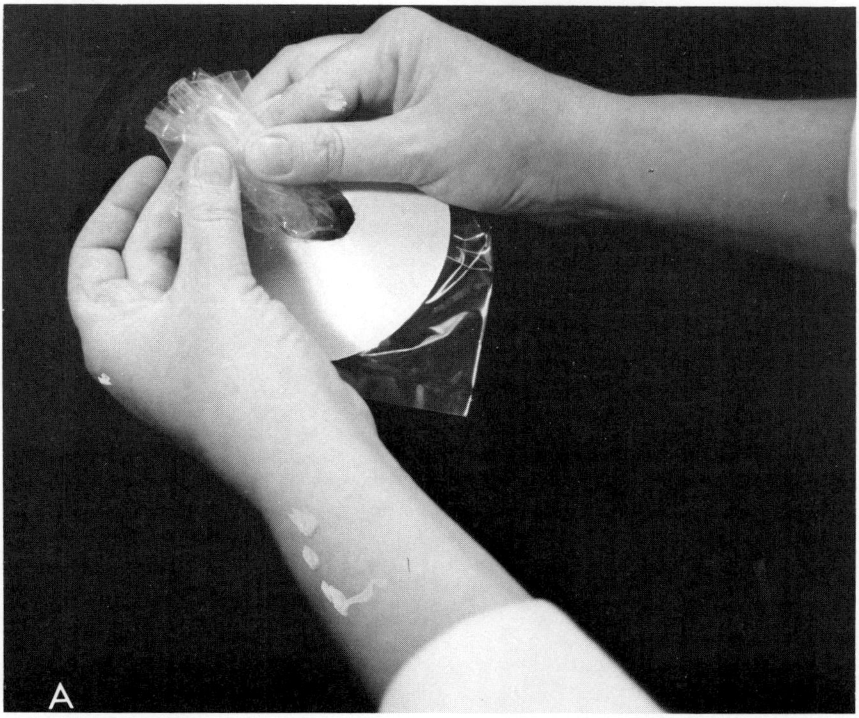

FIGURE 19-2. Technique for applying connector to open-ended bag.

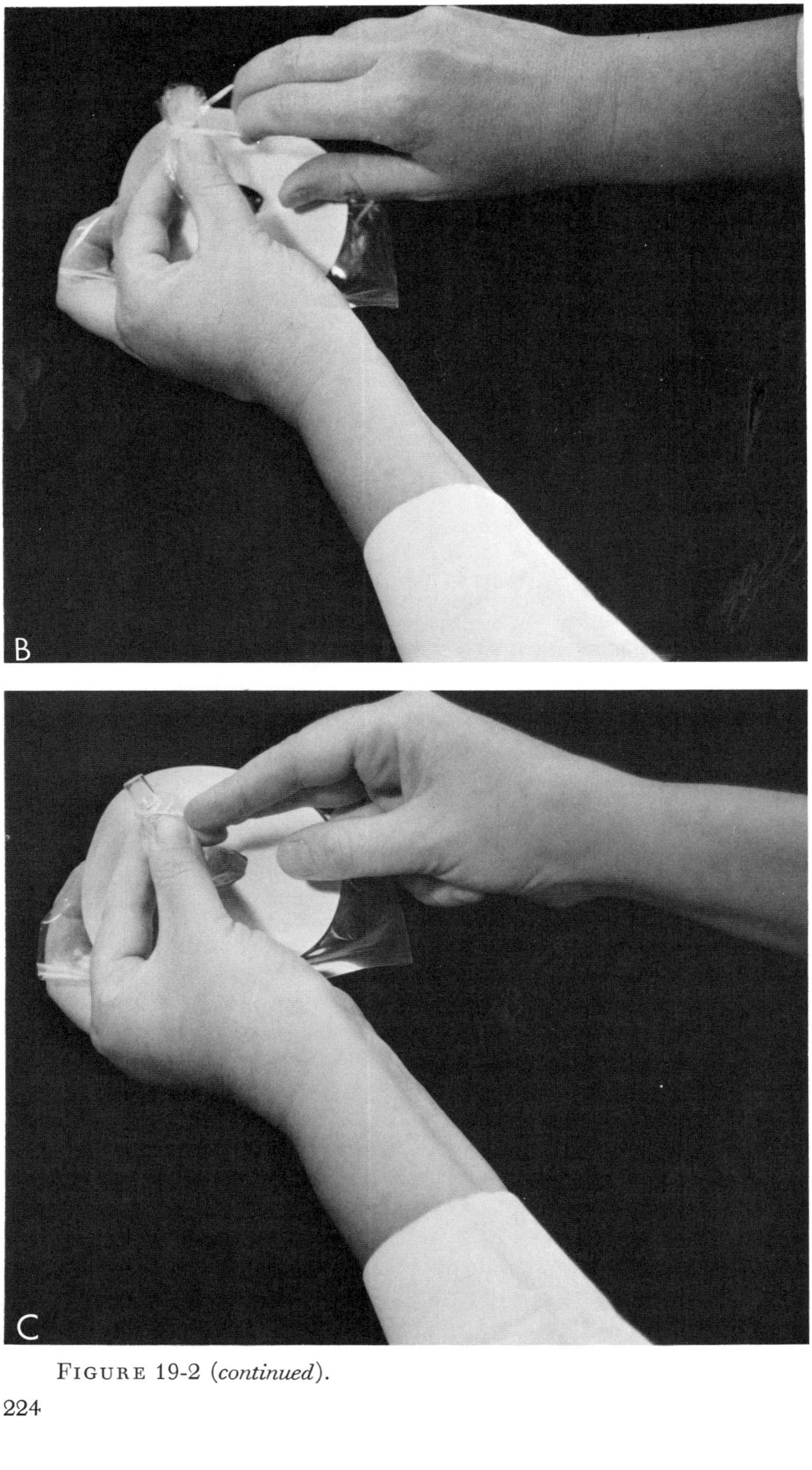

FIGURE 19-2 (*continued*).

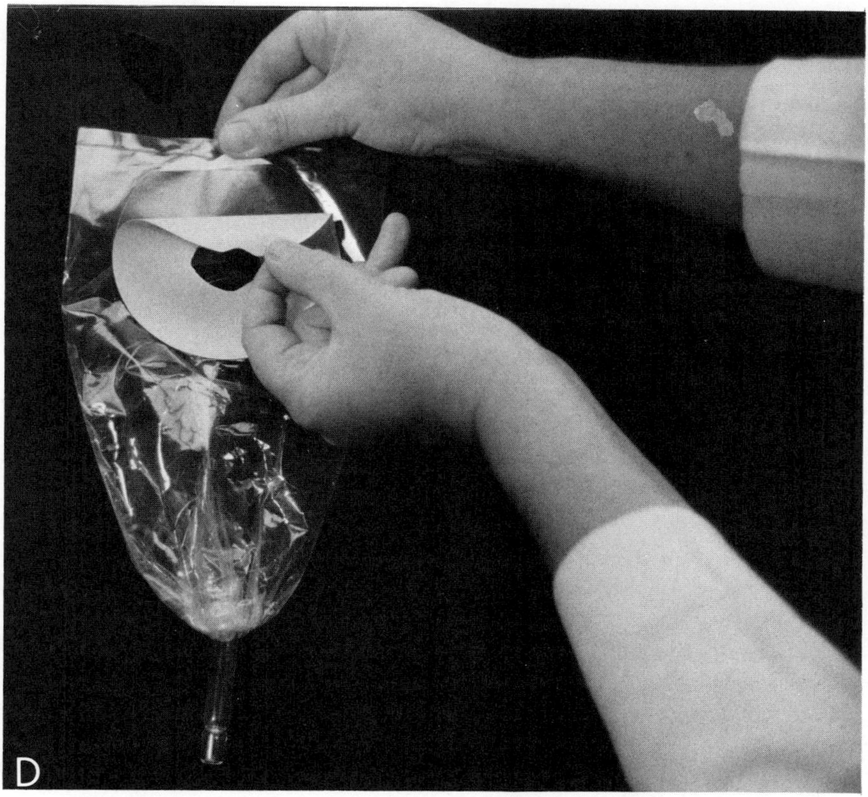

FIGURE 19-2 (*continued*).

to the dried skin before attaching the faceplate, since it not only improves adhesion but also coats and protects the skin.

Several modifications of this method can be tried should there be difficulty in maintaining a watertight seal. Applying a layer of skin cement to both the dried skin and the faceplate before attachment may give a tighter bond. The cement must be given time to become "tacky" for it to be effective. Another modification is the use of an interposed foam-rubber pad made of closed-cell, nonporous rubber. The pad is first cemented to the skin surrounding the stoma, after which the faceplate is glued to the outer surface of the pad. The pad has advantages in that it can be cut to fit any size or shape stoma and it molds itself easily to the abdominal contour. A common and useful size is one $3\frac{7}{8}$ inches in diameter and $\frac{1}{16}$-inch thick.

Temporary pouches should be left in place so long as there is no leakage. Of course, signs of skin or stomal irritation, requiring other measures, can easily be observed through the clear plastic. Probably the most common cause of skin irritation and breakdown in the stomal area is the too frequent changing of pouches. If the principles of application are followed carefully, however, bag changes can be kept to a minimum. Often, in the immediate postoperative period after construction of a urinary stoma, urine in contact with the skin seems to cause irritation. Usually this sensitivity subsides within 10 to 14 days. If the skin reaction is severe, a catheter may be introduced into the stoma. Skin irritation, if treated while still mild, subsides quickly when the area is kept dry and exposed frequently to a heat lamp. (See Appendix VII, page 386.)

Permanent Appliances

There are two types of permanent appliances commonly worn by patients with urinary diversion. The first and most frequently used is the ileal bladder pouch. Except for a valve outlet, it is identical with an ileostomy appliance. It is worn by patients with an ileal conduit or single ureterostomy. Because of the relatively large capacity of the pouch, a leg bag is unnecessary. The second type of appliance is worn by patients with bilateral cutaneous ureterostomies. It is commonly referred to as a cup appliance. In appearance it resembles a miniature straw hat approximately $3\frac{1}{2}$ inches in diameter, the brim of which is cemented to the skin around the stoma. Flexible rubber or plastic tubing drains urine from the crown to a leg bag. Because it is less bulky and light in weight, it is usually preferred when two appliances must be worn.

Pouch Appliances

The selection of the permanent appliance is a highly individualized matter. No two manufacturers' products are exactly alike. Differences may exist, for example, in the flexibility of the faceplate, the length and width of the pouch, the construction of the valve outlet, and the method of belt attachment. Although many of these variations seem minor, they can be decisive in determining whether or not the appliance is satisfactory for a particular patient.

Certain criteria should be met in the selection of a satisfactory appliance. The most important is that the appliance be leakproof for a minimum of 24 hours. The patient must be assured of a predictable period of time when he can carry on normal activity without fear of leakage. If there are no extenuating circumstances, and after the patient has mastered the application technique, a properly fitted device will adhere from four to seven days without leakage or skin irritation. On the other hand, when the patient is first learning ostomy care, he may need to change more frequently. In this learning period, the nurse will need to offer the patient much reassurance and encouragement, yet not inadvertently build unrealistic expectations. Some patients, because of stomal or dermal abnormalities, can never achieve a watertight seal for more than one or two days. With children the period a watertight seal lasts tends to be highly individual because of the greater difficulty in fitting the appliance properly and the child's greater activity.

A second consideration is that the appliance be inconspicuous under clothing. Women should be able to wear sheath skirts. The patient should be able to carry on his usual physical activity, even though this might include active sports, such as tennis, golf, or swimming. Finally, the appliance should be constructed of a material that is lightweight, impervious to odor, and easy to clean and maintain. The simpler the construction, the better. The ultimate goal, of course, is to have the patient completely able to care for himself except when a specific physical limitation makes this impossible.

The proper selection of the faceplate is essential if a leakproof seal is to be achieved. There are two basic types of construction. One if made of rubber throughout and, when constructed in a thin plate, is quite malleable. It is supported by a belt which fastens to a separate metal or plastic ring between the faceplate and the pouch. The other is rigid and consists of a metal ring vulcanized between two layers of rubber. Hooks protrude from the ring to serve as belt attachments. Because of its rigidity, the faceplate's curvature may have to be molded to accommodate variations in the contour of the skin surface around the stoma.

Faceplates on permanent adult appliances commonly range between $3\frac{1}{8}$ and 4 inches in diameter. Diameters in this range are usually satisfactory for the adult because of the large abdominal surface area. Among children, however, the smaller abdominal surface area requires that careful attention be given to the diameter measurement. Faceplates for child appliances are available in diameters beginning as small as 2 inches.

The position of the stoma and the topography of the abdominal surface are important in determining the flexibility, diameter, and convexity of the faceplate. One must observe the relationship of the stoma to the waist, midline, and neighboring bony structures in lying, sitting, and standing positions. If, for example, a rigid faceplate intrudes upon the iliac crest, it will not adhere properly. A flexible faceplate, on the other hand, will mold itself to surface irregularities. Such a plate can be trimmed with scissors to avoid protuberances. A flexible faceplate is better suited to points of movement, as when the stoma is close to either the waist or the groin. Because of the frequent creasing of skin in these areas, a rigid plate invariably pulls away. Generally, however, when no unusual conditions exist, most patients seem to prefer the rigid plate.

A stoma that is flush with the skin or slightly retracted will usually require a faceplate of moderate convexity. In these cases, it is also important that the lip of the opening under the stoma be as thin as possible to prevent urine droplets from pooling underneath. Such pooling may undermine the bond between the faceplate and the skin. If the patient has an unusually firm abdomen or is emaciated, a flat or shallow convexity is best. On the other hand, a large soft abdomen may require at least a moderate convexity. One can determine if the convexity is adequate by how long the seal remains watertight and by the faceplate's adherence to the skin. If a large area of the outer rim of the faceplate peels away from the skin, the convexity is too great. Some rigid faceplates are initially flat but are malleable and can be molded to the desired convexity with the fingers. With others, the convexity must be specified at the time the appliance is ordered.

The center opening of the faceplate is determined by the stoma measurement. Several manufacturers sell measuring gauges which are convenient to use and ensure greater accuracy. If such a gauge is not available, one can easily be made in the following manner: first, estimate the stomal diameter with a ruler; next, draw and cut out three circles on heavy paper or cardboard. The first circle should equal the estimated diameter, while the second and third circles should be $\frac{1}{8}$ inch smaller and $\frac{1}{8}$ inch larger, respectively. Using these circles, select the one that most closely fits the actual stoma. The final faceplate opening should then be $\frac{1}{8}$ inch larger than the actual size. This degree of clearance reduces the likelihood of stomal constriction and allows a small margin of error in centering the faceplate. If the stoma is mushroom-shaped (small at the bottom, large at the top), the size of the opening is the measurement of the broadest diameter of the stoma, rather than the skin opening itself.

Measurements should be taken and the appliance ordered so that the patient will have it for at least a week prior to his anticipated discharge from the hospital. Most patients can learn the use and care of their appliances within this period. Preferably, a member of the family should also be taught the procedure, particularly if the patient is very young or very old.

It is not unusual for the patient to be measured by the fifth or seventh postoperative day and to wear the appliance by the tenth day. Some edema of the stoma will usually be present for six to eight weeks following surgery. Since the first fitting is made soon after the operation, the opening of the faceplate may become too large, requiring remeasurement and the purchase of a new appliance within several months. When there is considerable reduction in stomal size, a foam-rubber pad cut to proper size and cemented between the faceplate and the skin is a valuable interim aid in order to prevent skin and stomal problems secondary to urinary contact upon the exposed skin surface.

The shape and the capacity of the collecting pouch are determined by the patient's general body build and urinary output. The capacity of the regular adult pouch is approximately 10 oz. Because of weight and increased bulk as urine accumulates, most patients prefer to empty the pouch when it is about half full. An adult with normal urinary output will usually empty the pouch every three to four hours. Pouches of larger capacity, up to 16 oz, are also available. Long, narrow pouches are better suited to tall, thin people. Shorter and wider pouches are available for the plump, stocky person.

Pouch capacity and shape are even more important in the selection of a child's appliance. Children with renal tubular damage may put out large amounts of dilute urine. A child with bilateral ureterostomies may have one kidney that produces large amounts of urine to compensate for diminished function of the other kidney. Fortunately, there is now a wide selection of pouches in many different sizes and shapes fulfilling the requirements for most situations.

In selecting the faceplate and pouch, one must consider the question of whether they should be purchased as a combined, one-piece unit or as a separate pouch and plate. In the one-piece appliance the pouch is permanently molded to the faceplate and is made of rubber throughout. The life of a rubber appliance will vary from three months to a year, depending upon the care it is given and the frequency with which it is worn. This time is further extended if two or more appliances are used alternately. One appliance worn continuously may soon acquire an offensive odor. Urinary salts may also crystallize on the inner surface, causing stomal irritation, as well as valve outlet obstruction.

Although the average patient can master the techniques of application of the one-piece unit, the person with limited eyesight may have difficulty centering the stoma within the faceplate opening. The patient who is not manually dexterous may find it difficult to manage, in fairly rapid sequence, the application of skin cement, holding a "wick" to the stoma, and the manipulation of the one-piece appliance during its attachment (Fig. 19-3).

The two-piece appliance consists of a separate faceplate and pouch. The faceplate is made of rubber with a protruding flange to which the pouch is attached. With proper care, these faceplates last indefinitely. Since the stoma can be examined daily by merely removing the pouch, the faceplate may be left in place from seven to ten days. The two-piece appliance has a further advantage in that, should the stoma size change, only the faceplate need be replaced. The pouch is made of semidisposable rubber or plastic material. Consequently, a clean pouch can be applied every day and, if properly cleaned and rotated, is reusable many times. The opening of the pouch fits snugly around the flange of the faceplate and is applied after the faceplate is cemented to the skin. A belt is attached to the metal or plastic ring that fits between the pouch and faceplate. The two-piece system also enables more accurate placement of the faceplate opening over the stoma. Finally, urine is less likely to leak onto the

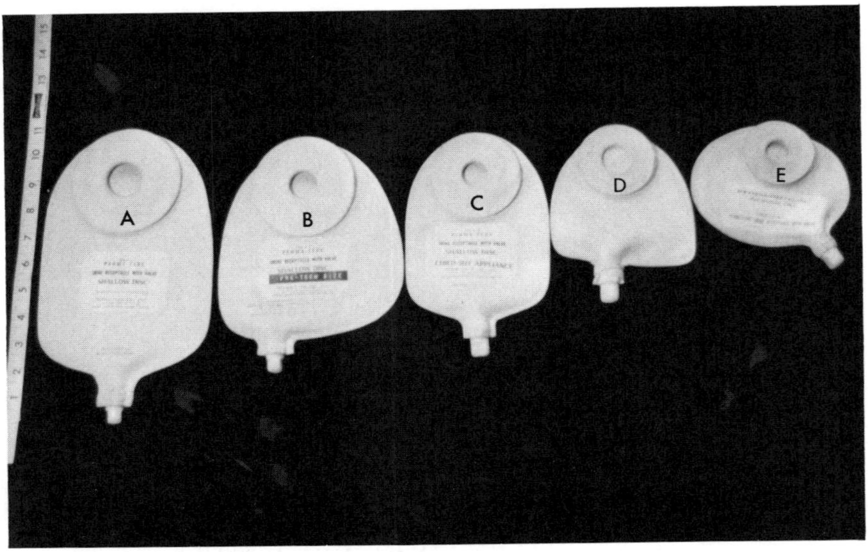

FIGURE 19-3. Perma type one-piece rubber appliance, with metal ring for belt vulcanized into faceplate. *A*, adult pouch; *B*, pre-teen pouch; *C*, child pouch; *D*, toddler pouch; *E*, infant pouch.

cement during application, since the "wick" may be kept in place until the faceplate is securely cemented to the body (Figs. 19-4 and 19-5).

Another decision in selecting appliance equipment involves the type of adhesive material to be used. The choice lies between liquid cement and double-faced adhesive discs. All cements are water-repellent and most contain zinc oxide to reduce skin irritation. Two layers of cement are usually applied to both the faceplate and the skin. It is important that both layers be thinly and evenly applied, using a brush applicator or the finger. The drying time between layers prescribed by the manufacturer should be closely observed. If the proper drying time has not elapsed or the layers are thick and uneven, one will usually encounter difficulty in achieving a watertight seal. Urinary drainage over the cement at any time during the application will also jeopardize the watertight seal. For this reason, it is advisable to have several "wicks" readily available to hold over the stoma.

FIGURE 19-4. United Surgical two-piece appliance. *A*, elastic belt; *B*, opaque plastic semidisposable pouch; *C*, rubber faceplate; *D*, metal locking ring to secure pouch to faceplate (includes hooks for belt); *E*, drying hanger used to separate side of pouch for fast drying and airing after washing; *F*, brush to clean inside of pouch and valve outlet; *G*, plastic valve inserted in pouch outlet; *H*, valve adapter for straight drainage; *I*, appliance completely assembled.

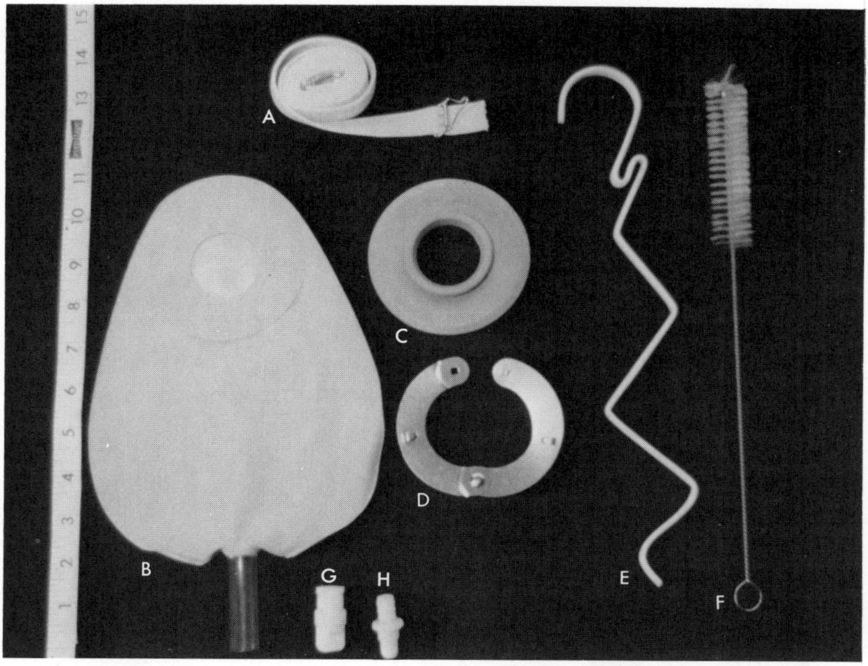
A
B
C
D
E
F
G
H

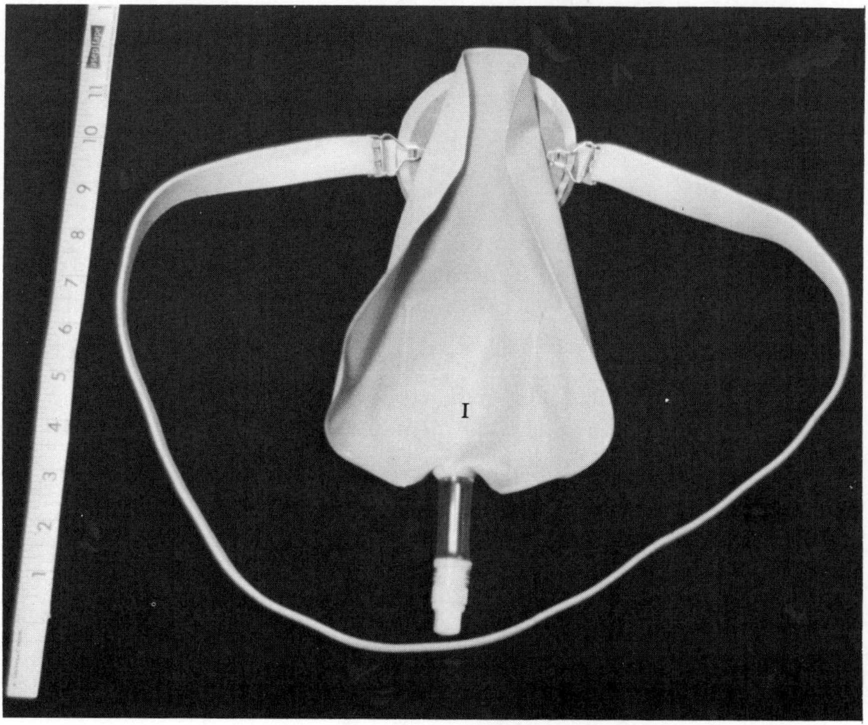
I

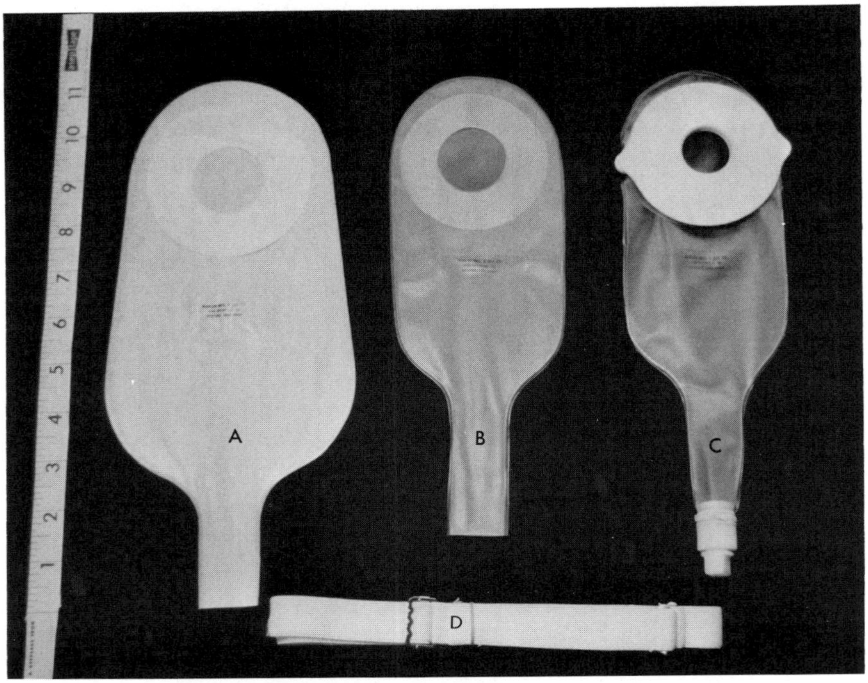

FIGURE 19-5. Marlen appliance. *A* and *B*, white and clear plastic disposable pouches; *C*, assembled appliance with faceplate, pouch, and valve outlet; *D*, elastic waistband that attaches to faceplate (hooks not visible).

A solvent is required to remove the cement. Each manufacturer sells his own brand. If the patient is known to have allergies, it may be wise to patch-test the skin with both the cement and the solvent before use. This is done by applying the material to a small area of skin on the forearm or abdomen. Should this area become reddened or begin to itch, a different product should be tried. Most skin irritations are temporary and may be due to excessive use of either the cement or the solvent or because of improper cleansing of the skin between applications.

Double-faced discs feature an adhesive surface on both sides of a thin paper base. They are ordered to match the diameter and opening of the faceplate. Each adhesive surface is protected by a paper covering which is simply peeled off at the time of use. Adhesive discs can be applied quickly and require a minimum of preparation and manual dexterity. As with skin cement, they must be applied to a clean, dry surface. The disc is first applied to the faceplate. For an even stronger bond, skin cement may be used to supplement the adhesive on the disc. Although discs usually do not adhere as long as cement, many patients prefer them because of their convenience. Not all appliance manufacturers supply double-faced discs, however. The effectiveness of skin cement and adhesive discs tends to vary from patient to patient, and often it is a matter of trial and error to find the most effective adhesive material (see Fig. 19-6).

All pouch-type appliances are designed to be worn with an elastic belt which serves to stabilize and support the faceplate. The belt seems to give the patient an added sense of security. The tension is adjusted so that there is firm support, without uncomfortable tightness or binding. The belt should encircle the body at the level of its attachment to the faceplate. If worn above or below the level of attachment, the constant upward or downward tension may displace the faceplate. Most manufacturers, upon request, will adjust the hooks of the faceplate up or down as necessary. A 1-inch, heavy woven elastic belt is satisfactory for most adult patients and is the type supplied with most appliances. The widths of children's belts vary from $\frac{1}{2}$ to 1 inch, depending upon the size of the child.

The patient should have at least two belts so that a clean, dry one is always available. Most patients, when bathing with the appliance on, prefer to wear the belt and change to a dry one afterward. A second one is also desirable in case the one worn should become soiled by drainage.

To change belts, the patient should support the appliance against his abdomen with his free hand. Some manufacturers provide belts with adjustable buckles. Others supply only a length of elastic. This is cut to the desired length and vertical slits are made to slip over the hooks on either side of the faceplate. The slits should be just wide enough to accommodate the hooks; otherwise, the elastic may tear and break.

Cup Appliances

Cup appliances consist of a faceplate or flange, which is cemented to the skin, and a dome with an outlet, which is connected by rubber tubing to a leg bag. There are two types of cup appliances commonly used. One of these consists of a flange and a dome of one-piece construction. It is made of fabric impregnated with rubber. The flange is thin and flexible. Either skin cement or double-faced adhesive discs are used to affix the appliance to the skin. In ordering the appliance, one must indicate the appropriate flange width, stoma opening, and dome height.

The second type of cup appliance is of two-piece construction. The faceplate is made of rubber. The dome of the appliance snaps to a flange on the faceplate. Skin cement or double-faced discs may be used for adhesion. Depending upon the manufacturer, it may be necessary to indicate the desired stoma opening (Fig. 19-7).

Cup appliances are designed primarily to transfer urine from the ureterostomy stoma to the leg bag. Because they have no pouch, they are

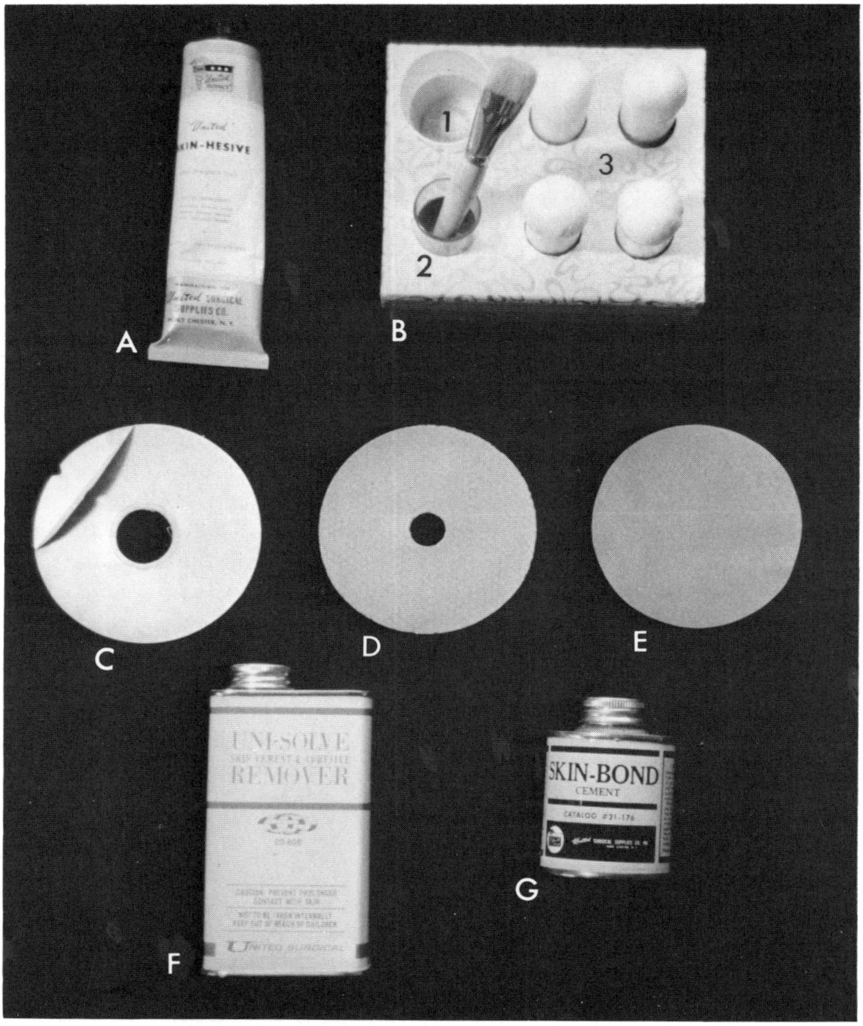

FIGURE 19-6. Skin adhesives and foam pad. *A*, skin cement in tube; *B*, tray made from small box, containing

1, paper cup for cement

2, brush for application of cement (purchased in dimestore)

3, 4 "wicks" made by folding 4″ by 4″ top of small plastic medicine bottle.

C, double-sided adhesive disc for use with permanent appliances, one side of backing folded back; *D* and *E*, nonporous rubber foam pad with and without precut center opening; *F*, commercial solvent; *G*, skin cement in can with lid applicator. (Products manufactured by United Surgical Co.)

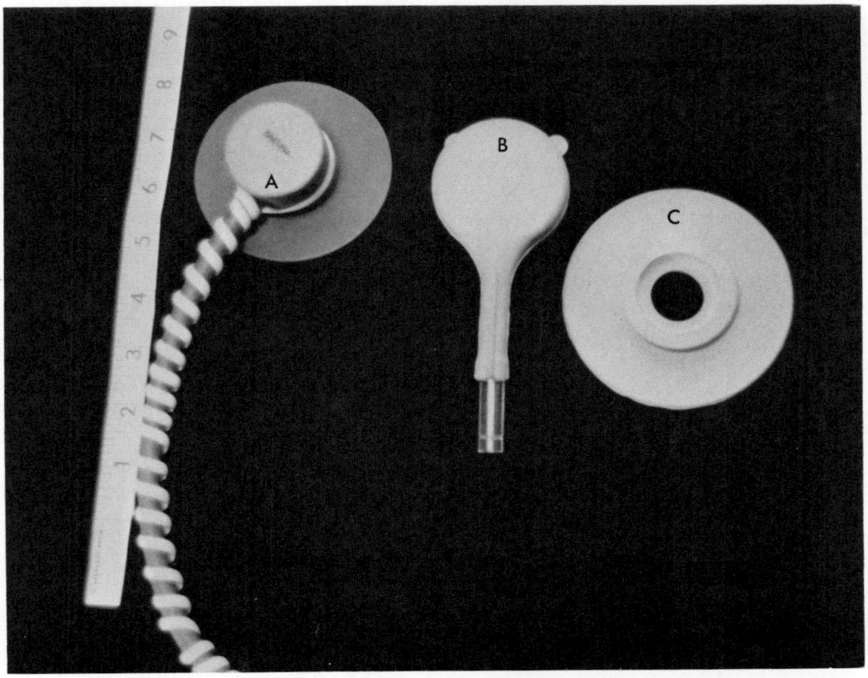

FIGURE 19-7. Cup appliances. *A*, one-piece Singer cup with nonkink coil, manufactured by C. R. Bard Co.; *B* and *C*, two-piece Whitmore cup, manufactured by United Surgical Co.

compact and lightweight. Also, since the faceplate does not support the weight of a pouch full of urine, a belt is usually unnecessary, although one may be worn if desired. Some patients prefer to use strips of adhesive tape around the flange of the cup to hold it securely in place.

Because of their size and weight, cup appliances are usually worn by patients with bilateral ureterostomies. In order to avoid wearing a leg bag for each cup, a Y connector may be used to connect each cup to a single leg bag. Some physicians, however, do not sanction the use of a Y tube because of the possibility of cross-infection. If the doctor has no preference, the choice of wearing one or two leg bags should be left to the patient.

The patient who wears a cup appliance should be advised that a vacuum may form in the dome of the cup. As urine passes from the dome through the tubing to the leg bag, air passes with it. The more shallow the dome, the quicker the air is evacuated. The valve at the top of the leg bag prevents air from equalizing the negative pressure. If the vacuum persists over a period of time, skin changes will occur. The earliest indication of a vacuum is a circumscribed, reddened, slightly elevated area the exact diameter of the appliance opening. As the condition progresses, the skin thickens, becomes irregular and hard. Encrustations and bleeding may develop because of the friability of tissue. These changes may also cause obstruction to the flow of urine from the ureterostomy.

With the one-piece cup appliance, some patients equalize the pressure by placing a small hypodermic needle through the top of the dome and taping the needle into place. It is also possible, upon request, to have a valve built into the dome. Another method of equalizing pressure is to detach the rubber tubing from the leg bag at intervals. To release the vacuum in the two-piece apparatus, one need only lift the dome from the flange enough to break the seal. Usually the vacuum should be released every four to eight hours. This will vary, however, from patient to patient. A depression in the center of the dome indicates the presence of a vacuum.

The rubber tubing connecting the cup to the leg bag should be just long enough to reach the bag without causing undue tension. A plastic coil that entwines the tubing and prevents kinking can be purchased. Kinking is most likely to occur in the area of the groin when the patient is sitting. It may be necessary, when applying the cup, to change the angle of the outlet to avoid kinking. Also, taping the tubing in the desired position is helpful. Usually, there must be extensive experimentation before the optimal positions for cup, tubing, and leg bag are determined.

Leg bags vary significantly in capacity, shape, and material. Capacity of the various leg bags ranges from 5 to 32 oz. The capacity should be such that the patient need empty the bag only every three to four hours. Plastic bags are rectangular in shape, worn on the thigh above the knee, and, though disposable, with proper care may be worn for six months or longer. Rubber leg bags are either oval or V-shaped. The oval shape, frequently referred to as a female leg bag, is worn on the thigh above the knee. The long, V-shaped leg bag, usually called a male leg bag, attaches above and below the knee. Most adult patients can wear the oval bag attached only above the knee, but the long bag must always be attached below the knee as well, usually at calf level. For this reason, the oval bag is preferred. If properly cleaned and alternated with another leg bag, these bags will last indefinitely. Although it is not difficult to find an appropriate leg bag for an adult patient, even the smallest available leg bag may be too large for a young child. For this reason, children are often fitted with pouch, rather than cup appliances (Fig. 19-8).

The patient should have at least two complete appliances to ensure proper cleaning, drying, and airing between uses. When ready to change the appliance, the pouch is first emptied of urine. The faceplate is gently detached from the skin using solvent applied with a gauze sponge or eye dropper. Once removed, the faceplate and pouch are rinsed in tepid

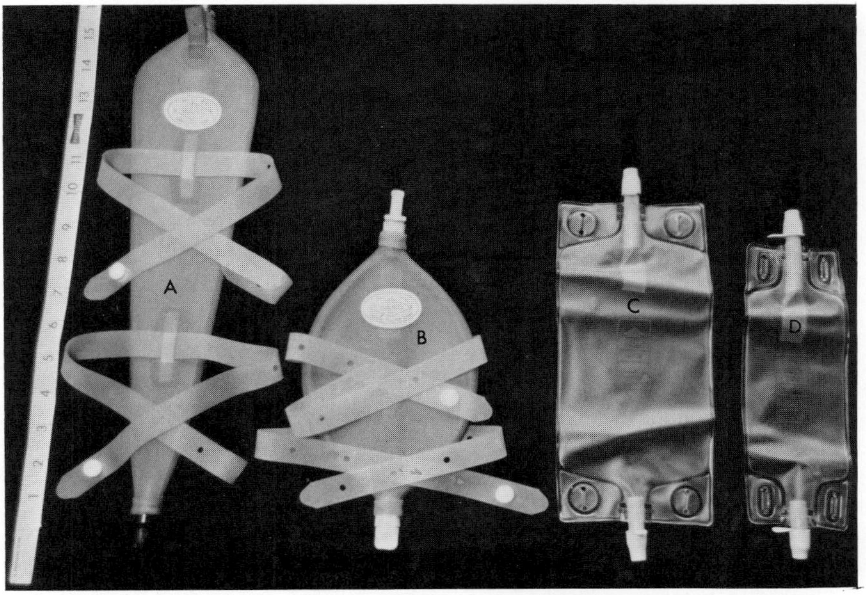

FIGURE 19-8. C. R. Bard leg bags. *A*, rubber, long (male); *B*, rubber, short (female); *C*, plastic, adult; *D*, plastic, child.

water, then scrubbed with a bottle brush using a mild soap and water. After this, the faceplate and pouch are again rinsed with tepid water and soaked for at least thirty minutes in a vinegar-water solution (1/4 cup vinegar to 1 qt water). The vinegar-water solution helps to remove urinary salts that collect on the inner surface of the pouch. This problem, as well as that of odor, is most apt to occur with the one-piece appliance. Should such encrustations form, every effort should be made to remove them, since the abrasive surface may contribute to stomal irritation and bleeding. Many patients never have difficulty with pouch encrustations, while others have a severe problem. For the latter, there are several suggestions. First, determine whether fluid intake is adequate for the individual, since concentrated urine tends to precipitate more salts than dilute urine. Second, have the patient rinse the pouch with the vinegar-water solution via the pouch outlet at least twice a day. The acidity of the solution should help to remove salts and also help reduce bacterial count of urea-splitting organisms that foster an alkaline urine and precipitation of calcium and phosphorus salts. Changing the pouch more frequently and rotating use among three or four appliances may also help to alleviate the problem. If encrustations continue to form after these measures, it may be advisable for the patient to switch to a two-piece appliance so the pouch can be changed as often as necessary.

After the cleaning and soaking process, the pouch is hung to dry and air. For best results, the sides of the pouch should be separated and the valve removed so that the outlet is open. A drying hanger can be purchased from the appliance manufacturer, or one can be easily fashioned from a coat hanger. To keep the rubber soft and pliable, the dry appliance is dusted inside and out with corn starch or talcum.

Excess skin cement can be removed from the faceplate by peeling it off using a rolling motion of the thumbs against the surface, very much as one removes excess rubber cement. Remove only as much cement as can be peeled off with the fingers. If used carefully, solvent can be used as long as it does not come into direct contact with the rubber. Solvent, if used to scrub the faceplate surface clean, will soon cause the rubber to become tacky and soft with curled edges. Any solvent that comes in contact with the rubber should be rinsed off immediately.

Leg bags and night drainage equipment are cleaned in the same way as the appliances. The patient should have at least two leg bags so that a clean one can be worn daily.

Teaching the Patient to Care for Himself

Once the patient is beyond the acute physical discomfort attendant to the immediate postoperative period, the nurse should begin a program to teach him ostomy care. His readiness to learn, however, will be determined by those myriad personality, socioeconomic, and cultural factors that make him the person he is and that subsequently influence his perception of the meaning of the surgery to his life pattern. Initially, the patient may seem to ignore any attention given to the ostomy, whether it be merely observing the stoma and its drainage or the more involved procedure of changing the dressing or the temporary bag. He may turn his head, close his eyes as if sleeping or, on the other hand, engage in a barrage of inconsequential small talk. Whatever his ploy, the nurse can be certain that he is fully cognizant of her presence and her actions. He will be quite alert to whether she is awkward and uncertain or skillful and confident in giving him care. He will be sensitive to any indications of rejection. It is essential during this period that the nurse, by her manner and actions, reinforce his physical and emotional strengths, rather than his liabilities. She must listen carefully and observe clues that indicate his fears and concerns. Only when she can begin to help the patient explore his feelings will he approach the level of readiness necessary to cope with the realities of living with a urinary ostomy.

The nurse can impart much information while giving daily nursing care. A written teaching plan, tailored to the patient's specific needs, should be formulated, including topics to be covered and tentative target dates. The plan should be available to all nursing personnel as well as to the doctor. It should be reviewed and evaluated daily by the nurse responsible for the patient's care. She should make specific note of goals accomplished and those not yet accomplished. Revisions of the plan of care of specific problems should be discussed in nursing team conferences. Such conferences are essential to the sharing of pertinent information and to ensuring that all nursing personnel are working toward the same goals.

It is also important that, along with the patient, a responsible family member be taught the whys and hows of ostomy care. Usually this will be the wife or husband, the son or daughter. When teaching this family member, the nurse should stress that the patient must be encouraged and allowed to assume complete responsibility for his own care, at least to the maximum extent of which he is capable.

It the patient is a child, both parents should be taught. The age of the child will determine the extent to which the parent will be responsible for care. With infants and toddlers, the parents will, obviously, be wholly responsible. It is extremely important that they understand that, as the child grows older and is able to assume more responsibility for his care, he be allowed to do so. By the time the child reaches adolescence, barring specific limitations, he should be completely independent in managing his care. Observation suggests that children adjust to the presence of the ostomy better than the parents. Many parents feel guilty, having made the decision to subject their child to so drastic a procedure. Many fear that the child can never become a happy, healthy, productive adult. As a consequence, some parents become overly protective and solicitous. If an optimal emotional environment is to exist for the child, it is imperative that the nurse and doctor be sensitive to the parents' feelings. Compassion and understanding, combined with reassurance and firm direction, will hopefully foster the desired parental attitudes.

An important adjunct to the patient's transition from hospital to home is the visiting nurse. Most patients are greatly reassured to know that they may expect her visit and that she will be available to give assistance and answer questions. No amount of teaching and reassurance will completely allay the patient's fears and doubts; however, a teaching program, thoroughly planned and systematically executed according to the patient's emotional and physical abilities, will certainly strengthen those factors necessary for his successful rehabilitation.

In Appendix VII are a number of questions frequently asked by patients, with the correct answers included. The reader is referred to this section for a comprehensive review of the essential information to be included in teaching the patient self-care. In Appendix VIII is a listing of a number of surgical appliance manufacturers and several helpful teaching manuals.

REVIEW QUESTIONS

1. Discuss those factors to be considered in selecting the temporary drainage appliance.
2. Describe a procedure for adapting the ileostomy-colostomy post-operative pouch for urinary straight drainage.
3. What is the purpose of a stoma pattern in cutting the pouch face-plate opening?
4. Identify those factors that may interfere with the adhesion of the temporary pouch. In what way could the nurse minimize these factors in fitting and applying the pouch?
5. Describe those steps you would take in order to prepare the pouch and stoma skin area for pouch application. List the materials you would need, and indicate your rationale for determining the sequence of the steps you will follow.
6. What factors contribute to irritation of the stoma skin area? Explain those measures the nurse should take to prevent skin irritation.
7. Discuss those factors the nurse should consider in selecting a permanent appliance, focusing specifically on the physical, psycho-social, and cultural characteristics of her patient.
8. Discuss faceplate construction relative to pliability, diameter, and contour, indicating patient factors that will determine selection.
9. What are the advantages and disadvantages of the one-piece pouch appliance, the two-piece pouch appliance?
10. Describe a cup appliance and indicate when it is used. What are the advantages and disadvantages of the cup appliance compared with the pouch appliance?
11. Explain why suction may occur inside the cup appliance, its possible effects, and how it may be prevented.
12. Discuss the preparation of both skin and faceplate for application, and indicate key considerations necessary to ensure a watertight seal.
13. Discuss factors to be considered in the selection and use of the following: skin cement; double-faced adhesive discs; commercial ostomy adhesive solvents, such as ether, benzene, and carbon tetrachloride; foam-rubber pads.
14. Outline a seven-day teaching program to prepare the patient for discharge. Include the following: application and removal of the appliance; care of the appliance and odor control; skin care to prevent irritation as well as treatment should it occur; health teaching regarding diet, activity, signs and symptoms reported to the doctor, recreation, and follow-up medical care.

CHAPTER 20
Surgery of the Urinary Bladder

OPERATIONS on the urinary bladder are accomplished through either an abdominal incision or the transurethral route, depending on the objective. The instruments, principles, and problems peculiar to transurethral operations are discussed in Chapter 22. Regarding bladder surgery, the latter technique is useful primarily for treatment and diagnosis of bladder neoplasia which can be reached with the transurethral instruments. Under favorable conditions, certain bladder calculi can be crushed by this route, using instruments known as lithotrites, and the particles evacuated. Invasive tumors, larger calculi, and plastic repairs of the ureterovesical junction and bladder neck are best handled by means of an open operative approach.

Any opening, intentional or otherwise, made into the urinary bladder is known as a *cystotomy*. Drainage of urine through such an opening is known as *cystostomy* drainage. *Suprapubic cystostomy* drainage is frequently indicated when the upper urinary tract has been damaged from long-standing prostatic obstruction with back pressure to the upper urinary tracts. This drainage, bypassing the blockage by the prostate, is maintained until the upper tracts improve sufficiently for definitive prostatectomy to be performed safely. The skin incision is made in the lower abdomen and may be midline, paramedian, or transverse. A cystostomy tube is preferably left in for drainage whenever the bladder has been opened for any reason. It is safer to drain the bladder by this method while healing takes place than to rely on urethral catheter drainage. The latter will not drain as well since one is limited to a smaller-caliber catheter. Furthermore, particularly in the male patient, there is the possibility of urethritis and prostatitis which may limit the time the catheter may be left in. At operation, the bladder is entered through its anterior wall, and the peritoneum is dissected off its dome. The drainage tube, usually a Malecot or Foley catheter, is placed in the bladder either at the upper end of the cystotomy incision or through a separate stab wound. After the bladder wall has been reapproximated, the site is preferably suspended to the anterior rectus fascia at the level of the tube to establish a secure sinus tract. Eventually, after the tube is removed, this sinus will close in a day or two if there is no distal obstruction. *Suprapubic cystolithotomy* is an opening of the bladder for removal of calculi. Bladder calculi are most often secondary to an outlet obstruction accompanied by urinary infection. An enlarged prostate is the commonest obstruction in these stone-bearing patients. Therefore, successful treatment will include not only removal of the calculi but also correction of causative obstruction.

Open plastic revisions of the bladder neck are being performed with greater frequency as these obstructions are recognized, particularly in children. Two examples are the Y-V revision of the anterior bladder neck and the "wedge resection" on the posterior neck. In the Y-V plasty, a V flap is outlined on the anterior bladder wall with the apex of the V at the bladder neck. A Y is formed by incising the anterior surface of the urethra for a centimeter or two distal to the neck. The apex of the V flap is sutured to the end of the urethral incision thus converting the Y to a V (Fig. 20-1). The result is a wider bladder neck by the insertion of the

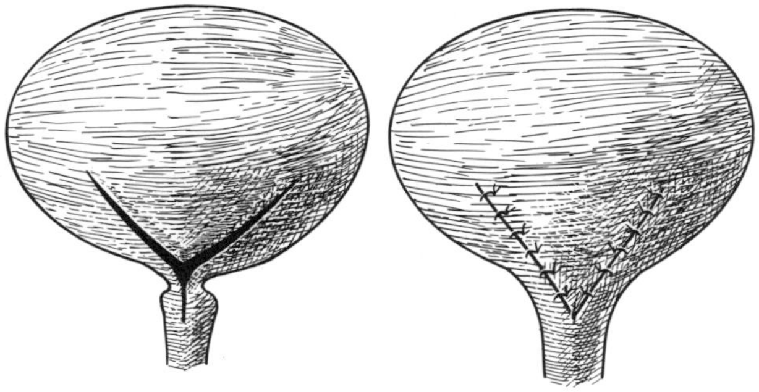

FIGURE 20-1. Anterior Y-V plasty of the bladder neck.

tongue of healthy muscular tissue through the scarred outlet. The second procedure, the posterior wedge resection, is simply that—the mucosa at the level of the posterior neck is incised and peeled back. A generous wedge of the neck is removed and the mucosa is sutured over this defect.

The Marshall-Marchetti operation is a procedure used for correction of stress incontinence. The most frequent cause for such incontinence is trauma, usually obstetric, with resultant weakness of the supporting structures at the bladder base. At operation, the urethra and anterior bladder wall are suspended by sutures in the adjacent vagina to the back of the symphysis pubis. Thus, a solid fixation point is achieved. This reconstructs normal anatomic relationships, permitting the bladder control mechanism to function properly. In the preoperative evaluation the urologist rules out other causes for incontinence, such as neurogenic dysfunction or urinary fistulas, congenital or acquired. A "stress test" is performed where the bladder is filled and its base supported with two vaginally inserted fingers on either side of the urethra. This simulates the final result of operative suspension. If, under these conditions, the patient can cough and strain without losing urine, the operation is advised. In 85 to 95 per cent of properly selected and studied patients, operation achieves acceptable urinary control.

Partial cystectomy or *segmental resection* is the removal of a full-thickness portion of the bladder. Such resections are usually performed for neoplasms that have invaded the muscle wall and are located sufficiently distant from the ureteral orifices and bladder base so that a wide margin of excision can be obtained.

Total cystectomy is the removal of the entire bladder. The usual indication for such an operation is cancer, although rarely it is for other reasons. Such total removal will necessitate urinary diversion by one method or another. *Simple cystectomy*, i.e., removal of the bladder alone by following its walls closely, is seldom performed. *Radical cystectomy*, by following the pelvic walls, is probably more effective in removal of cancer. This includes not only the bladder but adjacent pelvic organs and local lymph nodes. In men, the bladder, prostate, and seminal vesicles are removed en bloc with a wide surrounding peritoneal cuff. In women, the urethra, uterus, ovaries, and tubes are removed, as well as the anterior half of the vagina. The usual indication for radical cystectomy is invasive bladder cancer that cannot be eradicated by other means. Two such situations would be tumors located at the base of the bladder or tumors widely spread over the bladder mucosa.

Radical cystectomy is usually performed through either a transverse or a long longitudinal abdominal incision. The former incision extends from iliac crest to iliac crest just above the symphysis pubis. Since much pelvic peritoneum is excised and because of the large dead space, the incision will be drained generously and will be closed with through-and-through silver-wire stay sutures. The sutures are placed close together and in effect splint, stabilize, and support the incision. Small-lumen rubber tubing is frequently used to protect the skin from the cut ends of the wires. These sutures are usually left in for three weeks (Fig. 20-2). In the male patient, the prostate is often dissected off the rectum through a perineal incision which will be drained. In the female, dependent drains will be brought out through the remaining vagina.

At operation, prior to the removal of the organs, a bilateral pelvic lymph node dissection is performed, and frozen sections of any suspicious nodes are obtained. This node dissection is done primarily for diagnostic rather than therapeutic purposes, since cure is not often accomplished in the presence of positive nodes, regardless of what is done. This is in contrast to cancer of the breast, for example, where there is a 25 to 30 per cent five-year survival from removal of the breast and axillary lymph nodes in the presence of nodal metastases. Therefore, except for those instances where one or two nodes near the bladder may contain tumor, the demonstration of pelvic lymph node metastases at operation contraindicates cystectomy.

Cobalt radiotherapy often accompanies radical surgery in the treatment of bladder cancer. The therapy, given preoperatively and/or postoperatively, consists of a total tumor dose of 2000 to 4000 rads. If done preoperatively, usually one or two months are allowed to elapse before cystectomy, to allow local inflammation and tissue reaction to subside.

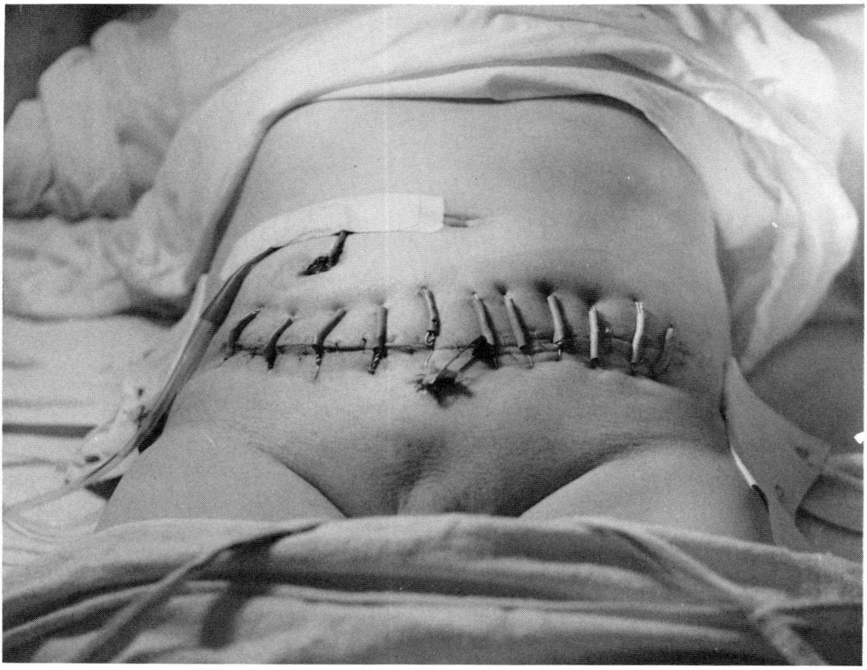

FIGURE 20-2. A postoperative radical cystectomy wound. The catheter splints the cutaneous ureterostomy draining the patient's solitary kidney.

Some doctors postpone cobalt therapy until after diversion and radical cystectomy because the resulting tissue changes make dissection at operation more difficult and seem to contribute to an increased incidence of postoperative complications, particularly wound infections and fistula formation secondary to poor healing. Currently, there is much speculation to determine the optimal treatment for bladder cancer. For this reason, the nurse is likely to see radical surgery and radiotherapy used in a variety of combinations and regimens.

Specific Nursing Considerations

Nursing care after suprapubic cystostomy is relatively uncomplicated. Usually one or two tissue drains will be in place. Wound drainage tends to be small to moderate in amount and subsides in several days. Bleeding is minimal and the drainage soon becomes serous in character. The major consideration is to make certain the position of the cystostomy tube is maintained and that drainage is adequate. The tube should be checked at least every two hours in the early postoperative period. After more extensive procedures, such as partial cystectomy or plastic revisions, the urinary drainage may be bloody for several days, gradually clearing by the third or fourth day. The cystostomy tube may be left in at least seven days and up to several weeks, depending on the type of surgery performed. There are several methods by which the doctor can decide if the tube can be removed safely. The tube can be clamped to determined whether the patient can void. If so, the time and amount of urination are recorded on an output sheet at the bedside. Using a container with legible markings, a pencil, and a watch, most adult patients can keep their own records. Since the tube in the bladder acts as an irritant, frequent voidings in small amounts do not represent the eventual true voiding pattern for the patient. However, the completeness of bladder emptying can be determined by unclamping the tube after urination and measuring the residual urine in the bladder. Another complementary method is to obtain a voiding cystourethrogram through the cystostomy tube. One can thus visualize healing of bladder suture lines and the adequacy of the bladder neck and urethra. A "postevacuation" film will demonstrate completeness of emptying.

After removal of a cystostomy tube, a dressing over the residual fistula is necessary to absorb urine and serous drainage until the tract heals. If distal obstruction is not present, urinary drainage will cease in a matter of one to three days. Should the physician decide that cystostomy drainage may be necessary for a protracted period of time, the nurse will instruct the patient on ambulatory care. This will include instructions for taping the tube in place, dressings, irrigation of the tube, and the maintenance of the drainage collection container. (See Appendix VI.)

Nursing care following a simple cystectomy is similar to that following any lower abdominal procedure. If urinary diversion has been performed previously, the management of the urinary drainage will be relatively simple. In the immediate postoperative period, temporary ostomy bags attached to straight drainage are used (see Chapter 19). As soon as the abdominal incision has healed sufficiently, the permanent appliance can be applied.

After a simple cystectomy, intravenous fluid therapy may be required for 24 to 48 hours, but the patients quickly progress to oral fluids and a regular diet in three to four days. Moderate amounts of wound drainage during the first two to three days may be expected, requiring several dressing changes daily. By the end of a week, however, drainage has ceased and the wound is usually healing well.

Radical cystectomy, on the other hand, may confront the nurse with formidable challenges to her judgment and skill. The complexity of nursing care will be increased if urinary diversion is constructed concomitant with the cystectomy and/or if the patient has undergone preoperative radiation therapy. If the combined procedure is performed, the nurse must care for a patient who has undergone a major surgical insult to his body. This includes the removal of a large bulk of tissue, an extensive area of denuded pelvis, and possibly several anastomoses involving the urinary and gastrointestinal tracts. Conceivably there are many possible complications, and a mortality of 10 per cent or greater following such operations is not unusual. These complications include breakdown of the various anastomoses creating urinary or fecal fistulas, wound infection and dehiscence, pelvic abscess formation, prolonged paralytic ileus with fluid and electrolyte imbalance. Adjuvant radiation therapy increases the possibility of poor healing and infection because of its effect on decreasing tissue vascularity.

Meticulous measurements and recording of intake and output are important. The intake will be solely by parenteral fluids until gastrointestinal function returns and oral feeding can be resumed. Output will consist of gastric and urine drainage, which can be measured fairly accurately, wound drainage, and insensible loss. Measurements of these outputs will determine, in large part, the optimal fluid and electrolyte replacement.

For the first week after operation, there is significant protein loss from the widely denuded area in the pelvis. This is not dissimilar to the patient with a moderately severe burn. The frequency of dressing changes and the estimated drainage loss per change should be recorded. When drainage is unusually large, it may be necessary to weigh the dressings. Great care must be taken in measuring urinary output. Should there be leakage around the temporary ostomy bag, the volume of urine lost should be estimated. Urine collection may become problematical because of stomal and wound edema, sutures, and wound drainage which interferes with the adhesion of the temporary postoperative appliance.

The patient will usually have some paralytic ileus, particularly if diversion is by ileal conduit, for at least five days postoperatively. During this period, the daily gastric drainage may be voluminous, with a significant loss in electrolytes. The nasogastric tube is irrigated several times daily to facilitate drainage and prevent intestinal distention. Such distention could compromise the intestinal anastomosis of an ileal conduit. Some surgeons prefer to use a gastrostomy tube to suction or straight drainage rather than a nasogastric tube. From a nursing standpoint, gastrostomy is more comfortable for the patient and nasal and pharyngeal irritation with pulmonary complications is lessened.

A guide to intravenous therapy will be not only the measurable output but also the weight of the patient. The patient will have been weighed in the operating room immediately before and after the operation. For the next 10 to 14 days the patient will be weighed daily. For most accurate weights, it is best if the patient is weighed nude at approximately the same time each day, on the same scale, by the same person (usually the doctor or professional nurse), usually with all dressings removed. Following radical surgery of this sort, there is a predictable weight loss due to protein catabolism at the average rate of 4 g per kilogram per day for at least the first 7 to 10 days; any other change is probably due to an excess or deficiency of water. The daily weight will be recorded by the doctor on a preplotted graph of projected weight loss (see Fig. 20-3). Generally if the weight is above the plotted line, the volume of intravenous fluids will be decreased. If the weight falls below the plotted line, the daily volume of intravenous fluids will be increased.

It is important that the nurse make certain that the patient receive the total volume of fluid ordered in the time prescribed. This is most easily done by calculating the volume to be absorbed hourly to reach the required total and titrating the intravenous drip accordingly. The intravenous drip should be checked hourly to make certain it is being absorbed at the desired rate. Blood is drawn daily for electrolyte levels, and intravenous correction is determined by the results.

Also of major importance is wound and skin care. When changing dressings, sterile technique should always be used. During the first week, the wire stay sutures tend to become encrusted with serum particularly where the suture comes through the skin. These encrustations not only prevent drainage around the suture but also serve as a nidus for infection. The care of wire sutures used on the urology service at The New York Hospital–Cornell Medical Center is carried out in this manner: Equipment needed includes a sterile dressing set (two clamps, approximately 12 2- by 2-inch gauze sponges, and cellophane), two sterile medicine glasses, hydrogen peroxide, povidone-iodine (Betadine), sterile applicators, and sterile abdominal pads. Hydrogen peroxide is poured into one medicine glass, providone-iodine into the other. Each wire is cleaned separately with peroxide, using a clean applicator for each wire. If the sutures are badly encrusted, a sponge saturated with peroxide is placed over the wires for several minutes. This makes it easier to remove the encrustations and is less painful to the patient. If the wires have rubber sheaths, they are turned with a clamp so that the underside can be cleaned. After the wound has been cleaned, it is exposed to a heat lamp for 20 minutes, after which povidone-iodine is applied followed by a dry, sterile

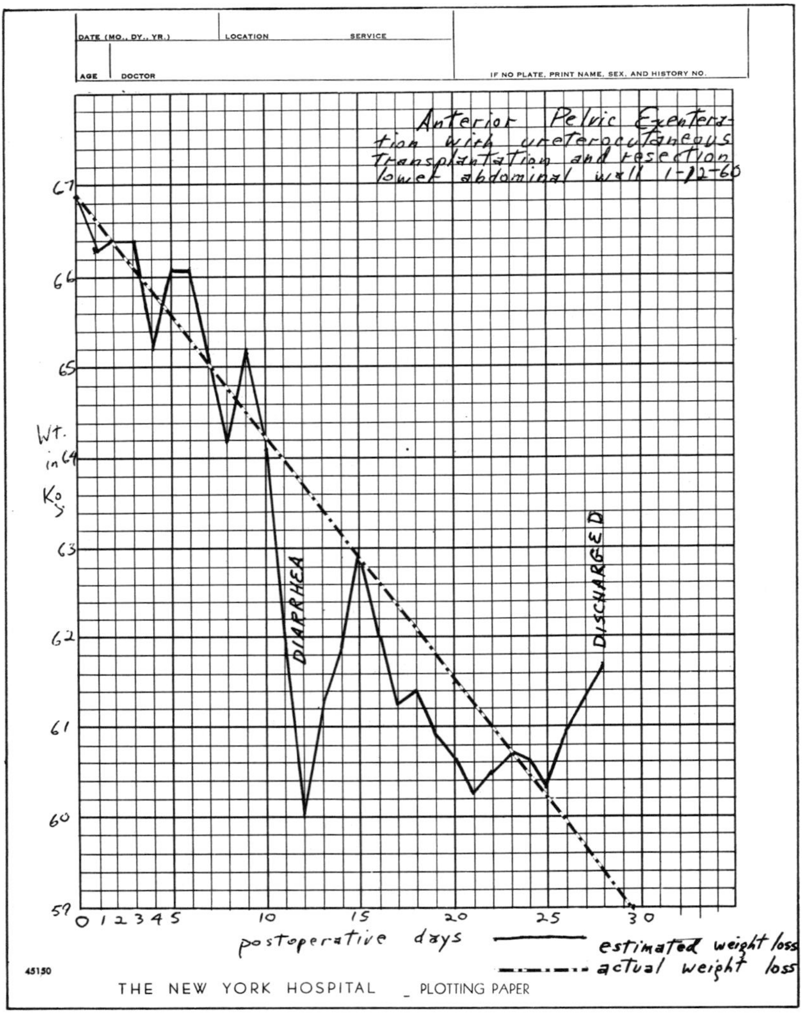

FIGURE 20-3. Typical weight-loss curve following major surgery (anterior exenteration for cancer of the bladder involving the anterior abdominal wall), which is used as a guide to fluid replacement therapy. The estimated weight loss is computed at 4 g/kg of body weight.

dressing. The procedure is usually begun on the third postoperative day and done three times daily until the wires are removed.

The care of perineal wounds is described in the discussion of perineal prostatectomy in Chapter 21 under "Specific Nursing Considerations." The female patient will not have a perineal incision but may have vaginal drains. These are left in place for five to ten days and shortened daily until completely removed.

The nurse should observe both abdominal and perineal drainage for any evidence of urine or feces. Should either appear on the dressing, it means a fistulous connection is present; and depending on the type and amount of drainage, appropriate measures will be needed to prevent skin breakdown. If there is suspicion of a urinary fistula the doctor may be able to demonstrate this with colored dye materials. For example, the appearance of blue perineal drainage after intravenous injection of indigo carmine will identify this drainage to be of urinary origin. If a gastrointestinal fistula is suspected, one can guess as to its origin by noting the time of appearance in the drainage of orally ingested charcoal. The higher the fistula, the more quickly will it appear. Once fistulas are suspected, additional appropriate x-ray studies may be ordered by the doctor.

Frequent coughing, turning, and ambulation as early as the doctor permits are necessary to prevent respiratory and circulatory complications. The anesthesia time, particularly if the combined procedures are performed, may have been anywhere from five to eight hours, increasing the possibility of pulmonary congestion and pneumonia. The patient also tends to minimize his pain by moving as little as possible.

During the first postoperative week, narcotics should be administered as frequently as the orders permit and the patient needs it, barring, of course, specific contraindications such as hypotension, shallow slow respirations, or stuporousness. Wound edema and intestinal distention often cause severe incisional pain during the first week. Thereafter the patient's narcotic requirement is usually less, but an order should be in effect since abdominal distention or wound care may cause severe pain. When the suture is ready for removal, the doctor cuts it with a wire cutter and quickly pulls the wire out with a clamp. There is minimal discomfort before and after removal, but at the moment of pull-through the distress is acute. A narcotic administered 30 minutes prior to removal has little effect in reducing the actual pain. However, it will allay the patient's anxiety and residual discomfort.

REVIEW QUESTIONS

1. Where the bladder has been incised, explain why cystostomy catheter drainage is preferable to a urethral catheter.
2. Before the cystostomy catheter is removed, what procedures may be employed to determine whether bladder emptying is adequate after voiding?
3. Describe the care of the cystostomy fistula after removal of the catheter.

4. Outline the factors the nurse must consider in preparing the patient to care for his cystostomy catheter at home.
5. Differentiate between a radical cystectomy in the male and in the female.
6. Describe the specific activities for which the nurse is responsible that assist the doctor in maintaining the patient's fluid and electrolyte balance after radical cystectomy.
7. Because the daily weight is important in determining daily fluid requirements, what factors should be considered by the nurse in obtaining the weight to ensure greatest accuracy?
8. Describe the care of the cystectomy wounds and what special circumstances make wound care so important?
9. Identify the location of urinary and intestinal anastomoses. Should either a fecal or urinary fistula occur, where might the nurse observe the drainage?
10. What simple procedure might the doctor use to verify whether the fistula was urinary or fecal? What particular observations would be relevant for the nurse?

CHAPTER 21
Surgery of the Prostate

THE majority of operations on the prostate gland are performed for relief of urinary obstruction secondary to benign enlargement. These operations are known as *prostatectomies.* If interpreted literally, the term is a misnomer, since the entire prostate is not excised. Rather the glandular hypertrophy is removed, leaving the prostatic capsule intact. This is in contrast to a total or radical prostatectomy when the entire prostate is removed with its capsule.

Although many ingenious surgical approaches for removal of benign hypertrophy have been devised, four are commonly used today: the suprapubic, retropubic, perineal, and transurethral methods. Each of these has its specific advantages and disadvantages. Consequently, urologists will use the operation best suited to the circumstances of the individual patient rather than employ one method exclusively. Regardless of the approach, the operator removes the hypertrophy by separating it from the "surgical capsule." As discussed in Unit I, the peripheral prostatic tissue is compressed as the new glandular element enlarges. This creates a distinct plane between the hypertrophy and the surgical capsule. Therefore, the surgeon identifies this plane and in open operations uses his finger or scissors to enucleate the enlargement. A simple analogy would be cutting into a lemon, inserting a finger to dissect out the pulp, and leaving the rind behind. The aim of the transurethral operation is the same, except that the hypertrophy is removed in small pieces with a wire cutting loop until the prostatic capsule is bared. Following prostatectomy, the bare surface of the capsule reepithelializes over a two-to three-month period, resulting in a wide-open, mucosa-lined, nonobstructing prostatic urethra.

The greatest problem during prostatectomy is to achieve adequate hemostasis. Although the major arterial supply can usually be identified and controlled with ligature or fulguration, venous oozing and bleeding from numerous small arterial vessels can sometimes pose a serious problem. The methods for control of bleeding in the recovery room and later are discussed in the section on nursing considerations.

At *suprapubic* (*transvesical*) *prostatectomy* the prostate is approached through an opening in the bladder. The enucleation of the adenoma is begun anteriorly in the prostatic urethra by splitting the mucosa in this area until the proper plane is encountered. The enucleation continues by developing this plane bluntly with the finger or with scissors dissection (Fig. 21-1). A circumferential incision of the mucosa at the bladder neck prior to the enucleation may prevent tearing of the mucosa. After

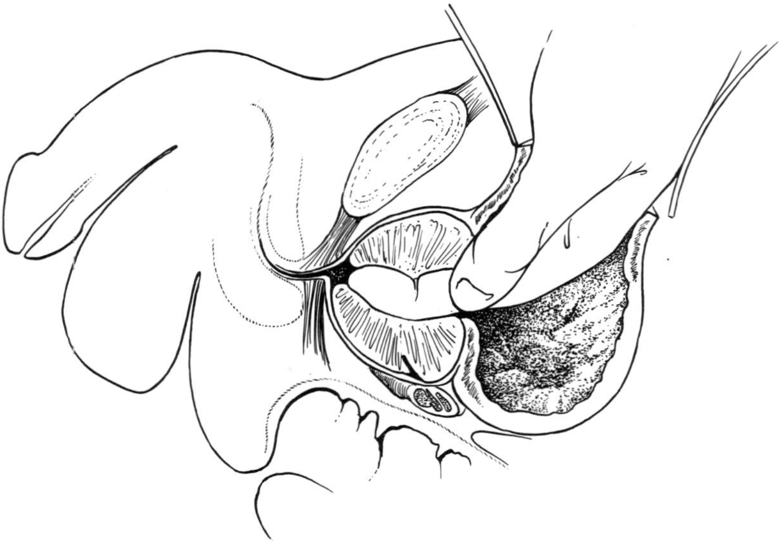

FIGURE 21-1. Suprapubic prostatectomy.

hemostasis has been accomplished, a Foley catheter is inserted through the urethra with its balloon expanded inside the bladder. The opening in the bladder is closed, and a suprapubic cystostomy catheter is inserted through a superior stab wound or the upper end of the bladder incision. Rubber tissue drains to the site of the bladder closure are brought out through the wound.

When a *retropubic prostatectomy* is done, the surgeon approaches the adenoma through an incision into the anterior prostatic capsule (Fig. 21-2). Therefore, the operator will retract the bladder upward and dissect out the extraneous fat behind the pubis and anterior to the capsule. The branches of the dorsal vein of the penis are carefully ligated and divided. The prostatic capsule is incised under direct vision down to the adenoma, using either a transverse or longitudinal incision, depending on the preference of the operator. Following enucleation of the adenoma, the major arterial supply entering the prostate posteriorly at five and seven o'clock can be sutured directly. After identifying the ureteral orifices, a generous wedge of the posterior bladder neck is often excised to prevent postoperative bladder neck contracture. A urethral Foley catheter

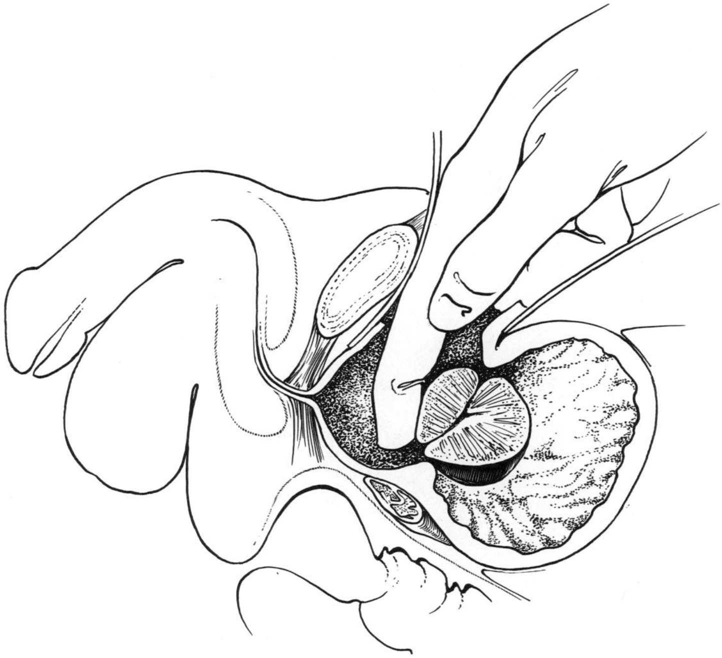

FIGURE 21-2. Retropubic prostatectomy.

is inserted and the prostatic capsule reapproximated. Many surgeons will also insert a cystostomy catheter for its advantage of additional drainage. Tissue drains down to the prevesical space are brought out through the incision.

The third open method is the *perineal prostatectomy*. With the patient in the extreme lithotomy position, a semicircular incision is made anterior to the anus, extending from just within one ischial tuberosity to the other. The rectum is separated from the prostate. Using a transurethral tractor, the prostate is rotated upward and the posterior prostatic capsule is exposed (Fig. 21-3). The capsule is incised, the adenoma enucleated, and hemostasis accomplished. After insertion of the urethral catheter, the capsular incision is reapproximated and the wound closed. As with the previous methods, rubber tissue drains leading from the capsular closure are brought out one end of the wound.

Properly performed, *transurethral operations* accomplish the same result—i.e., removal of the entire adenomatous hyperplasia. Since these techniques and their instruments are an entity to themselves, they will be discussed separately in the next chapter.

Cryosurgery of the prostate is presently an experimental procedure. It follows the principle that freezing of tissue results in its ultimate destruction. The technique requires the use of a specially designed urethral probe somewhat of the size and shape of a sound. The tip of the probe can be cooled to temperatures as low as −160°C by circulating liquid nitrogen through it. The freezing portion of the probe is placed in the prostatic urethra, and the adenoma is frozen solid. The lowering of

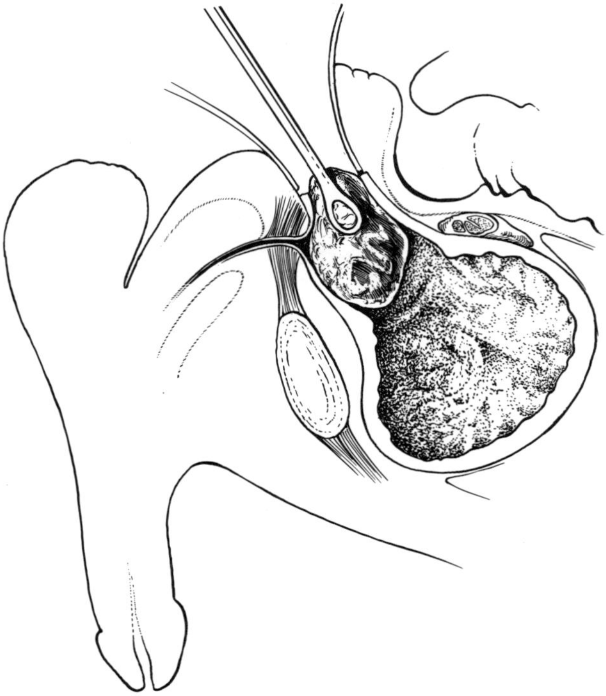

FIGURE 21-3. Perineal prostatectomy.

temperature is monitored by means of a needle thermocouple inserted into the prostatic capsule through the perineum. The prostate is frozen until the capsular temperature reaches −20°C. This will take from 5 to 15 minutes, depending on the bulk of the adenoma to be frozen. After this a heating unit is turned on for one or two minutes to warm the freezing element so that the urethral probe can be removed. Immediately thereafter, an indwelling urethral catheter is inserted.

To date, the principle advantages of this technique are a reduction in operating time and minimal blood loss during the procedure. Since the freezing can often be performed using heavy sedation and local anesthesia, these additional features make the operation attractive for the poor-risk patient. The technique has not been completely evaluated as yet, but there are several significant disadvantages. These include incomplete tissue removal necessitating an additional surgical session at a later date, prolonged discomfort and infection as the prostate sloughs (sometimes weeks or months), and the possibility of overfreezing causing injury to surrounding tissues. The latter injuries may include vesicorectal fistula and loss of urinary control.

There are many considerations in deciding on the method of operation for the specific patient. The least limiting factor should be the surgeon's ability to perform the various procedures. In most hands, adenomas larger than 50 g tend to be more suitable for an open procedure than a transurethral one. Suprapubic prostatectomy can be performed rapidly, but exposure of the fossa for the purposes of hemostasis is often poor. Despite various proposals for suturing the bladder neck, often only pressure, catheter traction, and sometimes packing the fossa can control the bleeding. The retropubic operation, although somewhat more time-consuming, has the advantage that the operator can see the bleeding points and place suture ligatures for hemostasis as necessary. Blood loss may be greater during the operation, but it is more reliable to control the bleeding at the operating table than to depend on indirect methods in the recovery room. Either of these abdominal approaches may be quite difficult in the overly obese patient. Consequently, the perineal operation may be the answer in such situations. Furthermore, of the open operations, the perineal incision is the most comfortable to the patient. Another advantage of the perineal approach is that a nodule suspected to be cancer can be accurately located and biopsied. If there is localized cancer, a radical prostatectomy can be performed. If not, and the patient has symptoms of prostate trouble, a simple prostatectomy can be done at that sitting. Disadvantages of the perineal operation include an inability to place the patient in the proper position (because of arthritis of the spine or hips, for example) and the major danger of injury to the adjacent rectum with the development of a fistula.

Interference with sexual ability following prostatic surgery may be an important consideration in deciding on the approach. Most patients will retain their preoperative ability to perform sexual intercourse (potency) after suprapubic, retropubic, and transurethral prostatectomies. The capacity to maintain an erection and to enjoy the pleasurable sensations of orgasm are usually retained. However, ejaculation will often be minimal because most of the producing tissue has been eliminated and especially because retrograde flow through the now large vesical outlet occurs. Following perineal surgery there is a greater interference with potency, a real consideration in the young and sexually active patient.

Fertility, the capacity to produce conception, is usually much reduced after any kind of simple prostatectomy because of the previously described retrograde ejaculation. If vasoligation has also been performed or the seminal ducts become obstructed, sperm cannot be ordinarily delivered, no matter how potent the individual—ergo, sterility.

The transurethral operations have the advantages of no external incision, less postoperative pain, and more rapid convalescence. The procedure is limited, however, by the size of the adenoma, by the caliber of the urethra for insertion of the necessary instruments, and, to a significant degree, by the surgeon's ability with this technique.

Radical prostatectomy is the en bloc removal of the entire prostate and the seminal vesicles. After the removal, the membranous urethra and bladder neck are sutured together. Such an extirpation can be done through either the perineal or the retropubic route. This operation is usually performed for cancer of the prostate evidently localized to the gland. Unfortunately, there are too few candidates for this operation, since such early cancer is not commonly discovered. Impotence after radical prostatectomy is almost invariably present, and some permanent weakness with urinary control is to be expected in 5 to 15 per cent of cases. During the first few postoperative months, inability to retain urine is very common.

Prophylactic *vasectomy* is performed by many surgeons as a part of prostatectomy. This greatly decreases the postoperative incidence of epididymitis and orchitis, which complications can be debilitating, quite painful, and sometimes serious. The retrograde spread of infection from the prostatic bed is prevented by interruption of the lumen of the vas. For medicolegal purposes, the patient should be told beforehand of the reason for vasectomy. Since most of these patients are at an age where further children are not sought, and since such ligation has no effect on potency, permission is rarely refused by the patient. The technique for vasoligation requires a short (1 cm) scrotal incision on either side, through which the vas is skeletonized, clamped, divided, and ligated (usually with excision of a short intervening segment). Closure is usually with catgut sutures, since the scrotal area is normally subject to superficial infection and the suture material will eventually dissolve spontaneously.

Specific Nursing Considerations

Immediately after operation, catheters are connected to clean, *empty* collection receptacles so that postoperative drainage can be observed and measured. Clear, amber urinary drainage immediately after prostatectomy is rare indeed! Excessive bleeding may follow any type of prostatectomy. The recovery room nurse plays an important role in estimating the amount of continuing blood loss and the general condition of the patient. Catheters may be connected to straight or decompression drainage, or through-and-through irrigations. The principles of these systems and their maintenance should be familiar to the nurse (see Chapter 15).

Since the urine may be grossly bloody, how can one determine the type and seriousness of blood loss? A bright red color suggests arterial bleeding. If this is accompanied by increased viscosity and occlusion of the catheter with bright red clots, the degree of blood loss is definitely significant and may be serious. Under these circumstances, the physician should be notified promptly. If hypotension and pallor appear, the call for the doctor must be on an emergency basis. While awaiting his arrival, blood should be called for and the patient placed in the shock position. If clots obstruct the catheters, they are gently irrigated with normal saline in the hope of easily opening them, being careful to obtain returns so as not to overdistend the bladder. Serious bright red bleeding without clot formation can occur in two situations. The first is with blood dyscrasias where there is an interference with the normal clotting mechanism. A defect of this nature will soon become evident to the astute observer. The second is hemolysis of the blood. Therefore isotonic solutions such as normal saline should be used for irrigation rather than distilled water, for example. This point becomes increasingly important when bleeding is heavy and large volumes of irrigating solution are needed.

Venous bleeding is characterized by a dark, deep burgundy discoloration. In excessive amounts, the viscosity of the drainage may also increase and black clots may form. However, this type of bleeding can be usually controlled by simple measures such as decompression (Fig. 21-4), intermittent irrigation, and/or mild traction on the transurethral Foley catheter. This kind of bleeding will gradually subside spontaneously unless unusual circumstances such as blood dyscrasia exist. The important point is to differentiate excessive arterial from venous bleeding, since the former may necessitate aggressive measures in the recovery room or even a return to the operating room for its control.

Orders for routine irrigation of catheters will vary from surgeon to surgeon. Urologic solution "G" should not ordinarily be used in the immediate postoperative period. It tends to interfere with clotting, is very irritating to raw surfaces, and may aggravate bladder spasms. Sterile isotonic saline, 5 per cent dextrose, or 1.5 per cent glycine is preferred. In general, if the catheters are draining well, they are best left alone even if the color of the drainage is impressive. Routine irrigation can cause more harm than good. Periodic milking of the catheters helps to keep them draining and does no harm. Should urinary drainage cease or diminish markedly, the catheter is probably obstructed with clot. Under such circumstances, the nurse can attempt to evacuate the clots using an appropriate irrigating solution and a 2-oz Asepto syringe. If clots reform rapidly or the catheters cannot be readily made to function properly, the doctor is called. If he is also unable to remove the clots, he may need a

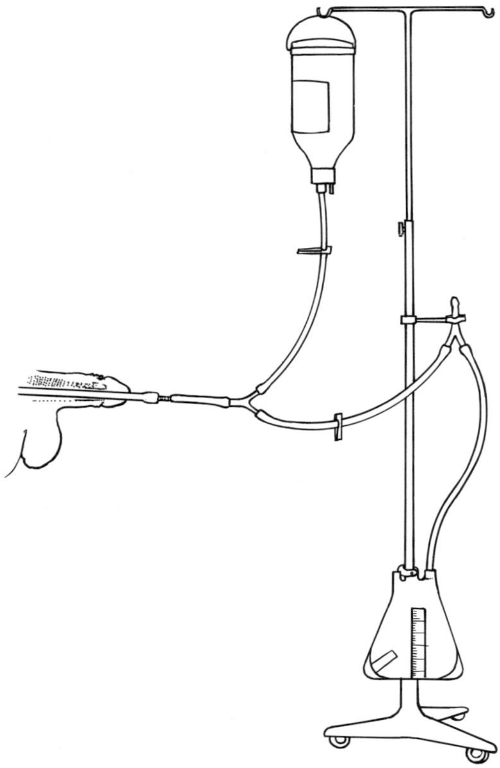

FIGURE 21-4. Decompression drainage with intermittent irrigation apparatus.

Toomey syringe. This syringe is made of glass or plastic, holds 50 ml of solution, and has a conical adapter tip. A rubber washer at the bottom of the barrel of glass Toomey syringes allows one to introduce fluid forcefully into the bladder without breaking the barrel. The plunger is pulled out rapidly to break up and suck out the clots. This rapid to-and-fro motion may need to be carried out many times until all the clots have been evacuated and the catheter is patent. Consequently, large amounts of isotonic saline (up to several liters) should be immediately available as well as extra basins. Such irrigations are emergency measures, but attempts should be made to maintain sterile technique. This procedure is painful to the patient so an analgesic can properly be requested.

Various manipulations of the urethral catheter can be employed to improve hemostasis. Most surgeons, on inserting a urethral Foley catheter, will inflate the balloon inside the bladder rather than in the prostatic fossa (Fig. 21-5). The prostatic capsule is allowed to contract, thus stopping

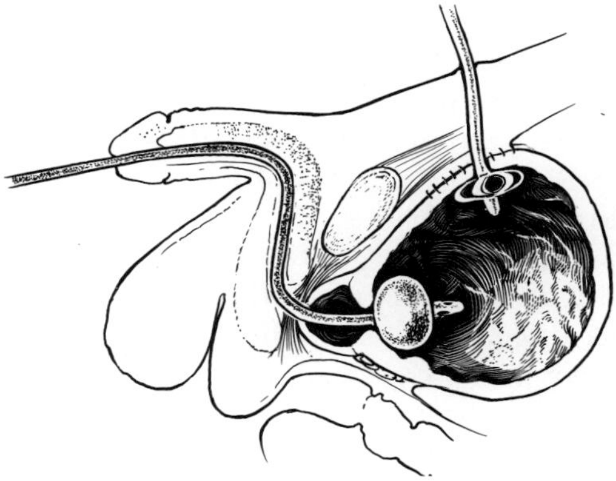

FIGURE 21-5. Postoperative open prostatectomy. Note positioning of urethral catheter.

a considerable amount of the venous oozing. This action is similar in nature to the hemostatic effect of the contracting postpartum uterus. Other operators, on the other hand, will inflate the balloon in the fossa for its direct pressure effects on the capsule. This method is less effective in controlling arterial bleeding and may be more uncomfortable to the patient. Often, catheters so placed will not irrigate or drain as well. A further advantage of placing the balloon in the bladder is that the prostatic arterial supply, which enters the capsule at the bladder neck, can be compressed by traction on the urethral catheter.

Catheter traction, used judiciously, may determine whether a patient's bleeding can be controlled adequately to tide him over or require his return to the operating room. The safest method is to tape the catheter under tension to the inner thigh. An alternate method where greater traction can be exerted is the use of the Hamer anchor. This is a wire frame inserted between the legs through which the catheter is threaded and anchored. Under all circumstances, traction should be applied and removed by a physician. The price paid for prolonged and excessive traction may be an eventual interference with urinary control. This interference may be quite marked and, in extreme cases, may be permanent. In the majority of instances, if arterial bleeding cannot be controlled by mild to moderate tension on the catheter, further pressure to the bladder neck will accomplish no more and is more prone to result in permanent sphincter damage. It is preferable not to maintain traction longer than four to five hours at a time. If a longer period is necessary, the traction is released for 10 to 15 minutes before reapplication. Although the nurse does not decide on or apply the traction herself, she should keep an accurate record in the nurse's notes of the period that the traction has been in use. If the length of use seems inordinately long, the physician should be reminded that it is still in use. The purpose of decompression drainage is to maintain a mild back pressure in the bladder to tamponade venous ooze. This is an ineffective technique for significant arterial bleeding. Through-and-through irrigation is used to maintain catheter patency when bleeding is heavy. The drawbacks and precautions in its use have been discussed in Chapter 15.

During the first few days after prostatectomy, the urinary drainage will become less bloody. By the fourth day, the color will be normally amber or minimally pink-tinged. The actual blood loss after the first 24 hours have elapsed will not be very great. However, the degree of bleeding in the recovery room and the measures used for its correction should be relayed to the floor nurse so that there will be continuity in the patient's care. The same techniques used by the recovery room nurse should be familiar to the floor nurse.

An accurate record of intake and output should be kept in the nurse's notes, particularly in the immediate postoperative period and especially if frequent irrigations are necessary. The nurse must carefully deduct the volumes of irrigating solution used from the total output so that the volume of urine produced can be recorded. Such measurements may be especially difficult to ascertain accurately in the patient who has bled heavily. If the urinary output falls below 30 ml per hour, the patient is observed for signs of renal shutdown and the physician notified. After 24 to 48 hours have elapsed, intravenous fluid therapy can be discontinued, and often before this time. By then, most patients are able to retain oral fluids and gradually resume their preoperative diet. Attention should be paid to resumption of normal bowel movements by appropriate laxatives in the first few postoperative days. The use of enemas during this time is discouraged, since massage by the enema may irritate the closely situated prostatic bed and incite further bleeding.

Wound care following open prostatectomy is similar to that following an abdominal operation except for the management of the urinary drainage. Wound drainage tends to be minimal, changing within one or two days from reddish pink to an amber serous drainage. Occasionally, even though the cystostomy tube is patent and properly positioned, some urine may drain around the catheter. This may seep through the cystostomy or capsular closures, which may not be completely watertight during the first few days. If this drainage is copious, the doctor will recheck the position of the tubes. Frequent dressing changes will be necessary under these circumstances to avoid skin maceration and infection.

After perineal prostatectomy, a male T-binder is used to support the dressing. Usually, beginning the second postoperative day, a regimen of special perineal care is instituted. Three times daily, this incisional area is cleansed with pHisoHex and water. The area is exposed to a heat lamp for 15 to 20 minutes. The procedure is completed with the application of an appropriate antiseptic (povidone-iodine, for example) and the dry sterile dressings are reapplied. Sitz baths are begun after removal of the drains. Perineal care and sitz baths are continued until the wound is healing well and perineal discomfort has subsided. An inflated rubber ring will make the patient more comfortable on sitting, since it will take pressure off the incision. Before any perineal prostatectomy, the patient may undergo bowel preparation consisting of a low-residue diet for several days as well as thorough mechanical cleansing of the bowel with cathartics and enemas. Postoperatively, the patient may be kept on a liquid or low-residue diet for several days to minimize bowel activity. When the patient needs to have a bowel movement, the dressing is removed. Afterward, the anal area is cleansed separately with soap and water. The incisional area is cleansed separately with pHisoHex and antiseptics followed by reapplication of sterile dressings. Since the anastomosis of the urethra to the bladder neck after radical prostatectomy is not necessarily watertight, urine may drain from the perineal wound. Frequent dressing changes will be required to keep the patient dry, as will more intensive perineal care and sitz baths. The nurse should also observe the drainage for any signs of fecal matter, since this may be the first indication of a rectal-urethral-perineal fistula.

Because there tends to be bloody drainage around the urethral catheter after any prostatectomy, the nurse must make certain the thighs and external genitalia are washed daily. Usually, washing with soap and water is sufficient. If, however, the drainage has dried, hydrogen peroxide applications to the area may first be necessary to loosen encrustations. Most patients can perform this cleansing if instructed how to do so and reassured that they will not injure themselves. A cotton ball or 2- by 2-inch gauze square saturated with hydrogen peroxide wrapped around the catheter at the urethral meatus is effective in removing crusts that form. Although the nurse may delegate perineal care to the patient or male orderly, it is her responsibility to make certain that care has been satisfactorily completed. The patient who is found with thighs, genitalia, and catheter covered with dried blood certainly causes one to question what other factors may have been overlooked in his care.

The type of pain experienced by the patient postoperatively will be influenced by the type of operation performed If an open procedure has been done, the patient will have incisional pain. After any prostatectomy, most patient, to varying degrees, complain of a desire to urinate and a desire to bear down as though to defecate. When such symptoms occur, it is important that the nurse not immediately ignore them as a natural consequence of operation and therefore to be tolerated by the patient. Should the patient experiencing these symptoms become quite restless and agitated, frequently request the nurse to check his catheter to see that it is draining properly, or ask to use the bedpan to have a bowel movement, the nurse, barring any contraindications, should administer the pain medication prescribed.

Another discomfort the patient may experience is bladder spasm. The pain is rapid in onset and subsides within a few minutes. It is manifested primarily as an uncontrollable urge to void. Such spasm occurs most frequently in the first two to four days after surgery and may be triggered by movement of the catheter, as when the patient is getting out of bed to ambulate. Spasm may also cause a sudden expulsion of bloody drainage from the urethral meatus. Usually, this amounts to no more than a few milliliters, but on a clean white sheet this amount can appear formidable. The patient needs reassurance that he is not bleeding excessively and that the spasms will subside within a few days. Narcotics are not very effective in controlling painful spasm. The doctor may order propantheline (Pro-Banthine) to be administered if bladder spasms occur hourly or more frequently. Many physicians, however, prefer not to order propantheline or similar antispasmodics for the elderly patient or the one with known cardiac disease, since such drugs may induce cardiac arrhythmias. The medication is discontinued when the catheter is removed, since the antispasmodic effect on the bladder may interfere with proper urination. In general, such drugs are relatively ineffectual.

If a cystostomy tube is in place, it will usually be removed around the tenth postoperative day. The order for removal of catheters is the choice of the surgeon. Many operators will remove the urethral catheter in the first two or three postoperative days, depending on how rapidly the urine clears of blood. The patient continues on cystostomy drainage. This is more comfortable to the patient since the urethral catheter is locally irritating and urethritis can develop. After eventual removal of the cystostomy catheter, a record of the time and amount of urination is kept. Appropriate dressings will be needed to cover the cystostomy fistula, which will usually stop draining urine within 48 hours.

If the cystostomy drainage persists, a urethral catheter may be reinserted and possibly connected to mild underwater suction, which keeps the bladder empty and allows the sinus to heal more rapidly. Such suction is occasionally necessary after radical prostatectomy when there is continued drainage of urine through the anastomosis. The apparatus is set up by the nurse but should be checked by the doctor. Ordinarily 2 to 4 cm of negative pressure suffice. Stronger suction can collapse the bladder wall onto the eyes of the catheter and may injure the bladder mucosa. The suction is maintained except for periods of ambulation until complete healing occurs.

Sometimes if a large urethral catheter or traction has been used, the patient may not have complete urinary control for several days following urethral catheter removal. In addition, he may have marked urgency which is not true incontinence. Should this urgency occur, the patient should be appropriately reassured that this is temporary and will improve rapidly. If necessary, gauze pads held over the penis and secured with a male T-binder can be used to prevent soiling. Exercises consisting of contracting and relaxing the perineal muscles and stopping and starting the urinary stream are helpful in reestablishing control. Following radical prostatectomy, control may be much slower in returning, occasionally taking weeks and months. Usually, the degree of control that the patient has at the end of one year is the maximum control he will have permanently. Few things are as demoralizing to a patient as urinary incontinence. The question arises as to when the patient should be given a urinal to wear. An important consideration is whether the patient will become so dependent on the urinal that he will cease to exert maximum effort to regain control. Some physicians, therefore, may wait several months before allowing the patient to wear a urinal. Certainly each patient and his individual circumstances need to be considered, but uncertain urinary control is a strong force to motivate the patient to exert maximum effort to achieve continence.

Devices for Urinary Incontinence

Unfortunately, although there are many collecting devices of various designs available, it is frequently difficult to find a urinal that is entirely satisfactory.

The basic design of commercially available male urinals is a plastic or rubber sheath into which the penis fits. A valve is located at the bottom so that urine can be emptied. If incontinence is greater than an occasional dribbling of a few milliliters, the outlet of the sheath can be attached to a leg bag or bedside collection container. The sheath is held in place by straps that run between the legs and attach to a waist band. Some sheaths are constructed to fit loosely over the genitalia. With this type, there is nothing to prevent leakage of urine when the patient is sitting or lying. The most satisfactory urinals are those with sheaths that fit the penis snugly. The two-sheath design consists of an outer, relatively loose-fitting one with an inner conical penile sheath. The inner sheath is trimmed with scissors to fit the individual patient. Trimming the inner conical sheath must be done with great care, since once the opening is too large, the penis will slip from the sheath and leakage will occur. A technique for determining the size of the opening is to measure the width of the penis with a piece of string. Half of this length less $\frac{1}{8}$ inch should be allowed the first time the cone is trimmed. The cone should always be cut perpendicular to the sheath. The rubber will tear if vertical cuts are made, thus making the opening too large and the apparatus useless. When the urinal is first worn, the patient should be checked every several hours for complaints of penile pain or evidence of swelling. Should this occur, the urinal is removed and trimmed again, this time by no more than $\frac{1}{16}$ inch. The process is repeated until the urinal fits comfortably and without urinary leakage or penile edema. The patient should have at least two urinals so that a clean one can be worn daily. The urinal is cleaned by being washed in mild soap and water and allowed to dry where air can circulate freely. Once dry, corn starch or talcum powder helps to keep the sheath soft and pliable. The preferred type of leg bag is one that is rectangular or oval in shape and can be worn on the thigh. The V-shaped male urinal, which extends from midthigh to midcalf, seems to be an unnecessary encumbrance (Fig. 21-6).

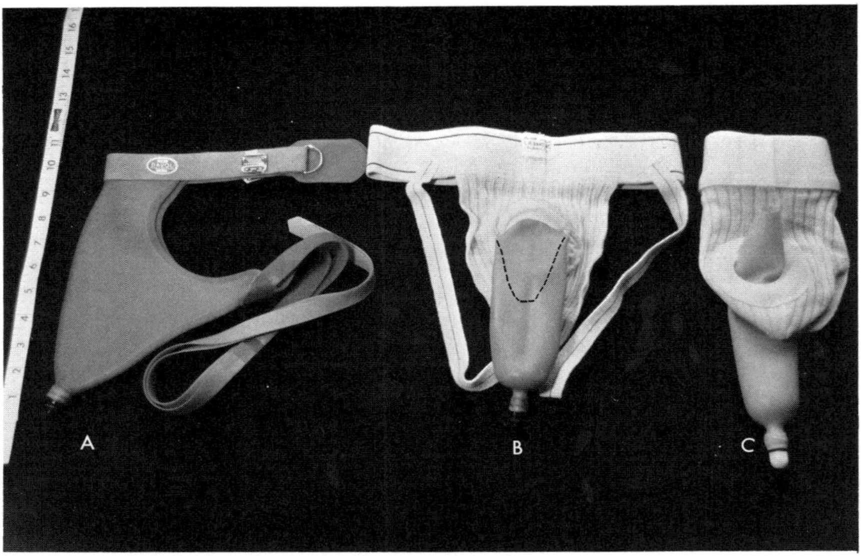

FIGURE 21-6. Male urinals for incontinence. *A*, Davol rubber urinal with loosely fitting inner sheath. *B*, C. R. Bard McGuire urinal. Dotted lines represent snug-fitting inner sheath. *C*, McGuire urinal with untrimmed inner sheath everted for purposes of demonstration.

Another method for controlling incontinence is the penile clamp. This consists of two hinged pieces of malleable metal lined with foam rubber. The clamp is placed on the penis and molded so that in the locked position it exerts only enough pressure to occlude the urethra. Care must be taken that the clamp not be so tight as to impair circulation or cause edema. It is equally important that the clamp be released every three to four hours so that the patient may void. If the clamp is not released, back pressure may cause distention of the posterior urethra and bladder. Its greatest disadvantage is that, over a period of time, a urethral diverticulum may develop at the point of pressure.

Condom drainage is still probably the most effective method for the incontinent male patient. The penis is placed in the condom. Adhesive tape is used to secure the condom to the skin. The distal end of the condom is attached to tubing which is connected to a leg bag or bedside container. A simple and leakproof method for attaching tubing to the condom is shown in Figure 21-7. Before applying the condom it is often necessary to shave some of the pubic hair to prevent discomfort from the adhesive tape. If there is evidence of edema or skin irritation, the condom should be removed immediately until the condition subsides. If there are no contraindications, changing the condom twice a week is sufficient. When removed, perineal care with soap and water and a sitz bath is desirable.

It has often been suggested to the authors that a temporary ostomy bag be used as a urinal for the male patient. It certainly seems feasible since it can be easily attached to straight drainage and has a convenient adhesive disc. However, the adhesives of many temporary bags are mounted on paper backing, the edges of which can be knifelike in sharpness. In areas where there are many creases and folds, as in the perineal area, lacerations may occur. If this method is tried, only bags with adhesive mounted on cloth backing should be used. In a few instances, temporary bags with a karaya gum ring and applied with skin cement have proven satisfactory.

The incontinent female patient's main recourse is to wear sanitary pads and some type of rubber or plastic pants. There are also waterproof pants available with absorbent, disposable liners. Many patients, male and female, prefer this method of protection because the pads and pants can be changed as necessary.

There are various rubber devices for the female patient that fit over the perineal area and are secured in place by straps to a waistband. Tubing drains urine to a collection receptacle or leg bag. Experiences of patients suggest that these devices are not worth the money invested.

The most distressing problem confronting the incontinent patient is that of odor. The smell of urine seems to quickly permeate clothing, bedding, furniture, and environment. The most effective ways of combating odors are scrupulous cleanliness and liberal use of commercial deodorants. Perineal care with soap and water may be necessary several times a day, as well as frequent changing of soiled clothing and bed linens. A rubber or plastic sheet is useful in protecting mattresses and chair cushions. Some deodorizing solutions, when used according to the manufacturer's instructions, may be added to washing solutions and applied to clothing. Special deodorizers, constructed with an electric blower fan, help to reduce room odors.

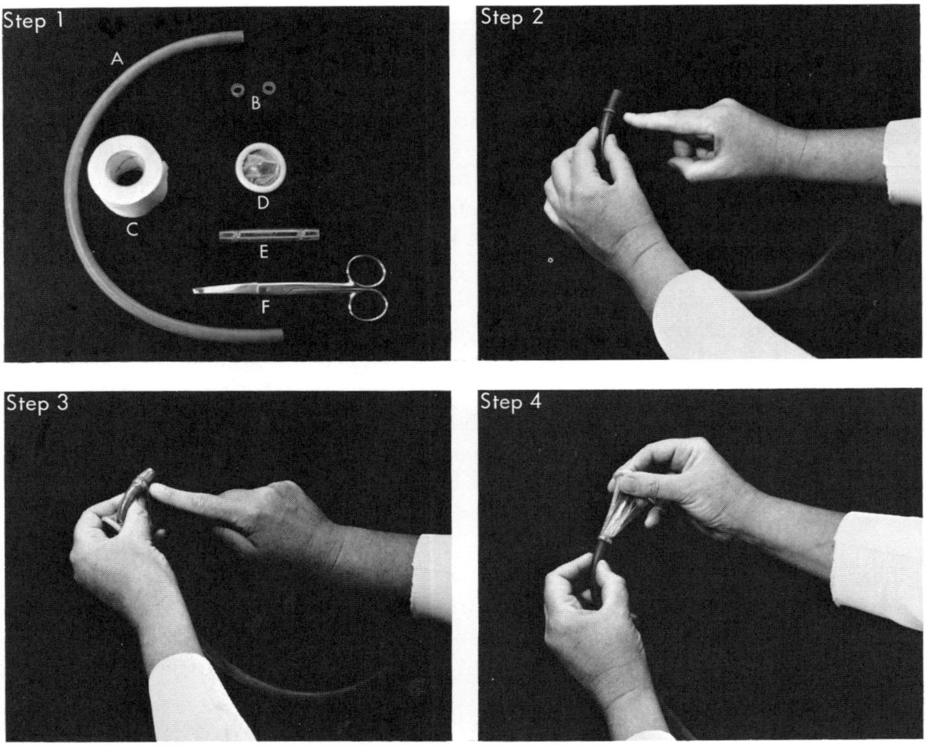

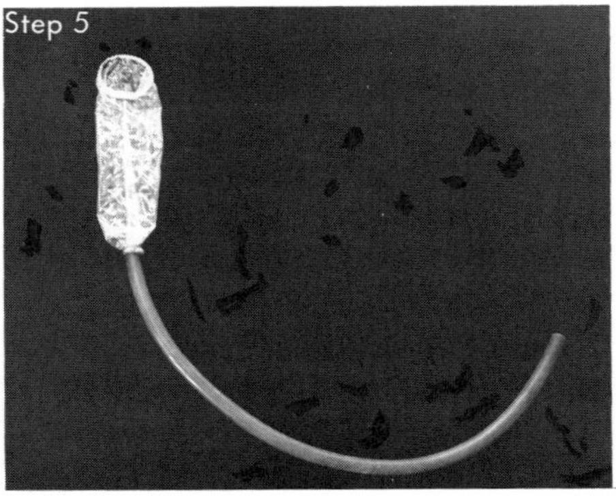

FIGURE 21-7.

Step 1: Necessary equipment
A, Rubber drainage tubing with two—
B, $\frac{1}{16}''$ bands cut from the end of tubing
C, Adhesive, 1 inch
D, condom
E, glass connector
F, scissors

Step 2: Place one of the bands approximately $\frac{1}{2}''$ from the end of tubing.

Step 3: Place the condom over the end of the tubing with the rolled edges of the condom inverted. Apply second band over condom until snug against first band.

Step 4: Pull condom forward over second band and doubly secure attachment by placing first band forward over second. Puncture hole in condom over lumen in tubing.

Step 5: Condom with drainage tubing ready for application.

REVIEW QUESTIONS

1. Describe the three "open" approaches to prostatectomy and the considerations relevant to selecting the approach.
2. Differentiate a radical prostatectomy from prostatectomy for adenoma of the prostate.
3. What is cryosurgery? What is its present status in prostatic surgery?
4. Describe in detail those characteristics of urinary drainage that the nurse would consider in evaluating the significance of postoperative hematuria.
5. Discuss the indications for irrigation following prostatectomy. What are the nurse's responsibilities in relation to this procedure?
6. When is catheter traction employed? What factors must the nurse consider when traction is in use?
7. Explain why enemas are avoided in the first few days following prostatectomy.
8. Describe the care of the perineal wound following perineal prostatectomy.
9. What is the purpose of time and amount urine measurement after catheter removal?
10. What measures may the nurse initiate that may assist the patient in regaining urinary control?
11. Describe a bladder spasm, and indicate why and when it is most apt to occur.
12. Discuss the use of propantheline (Pro-Banthine) and similar compounds in the treatment of bladder spasm, and indicate relevant factors to be considered by the nurse.
13. What are the alterations in sexual function to be anticipated following simple and radical prostatectomy?
14. Discuss the various devices available for the incontinent male patient. Identify those factors to be considered in selecting the device.

CHAPTER 22
Transurethral Surgery

TRANSURETHRAL surgical procedures comprise a major part of urologic surgery. These techniques require the use of highly specialized instruments and notable skill on the part of the operator for consistently satisfactory results. The transurethral excisions or resections are piecemeal removals of chips of tissue whittled under endoscopic vision. The actual cutting is accomplished with a high-frequency electrical current which passes through a wire loop applied to the tissue. The movements of the loop are controlled by the operator. Another method of transurethral resection, which does not use electricity for cutting, employs a cylindrical "cold" knife which cuts tissue as it is slid in and out.

A complete removal of the adenomatous hyperplasia within the prostate can be performed in this manner. The resectionist cuts off pieces of the enlargement until the entire prostatic capsule is exposed (Fig. 22-1). Properly done, the end result is the same as if an open enucleation had been performed. These operations are not as simple as they may sound, and there are many pitfalls. The surgeon must be able to orient himself in a changing topography. He must be able to differentiate between the cut surfaces of the normal and abnormal tissues, since overzealous resection leads to perforation with extravasation of irrigating fluids—serious complications particularly if not recognized immediately. On the other hand, incomplete resection is conducive to continued symptoms, persisting obstruction, and infection. Injury to the external urinary sphincter can too readily cause varying degrees of loss of urinary control. For obvious reasons, the bleeding vessels must be identified and coagulated precisely.

Many factors are considered before the decision is made to remove a prostatic adenoma by the transurethral route. The size of the adenoma is important. Even in the hands of experts, the complication rate rises with the larger adenomas (over 50 g), since the operating time is often extended, the blood loss greater, significant absorption of irrigating fluid enhanced, and the prospects of an incomplete removal increased. The caliber of the urethral lumen and the caliber of the instrument must be compatible because too snug a fit causes trauma which may well lead to postoperative urethral stricture. Sometimes a stricture is present preoperatively and prevents the proper insertion of the resectoscope. In such circumstances,

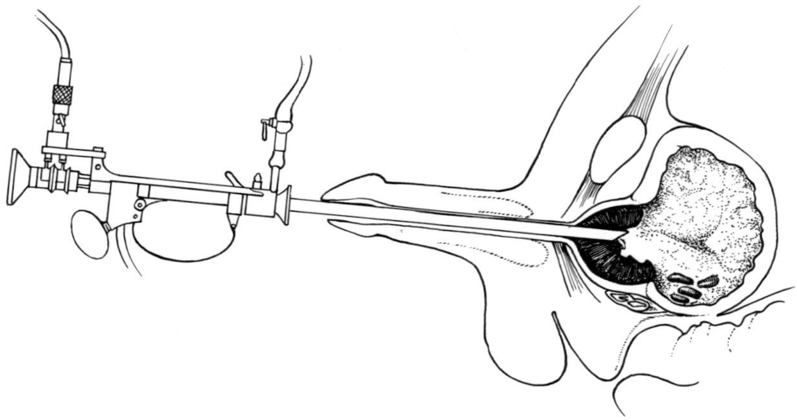

FIGURE 22-1. Transurethral prostatectomy.

the instrument can usually be inserted through an incision into the perineal urethra—perineal urethrostomy. If the patient's abdomen is large, the operator is likely to be inclined to the transurethral or perineal route.

A transurethral resection can often relieve obstruction produced by an incurable cancer of the prostate. Tissue planes may be difficult to identify, and landmarks are obscured, so a more than average hazard to the sphincteric mechanism exists. Furthermore, the surgeon may have difficulty controlling bleeding. Attempts to remove cancerous obstructions by open operation are usually plagued by magnification of these problems and by the added ones of wound infection and persistent fistula—so the transurethral procedure is generally preferred.

This route is also the choice for the total removal of bladder tumors that do not penetrate more than half the thickness of the musculature of the bladder wall. Papillomas and superficial carcinomas fall into this category. Slivers of the tumor are cut parallel to the bladder wall until the base of the tumor is reached. After the resected chips are evacuated from the bladder, separate biopsies are taken for several reasons: the pathologist can determine whether or not the tumor has indeed been removed in its entirety; he can define the depth of penetration; and he can at times better estimate the degree of malignancy from the basal tissue. These features help the surgeon decide on further treatment, if any. During transurethral operations on the bladder, the surgeon is working inside a hollow, distended viscus where the entire thickness of the wall may only be a few millimeters. Consequently, he must be able to visually differentiate the neoplasm, bladder muscle fibers, and perivesical fat.

Instruments and Equipment

The operating instruments used for transurethral surgery are modifications of the endoscope and are called resectoscopes. The essential addition is a movable "working unit" with which tissue is excised. In the most widely used instruments, this unit is a wire loop which can be activated with an electrical current. Numerous mechanical variations of this working unit are available: the Stern-McCarthy, Nesbit, Iglesias, and Baumrucker types, for example (Fig. 22-2, Table 22-1). The Stern-

TABLE 22-1
IDENTIFICATION OF COMMONLY USED RESECTOSCOPE ELECTRODES

COLOR OF INSULATION	INSTRUMENT DIAMETER	RESECTOSCOPE TYPE*
Yellow	24 French	Stern-McCarthy standard 24 and convertible models; Iglesias, Nesbit, and Baumrucker convertibles
Gray	26 French	Stern-McCarthy, Iglesias, Nesbit, and Baumrucker convertibles
Blue	28 French	Stern-McCarthy, Iglesias, Nesbit, and Baumrucker convertibles
Green	28 French	Stern-McCarthy multiple, Iglesias, Nesbit, and Baumrucker standard 28 French models
Black	28 French	Stern-McCarthy standard 28 French model
Brown	16 French	McCarthy and Nesbit 16 French models

* Cutting loops are available in wire diameters of 0.010, 0.012, 0.015, 0.018, and 0.020 inch. The 0.015-inch size is most commonly used for standard transurethral surgery.

McCarthy electrotome uses a rack and pinion to move the loop, whereas the Iglesias and Nesbit varieties use springs to facilitate the return of the loop by the operator's thumb. The gross components of the resectoscope consist of an electrically nonconductive sheath and its obturator (for insertion) and the working unit which fits into the sheath. These amazing instruments, proclaiming the wonders of technology and construction, are the direct descendants and fruition of the simpler observation instruments of many years ago. The most commonly used sheath is the 28 French size. Instruments are available in 26 and 24 French, and much smaller sizes for pediatric surgery.

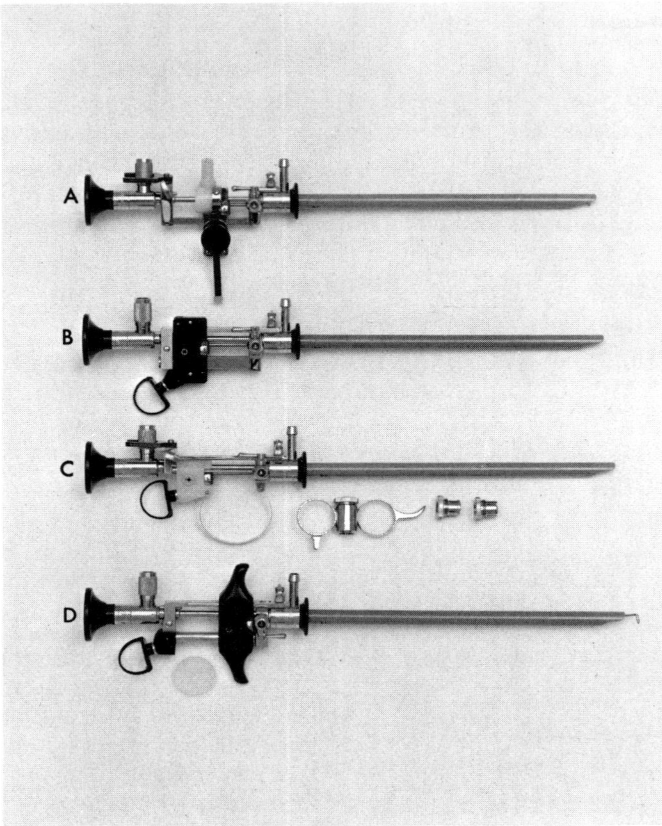

FIGURE 22-2. Four commonly used resectoscopes. *A*, Stern-McCarthy; *B*, Nesbit; *C*, Iglesias; and *D*, Baumrucker. (Courtesy of American Cystoscope Makers, Inc.)

The resectoscope is assembled by the nurse and checked by the doctor before introduction. The electrode loop must be seated deeply into the working unit and the screw tightened to ensure an adequate electrical contact. If any of the colored insulation is visible, the loop has not been inserted far enough into the unit. The telescope is next inserted and the working unit placed into the sheath. Looking through the lens, one must not see any portion of the lips of the sheath. If a full field is not seen, the telescope is adjusted accordingly. At times, the telescope will not seem to go far enough into the working unit because the rotating contact may be misplaced (it should be attached to the outer two of the three rings near the ocular). Excursions of the electrode are tested with the working unit inserted into the sheath. The wire must completely clear the lips of the sheath as it moves to and fro, particularly as it is drawn back. Otherwise, tissue will not be cut off cleanly, leaving many obscuring tags which will interfere with the progress of the resection. Furthermore, improper clearance can result in short circuiting and charring of the sheath. These instruments are handled with special care, since even a slight bend in any part will cause malfunction. Cleaning and sterilization techniques are essentially the same as for cystoscopic instruments in general.

A typical operative layout for transurethral surgery is shown in Figure 22-3. This includes a minor instrument tray so that vasectomy, urethral meatotomy, or perineal urethrostomy can be performed prior to resection. A set of Van Buren sounds to 30 French are available to dilate the urethra, if necessary, prior to insertion of the resectoscope. An

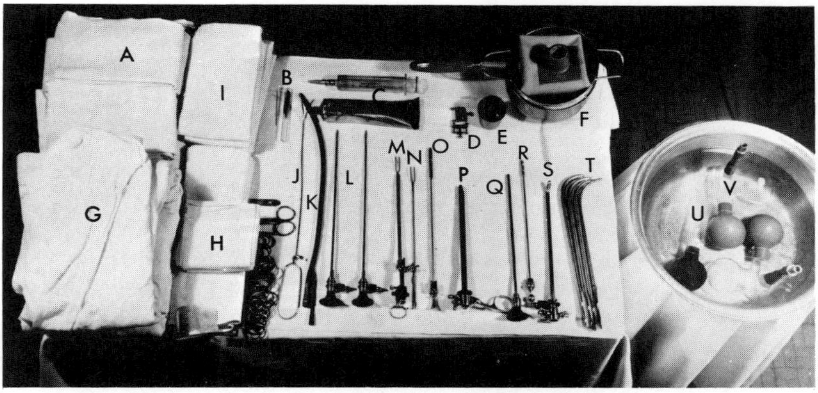

FIGURE 22-3. Transurethral setup.

A, drapes for patient
  1, towels
  2, lithotomy sheet
B, catgut (for vasectomy)
  Keith needle
C, 30-ml syringe
  KY jelly
D, Hoffman clamps
E, cup for mineral oil
F, large Monel basin with
  1, strainer
  2, O'Connor drape
  3, battery cord
  4, Wappler or Bovie cord
G, gowns, 3
H, towel with gloves and instruments
I, doctor's hand towels
J, catheter guide
K, #24, 30-ml Foley catheter
L, universal telescopes, 2
M, Nesbit resector
N, extra electrode
O, Timberlake obturator
P, Nesbit Bakelite sheath
Q, observation telescope BB } Brown-Buerger cystoscope
R, obturator BB } Brown-Buerger cystoscope
S, sheath for BB } Brown-Buerger cystoscope
T, urethral sounds
U, Asepto syringe
V, Ellik evacuators, 2

extra complete resectoscope is on the table or immediately available in case of any failure in the first instrument. Additional electrode loops and light bulbs (if a fiberoptic source is not used) are essential. The table also holds a 2-oz Asepto syringe, two Ellik evacuators for removal of the tissue chips, Bovie and light cords. A cystoscope is present for preoperative evaluation of the bladder. If the operating table does not contain a drawer to catch irrigating fluid and its contents, the nurse needs a stainless steel bowl and an ordinary kitchen strainer to catch bladder contents each time the bladder is emptied during the operation. Electrode loops are color coded for use in the various models and sizes of resectoscopes. Table 22-1 lists commonly used color codes for cutting loops.

Electrosurgical Equipment

The electrical currents used for transurethral surgery are generated by movable electrosurgical units similar to or identical with those employed in other branches of surgery, especially neurosurgery. Two commonly used units are the Wappler and Bovie machines (Fig. 22-4). These supply two basic types of current which can be used separately or variously blended. The first current is a high-frequency (1,000,000 to 3,000,000 cycles/second) tube generated one which, when applied through the loop, will cut tissue with minimal hemostatic effect. The second basic type of current is often called a "spark-gap" current, which coagulates tissue and is used primarily for hemostasis. The cutting current can be blended with varying degrees of coagulating current so that hemostasis can be accomplished while resecting tissue. Use of these blended currents has the advantage that the resectionist can cut tissue faster, since somewhat less time is spent in coagulating individual bleeders. A disadvantage, however, is that a larger surface of tissue is heated as compared to "spot" coagulation; also large vessels, the really important ones, are often not closed except by localized fulguration. Consequently, with the blending method there is more coagulated tissue that must slough before healing takes place, with an increased likelihood of delayed postoperative bleeding. The type of currents used and the settings of the machine are the preference of the surgeon. At times, an operator will use the combined currents while resecting the majority of the adenoma and switch to pure currents as the prostatic capsule is exposed.

Each current is turned on by the operator by depressing the appropriate pedal of a double foot switch. Conventionally, the left pedal controls the cutting current and the right one that for coagulation. Two electrical connections must be made from the machine to the patient so that a complete circuit is established. The insulated cord transmitting the current from the generating unit to the resectoscope is plugged into the jack marked "active" on the unit. A second cord is plugged into the jack marked "patient," with its other end clipped to a large conductive metal

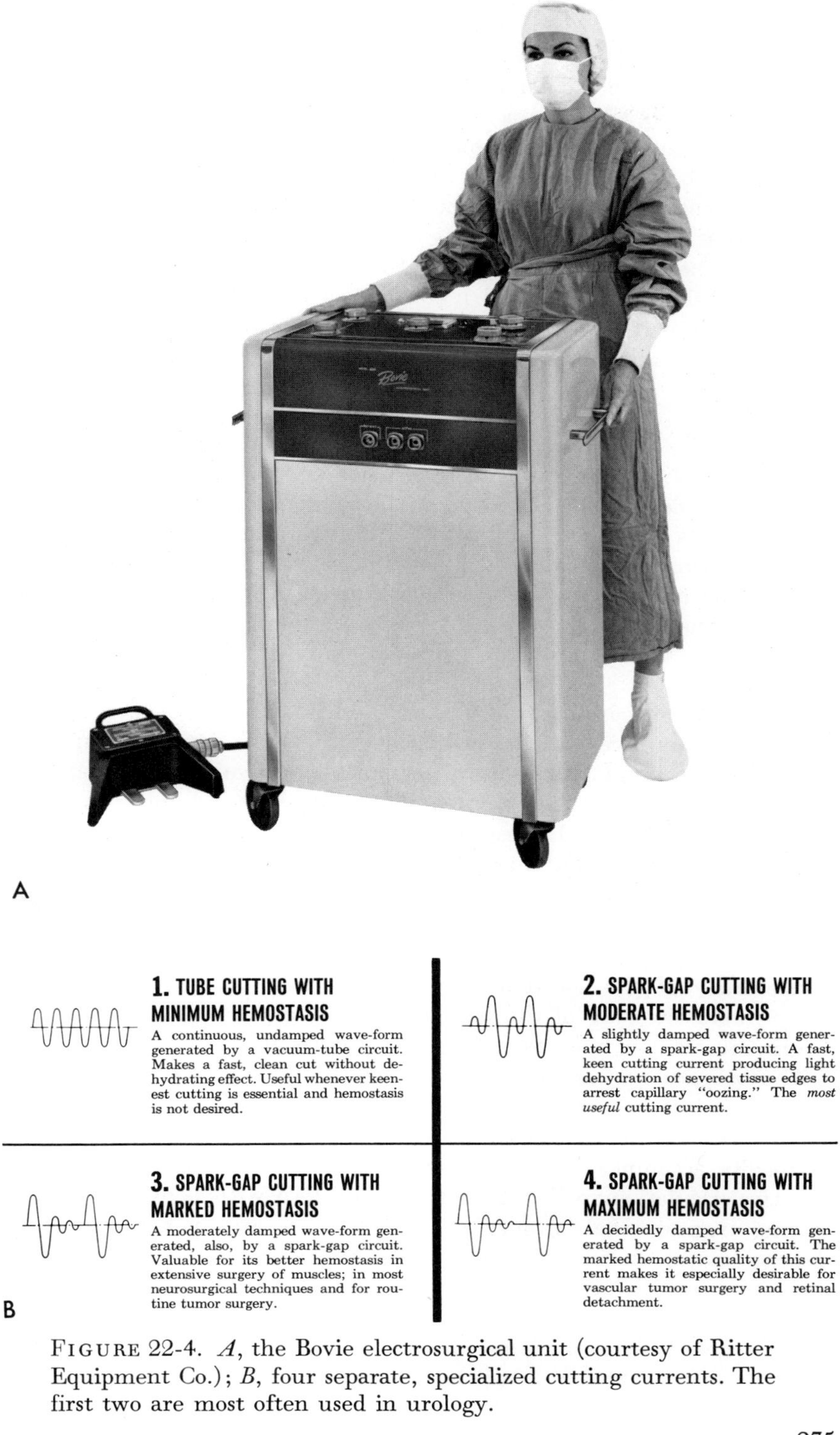

FIGURE 22-4. *A*, the Bovie electrosurgical unit (courtesy of Ritter Equipment Co.); *B*, four separate, specialized cutting currents. The first two are most often used in urology.

plate which is placed under the back or shoulders, thus completing the circuit. This plate must contact a wide surface of skin to prevent electrical burns. In addition, the plate should be moistened by use of an electrolyte solution, such as saline or jellies manufactured for this purpose, so that there is a good transmission of electricity over a large area. It is important to note that prior to disassembling the wiring at the conclusion of the operation, the unit must be turned off; otherwise, an accidental step on the foot switch can possibly burn the skin of the patient or the operator as the wiring is removed. Finally, the anesthesia used in such operations must be of the nonexplosive type.

Irrigating Solutions

Many liters of sterile irrigating solution may be used during transurethral procedures. Fluid constantly flows in past the area of resection to wash away tissue chips and blood so that the surgeon can see. As the bladder becomes filled and fluid flows in slowly, the field becomes obscured. The working unit is then withdrawn and the bladder is allowed to empty. The working unit is reinserted and the irrigating fluid is allowed to flow in again. This process is repeated many times until the operation is concluded.

Irrigating fluid is brought into the field through sterile tubing by gravity from an overhanging reservoir which may be of several types. These include permanently installed tanks, a Valentine flask that must be repeatedly refilled, or commercially prepared and interconnecting bottles. The height of the reservoir will vary with the preference of the surgeon: the higher, the more brisk the flow. Consequently, more fluid will be used during the procedure but the field will be clearer. Less fluid will be used if the column is lower, but vision may not be as clear. Usually a height of two feet above the level of the bladder suffices. The temperature of the solution should be normal body temperature. A considerable lowering of the patient's body temperature can follow the continuous exchange of cooler fluid, possibly resulting in shock.

The irrigating solution must not be one that conducts electricity, so that electrolyte solutions such as saline are never used. Such solutions will disperse the electrical current, so that cutting and coagulation cannot be readily accomplished. The solution should be one that, if absorbed into the circulation, will not seriously interfere with body metabolism. During transurethral surgery venous channels are opened which can absorb some of the irrigating fluid. Studies have shown that this rate of absorption can vary anywhere from near zero to 60 ml/minute or more.

Consequently, the ideal irrigating solution must be one that is optically clear, nonelectrolyte, not too expensive, and least injurious if absorbed in any quantity. Sterile water has the greatest clarity and is the least expensive. Its greatest drawback is that it is hypotonic to body fluids, so that absorption (in fact, an intraveneous infusion) can result in hemolysis of red blood cells followed by renal shutdown from ischemic nephrosis. Some experienced resectionists still use water because of its excellent optical qualities and feel that the danger of intravascular hemolysis is generally insignificant if the total resection time is kept to one hour or less. Isotonic glucose in water (5 per cent) can be used, but the clarity is not quite as good as water and spilled solution becomes sticky. Rising blood sugar levels during resections have been reported while using glucose. Isotonic, nontoxic amino acid solutions are now most commonly used for transurethral surgery and are the safest. These can be obtained in sterile bottles ready for use. Although large quantities will be required by a busy urologic service, their greater cost is offset by increased safety to patients and reduced personnel time spent in preparing and delivering sterile solutions.

Surgery

Ideally, a nurse should be scrubbed and gowned at operation since she can greatly expedite the procedure. If a drawer is not available on the operating table, she must be ready with a pan and strainer to catch the bladder contents each time the working unit is withdrawn. Furthermore, she must have an evacuator properly prepared each time the surgeon needs it to remove retained chips from within the bladder cavity. An Ellik evacuator is very useful (Fig. 22-5). By means of the evacuator's hourglass construction, bladder contents can be irrigated back and forth and the chips trapped in the lower part of the hourglass. For the evacuator to be effective, the nurse must be sure that no air is inside.

Problems During Operation

Problems that can arise during surgery are malfunctioning instruments, bladder perforations, hemorrhage, and problems related to excessive absorption of irrigating solutions.

Instrumental problems include inadequate illumination. This subject has been covered in the section on cystoscopic maintenance. Failure of the electrode loop to cut or coagulate most commonly is due to a poor connection somewhere, particularly in the seating of the loop or an actual break in the loop. One must look for a breakdown in the electrosurgical unit or a shortcircuit within the resectoscope itself. Finally, the generating unit must be not only turned on but also connected to the main power supply! Tracking down the source of this difficulty can prove exasperating, particularly if it arises after the operation has begun and substitute equipment is not immediately at hand.

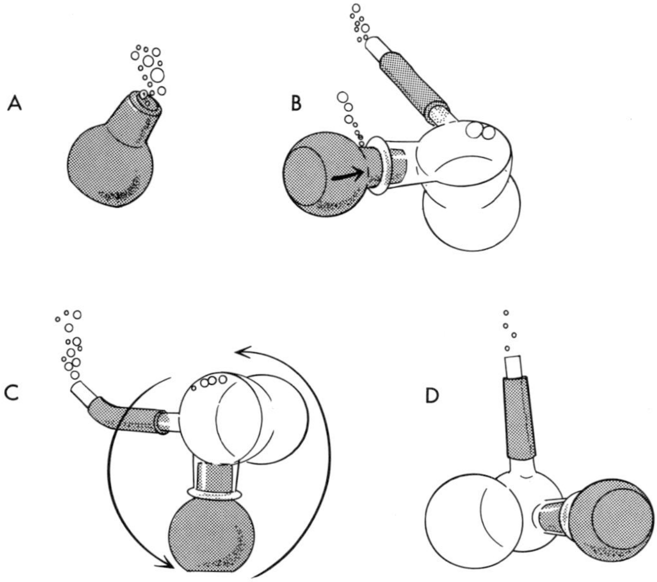

FIGURE 22-5. Filling the Ellik evacuator. *A*, the bulb is filled with water; *B*, the bulb is connected to the glass trap; *C* and *D*, the evacuator is turned with the outlet uppermost until all air bubbles are removed.

Perforation and extravasation may either be intraperitoneal or extraperitoneal, depending on the location of the injury. This can be insidious and may be suggested by a seemingly inadequate return of irrigating solution from the bladder each time the working unit is withdrawn. As the operation progresses, the abdomen may become gradually distended until the extravasation becomes too obvious to all. Shock tends to develop. The consequences of extravasation are usually not severe if the complication is recognized and treated promptly. The treatment is prompt drainage by means of a suprapubic cystostomy and insertion of drains. Often it is necessary also to inspect the peritoneal cavity to be sure than an intraperitoneal leak has not occurred. This complication, fortunately, is not common but it can occur even in the most experienced hands. Consequently, transurethral surgery should be performed in or near an operating room where everything is available for a cystostomy and abdominal exploration.

A complication that is sometimes difficult to prevent is the *hyponatremic reaction* (actually an acute water intoxication). This is secondary to marked absorption of the nonelectrolyte irrigating fluid into the circulation, causing a relative dilution of sodium in the body extracellular fluid. At first the blood pressure is well maintained and may even be elevated to alarming levels. Characteristically, this phenomenon is accompanied by a slowing pulse rate. Soon the patient will look pale despite the normal or elevated pressure. Often the blood loss has not been alarming or has been replaced adequately. Intravenous saline has usually not been given. The respirations tend to become damp.

Unrecognized, the situation may progress rapidly to profound shock not readily responding to transfusion, followed by pulmonary edema, coma, and death. Treatment begins with prompt recognition (confirmed shortly by determination of the serum sodium), immediate and drastic slowing of intravenous fluids, and the prompt administration of hypertonic saline solution (3 to 5 per cent). Usually 200 to 400 ml of 5 per cent solution will be needed. Accordingly, hypertonic saline should be in the operating suite and also in the recovery room. General supportive measures including management of acute heart failure may be necessary. Convalescence is marked by a profound diuresis. Prevention is by avoidance of the factors conducive to the introduction of fluid into the prostatic vessles—minimum operating time, especially near the end of the resection when capsular venous sinuses may be opened, irrigation at low pressure, gentleness, and an awareness of this possibility.

Cold Punch Prostatectomy

Transurethral surgery by the cold punch, contrary to the implications in its name, is a method wherein the expert resectionist can perform as complete a removal as can be achieved with electrical cutting. The instrument and the technique are somewhat different. The Thompson resectoscope is the best known model of this type. Basically, the sheath has a window, a fenestra within which tissue is engaged and then cut off by a sliding tubular knife. The cut tissue is removed via a large outlet valve connected to suction. Bleeding points are coagulated electrically by an electrode inserted in the instrument. The field of vision is notably different from that of the previously described resectoscopes. Rarely is a urologist adept in the use of both types of instruments—it is hard enough to learn the use of one!

Specific Nursing Considerations

The care of patients after transurethral surgery is similar to that following open prostatectomy except there is no external incision which requires care. Unless a preliminary cystostomy has been performed, urinary drainage will be totally dependent on the indwelling urethral catheter. This catheter is placed to straight drainage under average conditions.

Some surgeons employ low decompression with or without an intermittent irrigation. Through-and-through irrigation is not possible unless a cystostomy tube is in place or a special double-lumen urethral catheter has been inserted. The use of these double-lumen catheters is not particularly rewarding: the diameters of the channels are necessarily narrower, so drainage is not as free as with a comparably sized single-lumen catheter; the irrigations may seem to function well, giving a false sense of security, when actually the bladder is overdistended with clots. A catheter that is draining well is ordinarily best left alone and not irrigated routinely. If drainage stops or the bladder is distended, gentle irrigation is tried. Often the dislodging of a small plug in the catheter is all that is needed. Occasionally a mere squeeze of the tubing may suffice. If 5 or 6 oz have been introduced but the returns are inadequate, the physician is best called. More vigorous methods should be left to the urologist's direction.

The nurse must be alert to the signs of hyponatremia, as previously described: unexplained hypertension and bradycardia followed by a sudden profound hypotension, cyanosis, and pulmonary edema.

Ambulation after transurethral surgery is usually begun on the first postoperative day, if not some hours after operation. On the first postoperative day, the patient is usually able to take an adequate volume of fluids by mouth and rapidly progresses to his preoperative diet. By the third day after operation, the drainage is grossly clear in most instances, and the catheter is removed 24 to 48 hours later. The patient is given a measuring cup and instructed to keep a written record of the time and amount of urination. If this is satisfactory and other indications are favorable, he is discharged from the hospital several days later. Patients can often be sent home safely one week after a transurethral operation. They are best told that during the first few weeks after operation urgency, frequency and burning are expected but should diminish. The patient should also be told that there may be some gross hematuria off and on for up to four weeks after operation secondary to sloughing of coagulated areas in the fossa. Rarely is it physiologically (as opposed to psychologically) alarming, but the patient is advised to notify the doctor promptly if it is persistent or associated with the passage of clots.

REVIEW QUESTIONS

1. Describe factors to be considered by the surgeon in deciding whether to resect a prostate adenoma transurethrally.
2. Diagram and label the parts of a resectoscope. Indicate those features to be checked by the nurse to determine that the instrument is working properly.
3. What special precautions are necessary for patient and personnel

during transurethral surgery because of the use of an electric current? Explain.

4. Explain the advantages and disadvantages in the use of the following fluids during transurethral surgery: distilled water, normal saline, isotonic glucose in water, isotonic nontoxic amino acid solutions.
5. Explain why transurethral surgery is best performed in or near the operative suite.
6. Discuss hyponatremia: what it is, why and when it occurs, signs and symptoms, treatment.
7. What are the salient factors to be considered in planning nursing care for the patient during his hospitalization for transurethral surgery? Outline care under the following headings: time period, objectives of care, rationale underlying objective, specific nursing activity.

CHAPTER 23

Surgery of the External Genitalia

Surgery of the Penis

THE most commonly performed operation on the penis is the excision of the prepuce (*circumcision*). In fact, circumcision is the only elective surgical operation frequently performed by operators without a medical education! Besides medical indications, religious and traditional ones are important. Medical contraindications do exist and, in their presence, essentially all religious authorities permit omission or postponement of the rite. This is particularly true of hemorrhagic disorders such as hemophilia and purpura or in the presence of penile deformities. The preputial skin is usually valuable in the correction of hypospadias, and so this skin should not be sacrificed from the medical viewpoint.

The usual medical indication is *phimosis*. This is a ringlike tightening of the end of the foreskin so that it cannot be readily retracted to expose the glans. Newborn males *normally* have adherence between the inner surface of the prepuce and the glans penis—this is not phimosis. This adherence gradually resolves over the first year and ordinarily requires no treatment. Under the circumstances of true phimosis, smegma will collect beneath the prepuce. Such collections can cause irritation and an unpleasant odor. With such poor hygiene there will be irritation, infection, and further contraction of the phimotic ring. In extreme cases, the opening can contract to such a degree that there will be difficulty with urination. Another form which may necessitate urgent surgical treatment is *paraphimosis*. In such a situation, the foreskin retracts below the corona of the glans and cannot be reduced. This results in a vicious cycle of swelling of the glans and further tightening of the paraphimotic ring with increasing inflammation. Under these conditions, an emergency *dorsal slit* of the prepuce may be done to release the pressure, splitting the foreskin down to and through the ring. After the acute inflammation subsides, an elective circumcision is performed at a later date.

Presently there is controversy regarding the justifiability of *routine* circumcision of newborn male infants. One argument is that hygiene in this area is improved. However, in most instances, a normally retractible foreskin can be kept clean without difficulty. A second argument is that circumcision will prevent cancer of the penis in later life. This is indeed true in that such cancers have rarely been reported in men who were circumcised in infancy. On the other hand, cancer of the penis is uncommon in this country and there is a significant cure rate. Finally, the argument that circumcision will decrease the incidence of uterine cervix cancer is very speculative.

Although the operation seems simple enough, drastic deformity can result if improperly done. These deformities include injury to the glans, urethral fistula, and too extensive a removal so that there will be interference with normal erection in adult life. Circumcision can be performed by several techniques, all requiring care. After excision with scissors or knife, the skin on the shaft is sutured to the cut edge of the mucosal side with fine interrupted catgut sutures. Another method is the use of specially constructed bell-shaped clamps which fit under the foreskin over the glans. A second clamp is placed over the skin, tightened down, and the prepuce cut.

Partial and total *amputations* of the penis are usually performed for cancer. Generally, the cancer-bearing segment of the penis is excised with at least a 1.5-cm margin. Local recurrences of the cancer are uncommon if the amputation is performed in such a manner. Although these tumors tend to grow slowly, many surgeons excise the local (inguinal) lymph nodes during the same hospitalization. Others prefer to wait until palpable suspicious nodes are present, since not all metastasize and since groin dissections are not minor matters. The first echelon of lymphatic spread is to the inguinal and femoral nodes, followed by the nodes inside the pelvis.

The operation for nodal excision is known as the *inguinal* or *groin dissection.* The incision begins medial to the anterior superior iliac spine and is carried downward and medially across the inguinal ligament on to the inner thigh. A rectangular block of subcutaneous tissue including the underlying fascia of the thigh is excised. This fat contains the superficial inguinal lymph nodes. Dissection of tissues in the femoral canal, particularly medial to the femoral vein, will remove the deep nodes. Although the terminology is variable, such an operation is classified as a simple groin dissection. By dividing the inguinal ligament or making an incision above it, the femoral vessels can be followed upward and retroperitoneally, so that the node-bearing areolar tissue on these vessels can be removed (external iliac artery and vein). The tissue along the internal iliac (hypogastric) and obturator vessels is similarly explored. By entering the bony pelvis, the operation is thus converted to a truly radical dissection. Postoperatively, the skeletonized femoral vessels, if covered only by skin, can be eroded by infection, particularly if the overlying skin should slough. Cutaneous necrosis is not rare after this operation. To minimize this possibility, the upper end of the sartorius muscle is detached from the anterior superior iliac spine and moved medially to cover these vessels. Closure of the skin may require some ingenuity, particularly if a large area of skin is removed with the specimen because of neoplastic involvement. Although free skin grafts can be used, one valuable technique consists of the removal of the testicle from the end of the spermatic cord on that side, placing the freed cord into any potential dead space in the groin or thigh. The spread-out half of the scrotum is then attached to the wound edges to cover the cutaneous deficiency.

Surgery of the Urethra

Surgery of the urethra is usually performed for strictures and congenital malformations. Stenosis of the urethral meatus is corrected by *meatotomy*. The meatus is enlarged by a ventral midline incision, and the urethral mucosa is sutured out to the skin edges on the glans with fine interrupted catgut sutures. If the meatus is simply cut open and not sutured as described, the opening tends to contract again.

Innumerable operations have been devised for the correction of urethral strictures. The selection of operation depends in part on the location and length of involvement. For a short stricture (1 cm or less), excision followed by anastomosis of the adjacent ends of urethra may be sufficient. For longer segments, a two-stage repair such as the Johansen technique is often used. At the first stage, the length of strictured urethra is incised longitudinally until healthy tissue is reached at either end. The stricture is laid open and its edges are sutured to the adjacent penile skin (Fig. 23-1). The second stage is carried out after a minimum of four to six months. The reason for this delay is to get a maximum subsidence of inflammation

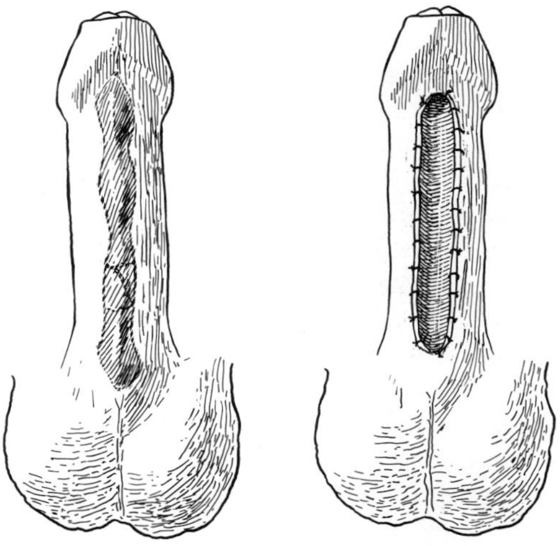

FIGURE 23-1. First stage, Johansen repair for urethral stricture.

in the tissues before reconstruction is attempted. At the second operation, a wide strip of penile skin is outlined between the healthy ends of urethra, incorporating any intervening urethral remnants. This strip will be the base of the reformed urethra. Lateral to the strip, flaps of penile skin are mobilized and sutured over the strip, thus burying it (Fig. 23-2).

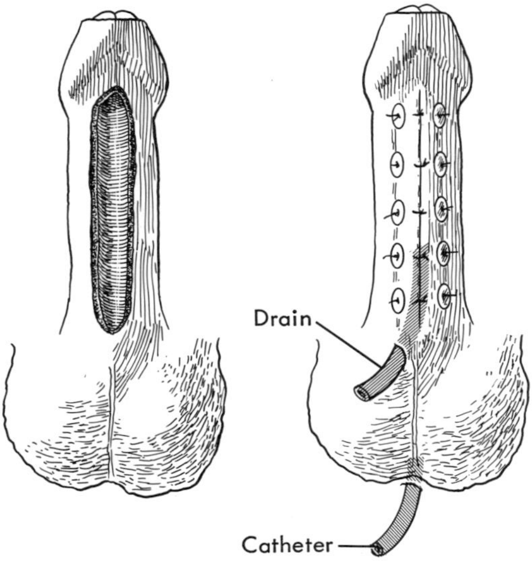

FIGURE 23-2. Second stage, Johansen repair for urethral stricture.

Eventually the underside of the flaps reepithelializes to form the new urethra. During the 10 to 14 days necessary for the suture line to heal, the vesical urine is diverted by a catheter inserted either via a perineal urethrostomy or a suprapubic cystostomy.

The commonest congenital anomaly of the urethra is *hypospadias.* Here the urethra ends short of its usual location in the glans penis. The milder forms with the urethral opening low in the glans require no treatment. With the more severe forms, the urethral opening may be located as far back as the perineum. In the newborn infant with severe perineal hypospadias and a bifid scrotum, a differentiation as to the sex of the child may be impossible on inspection alone. Accompanying the hypospadias, there will be a ventral curvature of the penile shaft (*chordee*), especially notable on erection. This downbending is caused by inelastic fibrous tissue which replaces the missing segment of urethra, acting like the string of a bow to pull the penis down. Major degrees of chordee need correction, since the penile curvature can interfere with eventual sexual intercourse. If the urethra is too short, the boy may have to sit to void and the man may have reduced fertility. Finally, the cosmetic appearance may have psychologic repercussions.

Correction of chordee and hypospadias is usually carried out in two or more stages, although surgeons are constantly searching for a satisfactory repair in one stage. Generally, a six-month period should elapse between each stage for the reason previously outlined in the discussion of urethral strictures. The chordee is corrected at the first stage by excising the ventral fibrous tissue. Mobilized dorsal preputial skin is often transplanted to fill the ventral skin defect resulting from the straightening. At the second stage a new urethra is constructed by one of many techniques at the surgeon's disposal. Some of the more popular operations include the buried skin strip procedure of Denis-Browne, the use of buried tubes of penile skin, and the application of free tubular grafts of skin or bladder mucosa. A third stage is not infrequently needed to correct deficiencies such as fistula or stricture formation, so the family should know beforehand of such a possibility.

Epispadias is a much rarer anomaly of the penis and urethra wherein the corpora cavernosa are partly separated and the urethra lies open on the dorsum of the penis. With more severe forms, the external sphincter and bladder neck are involved so that the patient is incontinent. The most common form of epispadias is that associated with exstrophy of the bladder. The epispadias is corrected by suturing the edges of the urethra together and rolling the separated corpora together over it. When incontinence exists, the procedure is more complex and the results often less satisfactory.

Surgery of the Scrotal Contents

A *hydrocele* is an excessive accumulation of serous fluid around a testicle. Normally, there are 1 or 2 ml of clear fluid between the tunica albuginea covering the testis and the tunica vaginalis lining the scrotum. A hydrocele develops when more fluid is produced than that absorbed in this space. This accumulation rarely causes any symptoms other than from its size, weight, and appearance. A mild to moderate hydrocele is common in newborn males; the majority subside in a month or two without treatment. A hydrocele can develop acutely in the presence of epididymitis or torsion of the testicle or its appendages. The majority develop slowly. The most important point is managing a hydrocele is for the doctor to differentiate the mass from a neoplasm of the testis and to be satisfied that an associated neoplasm does not exist. An example of the latter situation is when a fairly tense hydrocele has developed rapidly during a period of a few weeks without obvious cause. If the testis cannot be palpated easily through the hydrocele, exploration of the scrotum may be indicated simply to visualize the testicle.

The best treatment for a hydrocele is surgical excision of the sac (*hydrocelectomy*). This can be done through either a scrotal or an inguinal incision. The latter is preferred when there may be associated problems such as an inguinal hernia or possible neoplasm of the testis. Various other benign conditions of the scrotal contents, such as spermatocele and epididymal cysts, are also treated by excision if any treatment is indicated. Aspiration of hydroceles affords only temporary relief, since the fluid will simply reaccumulate, and there is a real danger of introducing infection. Aspiration and injection of caustic compounds to destroy the lining of the sac is to be condemned as uncertain, painful, subject to infection, and conducive to a long convalescence.

Varicocele is a collection in the spermatic cord of dilated tributaries of the spermatic vein. Varicoceles strongly favor the left side. Treatment is only rarely indicated from symptoms arising directly from the varicocele. However, in certain selected instances of subfertility, ligation of these veins is followed by enough improvement in the sperm count for successful conception to occur. The operation is performed by interrupting the spermatic veins in the inguinal canal.

Orchiectomy, the removal of a testis, can be carried out through either a scrotal or an inguinal incision. The commonest indication for this operation is in the endocrine treatment of prostatic cancer where both testes are removed. The testicle can be either removed along with the epididymis in a guillotine fashion or excised separately, leaving the epididymis behind. The only advantage of the latter method is that some bulk is left behind in the scrotum to soothe the ego of the castrated patient. A testicle suspected of neoplasm is best explored through an inguinal incision. The spermatic cord is mobilized at the internal inguinal ring and the blood supply to the testicle temporarily occluded using a bulldog or rubber-shod clamp. This occlusion will prevent spillage of tumor cells into the bloodstream as the testis is brought out of the scrotum into the operative field. At this point, the surgeon must decide whether or not to remove the testicle. A biopsy or incision into malignant testicular tumor is to be avoided if at all possible. Such maneuvers invite local spillage, recurrence, and metastases to inguinal nodes. Consequently, if the exposed testis is still suspected of neoplasm, the specimen, consisting of the testis, epididymis, and attached spermatic cord, is usually removed, particularly if a good organ exists on the other side.

Orchiopexy is an operation to bring an undescended testicle into the scrotum. The majority of undescended testes are located in or about the inguinal canal, and most are associated with a congenital inguinal hernia. Consequently, the operation is performed through an inguinal incision. In most instances, the incomplete descent is caused by a relative shortness of the spermatic vessels. After the testis has been dissected free of surrounding tissues, the spermatic vessels and the vas deferens are traced toward their origins. At times, retroperitoneal mobilization of the vessels must be carried to the kidney to achieve sufficient length. The indications and technique for vas ligation have been described in Chapter 21.

Specific Nursing Considerations

Nursing care after circumcision is not complicated. A simple effective bandage is the indian flap dressing (Fig. 23-3). The hanging gauze sponge prevents excessive chafing by the bedclothes. Another dressing consists of a strip of petrolatum gauze wrapped around the penis at the suture line. Sometimes the strip is tied down to the incision with long ends of the sutures, a neat-looking arrangement which tends to be painful. The main purpose of wrapping is to achieve better hemostasis by pressure. However, such hemostatic measures should ordinarily not be necessary. Removal of an adherent dressing of this type may be quite

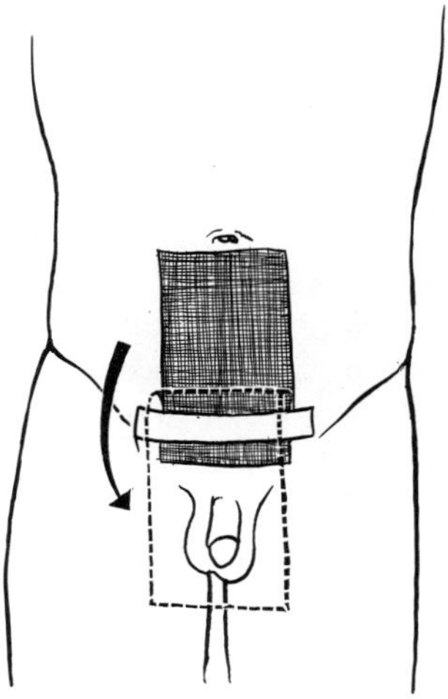

FIGURE 23-3. Indian flap dressing.

uncomfortable to the patient, so preliminary soaking with saline will be greatly appreciated. By 48 hours after operation, the most dressing needed is a pad inside snugly fitting shorts or an athletic supporter. Patients may take a bath or shower at once, and they are advised that the catgut sutures will fall out spontaneously over the next two or three weeks.

Nursing care after penile amputations is rarely complicated. Actual hemorrhage, while uncommon, can be controlled by local pressure and the surgeon called. During the first few days after partial amputation, there may or may not be an indwelling catheter to drain the bladder while the suture line between the end of the severed urethra to the stumps of the corpora cavernosa heals. Dressings should not obstruct the urethral outlet. On the other hand, proper attention and care promote the healing of groin dissections. The skin flaps have been intentionally denuded of subcutaneous tissue and are thus partially deprived of their blood supply. Skin sloughing to some degree is almost usual. To minimize this complication, drainage is usually employed, sometimes with attached suction. A pressure dressing further reduces the prospect of serum accumulations which raise the skin flaps off the underlying tissues and thus interfere with healing. By the end of the first postoperative week, it will be obvious whether there will be primary healing or if some necrosis of the flaps is to be anticipated. Should the latter be the case, the surgeon will debride the necrotic areas and order saline soaks until there is a healthy bed of granulation tissue. When this has occurred and there is no further demarcation of the wound, split-thickness skin grafts are often applied. Major hemorrhage may occur in the early postoperative course if the principal divided vessels have not been secured. Firm pressure can temporarily control this—even if from the main femoral artery—while awaiting the doctor. If the large vessels become exposed in the later postoperative course, sudden massive hemorrhage is a constant threat that must be immediately met! When this happens, there is no time to search for sterile gloves. The hand is pressed hard enough on the wound to control the bleeding while the doctor is called.

Any surgery of the penis or scrotum can be followed by impressive swelling of the loose subcutaneous tissues during the first postoperative week. However, sloughs almost never occur from swelling alone, though the appearance may be alarming, particularly if discoloration from blood extravasation coexists. Actual hematomas are discolored and their swelling is firm or hard. Oozing of blood and serum from suture lines may cause crusts to form which can stick annoyingly to dressings. For the first several days after reconstructive procedures, particularly for hypospadias, many surgeons will suspend the penis to the anterior abdominal wall by means of a suture taken through the glans. This maneuver reduces maceration and crust accumulation and induces healing in an over-corrected state.

One satisfactory dressing consists of a wide-caliber Penrose drain or condom which is slipped directly over the penis. A suitable pressure dressing is applied over this, often with elastic adhesive strips. An advantage of this dressing is that, when it is cut, there will be no adherence to the suture line. After the dressings are off, the doctor will remove crusts daily after they have been softened with hydrogen peroxide soaks. Such meticulous efforts toward cleanliness will go far to prevent localized areas of suppuration which may cause wound breakdown and fistula formation. Exposure of the suture lines to a heat lamp several times a day will also increase circulation and keep the wound dry. A 60-watt electric light bulb in a gooseneck lamp held about 15 inches from the wound is sufficient. Obviously, the arrangement must be watched to prevent burns, especially with overactive children. After the first week, the wound can be kept clean with soap and water.

A dressing useful after operations on the scrotal contents, such as hydrocelectomy, is the military strap dressing (Fig. 23-4). This dressing

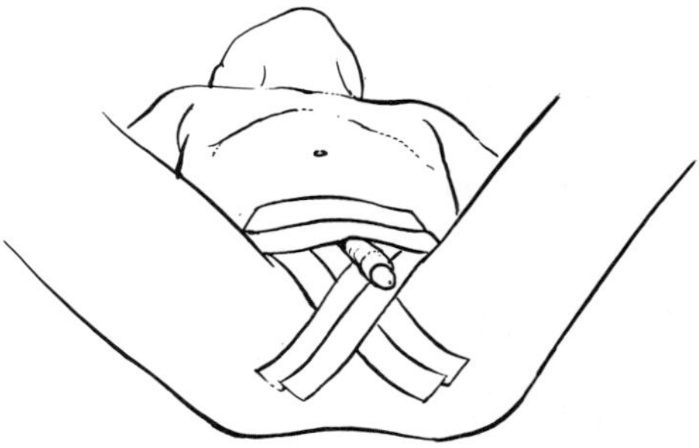

FIGURE 23-4. Military strap dressing.

securely immobilizes the scrotum and is also useful in the treatment of acute inflammatory disorders such as epididymitis. Although this method of bandaging may appear impressively cumbersome, patients are quite comfortable with it. The application of cold in the form of an ice bag also helps to reduce swelling and discomfort. After the first 48 hours following operation, such measures are usually no longer necessary. By that time bulky dressings can generally be removed and replaced with an athletic supporter.

Postoperative care following orchiopexy is related primarily to the method used for anchoring the testis in the scrotum. Ideally, if the relocated testis lies freely in the scrotum without tension, there are no special considerations in aftercare. Often, however, the testis has been brought down under some tension. Most often two to seven days of traction are all that are necessary. One method used to apply traction is via a rubber band tied to a stout suture taken through the scrotum and lower pole of the testis. The rubber band is made mildly taut by taping or suturing its other end to the inner thigh (Fig. 23-5). Should traction for several months be necessary in the opinion of the surgeon, the Torek procedure may be used in which the testis is sutured through an opening in the lower scrotum to the fascia of the inner thigh. Several months later, a second operation is carried out to take down that anastomosis. During the interval between the two procedures, the child must be kept relatively inactive, avoiding contact sports, bicycle riding, and other activities that may injure the immobile testicle.

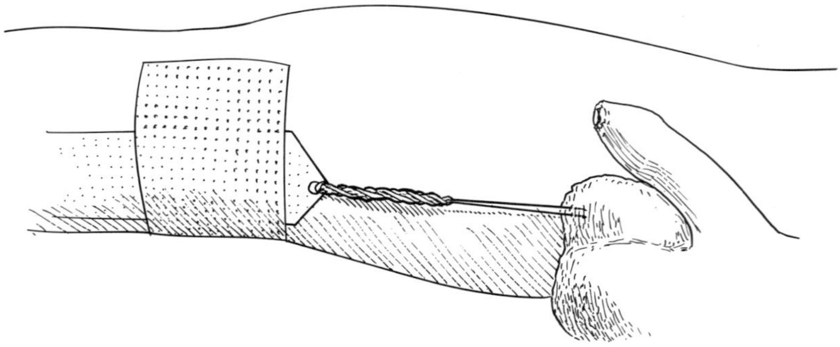

FIGURE 23-5. A method to apply traction to the testis following orchiopexy.

REVIEW QUESTIONS

1. Define phimosis and paraphimosis.
2. What should the nurse teach the mother of an uncircumcised male baby relative to genital hygiene?
3. Describe hypospadias, chordee, epispadias.
4. Describe the factors that may affect wound healing after groin dissection. Under what circumstances should the nurse be particularly alert to the possibility of hemorrhage? What should she do if hemorrhage occurs?
5. Describe wound care following circumcision.
6. Outline a sterile dressing procedure, including equipment that will be appropriate for caring for genital wounds, keeping in mind that wounds may be encrusted and dressings adherent.
7. Why may physical activity be limited following a Torek procedure? What are the nursing implications in planning for the patient's discharge?

REFERENCES—UNIT III

Alexander, Edythe, Wanda Burley, Dorothy Ellison, and Rosalind Valleri: *Care of the Patient in Surgery*, 4th ed. C. V. Mosby Co., St. Louis, 1967.

Ansell, Julian S.: "Catheter Care," *J Urol*, **89**: 940–44, 1963.

Ansell, Julian S.: "Nephrectomy and Nephrostomy," *Amer J Nurs*, **58**: 1394–96, 1958.

Barnes, Roger W.: "Prostatic Tumors, Part I, Surgical Treatment," *Amer J Nurs*, **56**: 982–85, 1956.

Beal, John M., ed.: *Manual of Recovery Room Care*, 2nd ed. The Macmillan Co., New York, 1962.

Blandy, John: "Urinary Bladder Substitution and the Nursing Care Involved," *Nurs Mirror*, **122**: 5–7, 1966; **122**: 7–10, 1966.

Christopher, Nancy: "Postoperative Care Following Nephrectomy," *Canad Nurse*, **59**: 838–39, 1963.

Chute, Richard: "Preoperative and Postoperative Care of Aged Patients Undergoing Urologic Surgery," *JAMA*, **148**: 184–87, 1952.

Creevy, C. Donald: "Ileal Diversion of the Urine," *Amer J Nurs*, **53**: 530–33, 1959.

Ellis, William J., and John T. Grayhack: "Sexual Function in Aging Males After Orchiectomy and Estrogen Therapy," *J Urol*, **89**: 895–99, 1963.

Euty, F. Harold: "Fibrinolysis: A Complication of Transurethral Resection of the Prostate Gland," *J Urol*, **91**: 671–75, 1964.

Frenay, Sr. M. Agnes Clare: "A Dynamic Approach to the Ileal Conduit Patient," *Amer J Nurs*, **64**: 80–84, 1964.

Glenn, Frank, S. W. Moore, and John M. Beal, ed.: *Surgery in the Aged*. McGraw-Hill, New York, 1960.

Glenn, James F., and William H. Boyce: *Urologic Surgery*. Hoeber Medical Division, Harper & Row, New York, 1969.

Gregg, Dorothy: "Anxiety—A Factor in Nursing Care," *Amer J Nurs*, **52**: 1363–65, 1952.

Gregg, Dorothy: "Reassurance," *Amer J Nurs*, **55**: 171–74, 1955.

Hudson, Perry B., and Arthur Purdy Stout: *An Atlas of Prostatic Surgery*. W. B. Saunders Co., Philadelphia, 1962.

Jackson, Arlene F.: "Cancer of the Bladder," *Amer J Nurs*, **58**: 249–50, 1958.

Kasselman, Mary Jo: "Nursing Care of the Patient with Benign Prostatic Hypertrophy," *Amer J Nurs*, **66**: 1026–30, 1966.

Keitzer, Walter A., and Carlyle Benavent: "Bladder Neck Obstruction in Children," *J Urol*, **89**: 384–88, 1963.

Kerr, W. K., C. J. Robson, J. L. T. Russell, and J. P. Bourque: "Collective Review of Urinary Tract Diversion. Canadian Academy of Urological Surgeons," *J Urol*, **88**: 644–52, 1962.

King, J. M.: "Ileo-cutaneous Ureterostomy," *Nurs Times*, **57**: 1531–34, 1961.

Kouzen, Ruth: "Guide for Geriatric Care," *Amer J Nurs*, **57**: 1166–67, 1957.

Kunin, Calvin M., and Regina C. McCormack: "Prevention of Catheter-Induced Urinary Tract Infections by Sterile Closed Drainage," *New Eng J Med*, **274**: 1155–61, 1966.

Lapham, D. M.: "Odor Control in Long-Term Care Facilities," *Nurs Homes*, **16**: 20–23, 1967.

Litil, Edward: "Mental Reaction to Trauma and Hospitalization in the Aged," *JAMA*, **162**: 1522–24, 1956.

MacKinnon, Harold A.: "Urinary Drainage: The Problem of Asepsis," *Amer J Nurs*, **65**: 112, 1965.

Marshall, Victor F., Russell W. Lavengood, Jr., and Daniel Kelly: "Complete Longitudinal Nephrolithotomy and the Shorr Regimen in the Management of Staghorn Calculi," *Ann Surg*, **162**: 366–73, 1965.

Metheny, Norma M., and William D. Snively: *Nurses Handbook of Fluid Balance*. J. B. Lippincott Co., Philadelphia, 1967.

Miller, Opal: "Nursing Care after Pelvic Exenteration," *Amer J Nurs*, **62**: 106–107, 1962.

Morrissey, Alice B.: "The Procedures of Urinary and Bowel Rehabilitation," *Amer J Nurs*, **51**: 194–97, 1951.

Mossholder, Irene B.: "When the Patient Has a Radical Retropubic Prostatectomy," *Amer J Nurs*, **62**: 101–104, 1962.

Obermeier, William B.: "Crotch Care," *Amer J Nurs*, **57**: 618–20, 1957.

Paquin, Albert J., Jr., Victor F. Marshall, and Bernard Nathanson: "Studies on a Practical Method for the Determination of Operative Blood Loss," *Ann Surg*, **141**: 53–61, 1955.

Patricia, Sister M., and Loyola C. Floyd: "Nursing Care in Prostatectomy," *Canad Nurse*, **59**: 833–35, 1963.

Purdey, Angus: "Prostatic Tumors, Part II, Nursing Care," *Amer J Nurs*, **56**: 986–87, 1956.

Pyrah, L. N.: "The Rectosigmoid Bladder as a Method of Urinary Diversion," *J Urol*, **90**: 189–92, 1963.

Reams, Gerald B., and Elma J. Powell: "Postoperative Catheterization—Yes or No?" *Amer J Nurs*, **60**: 371, 1960.

Robertson, Carolyn A.: "Manual Expression of Urine," *Amer J Nurs*, **59**: 840–41, 1959.

Saxon, Jean: "Techniques for Bowel and Bladder Training," *Amer J Nurs*, **62**: 69–71, 1962.

Schneider, David H.: "Aseptic Closed Urinary Tract Drainage," *J Urol*, **74**: 158–61, 1955.

Soller, Genevieve R.: "The Aging Patient," *Amer J Nurs*, **62**: 114–17, 1962.

Spellman, Robert M., and Mary Helen Swanwick: "The Management of Cutaneous Ureterostomies," *Amer J Nurs*, **55**: 800–803, 1955.

Spence, Harry M.: "Genitourinary Injuries," *Amer J Nurs*, **55**: 970–73, 1955.

Stolov, Walter C.: "Rehabilitation of the Bladder in Injuries of the Spinal Cord," *Arch Phys Med*, **40**: 467–74, 1959.

Sweetser, Theodore H., Eldon B. Berglund, Tague C. Chisholm, and Genevieve S. McCarr: "Care of the Child with Exstrophy of the Bladder," *Amer J Nurs*, **58**: 1115–17, 1958.

Taufic, Marjorie R.: "Nursing the Patient after Nephrectomy," *Amer J Nurs*, **58**: 1397–98, 1958.

Thomson, Gretchen: "After Renal Surgery," *Amer J Nurs*, **61**: 106–107, 1961.

Tollefson, Dorothy M.: "Nursing Care of the Patient with an Ileac Diversion of the Urine," *Amer J Nurs*, **59**: 534–36, 1959.

Turck, Marvin, Bernard Goffe, and Robert G. Petersdorf: "The Urethral Catheter and Urinary Tract Infection," *J Urol*, **88**: 834–37, 1962.

Walsh, Michael A., Marion Ebner, and Joseph W. Casey: "Neo-Bladder," *Amer J Nurs*, **63**: 107—10, 1963.

Walzak, Myron P., Jr., and Albert J. Paquin, Jr.: "Renal Pelvic Pressure Levels in Management of Nephrostomy," *J Urol*, **85**: 697–702, 1961.

Whitmore, Willet F., Jr., and Theodore Bongart: "A Device for the Management of Cutaneous Ureterostomy," *J Urol*, **74**: 603–606, 1955.

Wolf, Roger C.: "Can New Laws Solve the Legal and Psychiatric Problems of Voluntary Sterilization," *J Urol*, **93**: 402–406, 1965.

UNIT IV

Acute and Chronic Renal Failure: General Principles and Nursing Considerations

CHAPTER 24
Uremia and Renal Failure

UREMIA is a clinical syndrome that is the manifestation of a severe loss of total renal function. An elevation of the blood urea nitrogen level alone is defined as *azotemia* and does not necessarily imply significant renal failure per se. For example, urea is infused into patients for divided renal function studies under osmotic diuresis. Such patients will have temporary elevations of their blood urea nitrogen secondary to the infusion but do not develop the uremic syndrome on this basis. Another example is the azotemia following breakdown of digested blood in the intestinal tract after a major gastrointestinal hemorrhage. Not all the chemical factors contributing to the uremic syndrome have been defined. Besides retention of the recognizable end products of protein metabolism such as urea and creatinine, relatively minute amounts of organic acids, indoles, phenols, and other unidentified toxic substances contribute to the patient's illness.

The clinical picture may develop acutely, as when there is a severe insult to previously normal kidneys, or gradually, as in end-stage renal disease. The term *end stage* refers to any slowly progressing disorder, whether it be chronic pyelonephritis, glomerulonephritis, nephrosclerosis, or other disorders. The ability of a patient to tolerate his uremia depends in large part on the rapidity of the change. A sudden marked decrease in kidney function is usually tolerated poorly and the patient may deteriorate rapidly. The problem is often compounded by the disorder that initiated the renal failure in the first place. On the other hand, a long-standing renal insufficiency with a profound but more gradual deterioration is often tolerated surprisingly well.

Chronic Renal Failure

Chronic renal failure is characterized by derangements of the normal renal function described in Unit I of this text. As renal function declines, the kidneys lose their ability to concentrate water, so that large volumes of urine may be excreted with a specific gravity equal to that of the plasma and sometimes lower. Severe disturbances in electrolyte metabolism are common. In advanced renal failure the kidney's control of sodium excretion is poor and does not necessarily vary with the patient's intake as it would in a normal person. Often, there will be excessive excretion of sodium in the urine which may cause a lowering of body sodium (hyponatremia). This, however, is not the only cause for hyponatremia in uremia.

An inability to excrete potassium may bring about an elevation in circulating potassium ion (hyperkalemia) with subsequent increased irritability of the myocardium. Impairment of the renal tubules in excretion of hydrogen ions and resorption of bicarbonate results in an acidosis. The major source of metabolic acid and phosphorus is protein. An increase in blood phosphorus levels is accompanied by a decrease in calcium values. The latter changes may stimulate excess parathormone production by the parathyroid glands with a resultant secondary hyperparathyroidism and increased resorption of bony calcium.

The anemia of chronic uremia is not completely understood. There seems to be a nonspecific depression of bone marrow function, and hypothetically there may be decreased erythropoietin production by the failing kidneys. In addition, there will be anemia from blood loss secondary to the bleeding diathesis common to uremic patients. Finally, the rate of normal red blood cell destruction is increased.

Clinical Picture

The syndrome of chronic uremia is manifested in many ways. The patient is obviously ill. Generally he will appear sallow and may have a yellowish cast to his skin. He will tire easily, may frequently complain of headache, and often his mentation is dulled. Characteristically he will be anemic, anorectic, and may have persistent diarrhea. Dependent edema is not unusual. The breath will have the characteristically unpleasant uremic odor. There may be signs and symptoms of hypertension and congestive heart failure. There may be muscular twitching, weakness, and peripheral neuropathy with paresthesias. As the situation deteriorates, the aforementioned signs worsen. The skin becomes darker as urinary pigments are deposited there in increasing amounts. The patient becomes markedly cachectic and tetany may become uncontrollable despite vigorous calcium supplements. Often, massive, uncontrollable hemorrhage from the gastrointestinal tract is a terminal event, presumably because of an unexplained increase in capillary fragility with a generalized increase in bleeding tendency.

Treatment of Chronic Renal Insufficiency

The first step in the treatment of chronic renal insufficiency is to identify its cause. The depth of urologic investigation must be guided by clinical judgment. The hope is that a surgically relievable obstruction can be found so that there may be a possibility of some recovery of renal function by improving urinary drainage, as with hydronephrosis. If small kidneys without significant outflow obstruction are present, it is unlikely that any surgical measures on the patient's own urinary tract will change the outlook. Consequently, other modalities such as an artificial kidney or renal transplantation will be considered.

Although the treatment of chronic uremia is essentially palliative, many of the consequences of renal failure may be partially overcome by dietary, fluid, and drug management. In many patients, additional years of useful life may thereby be attained. Since, as previously mentioned, dietary protein is a major source of phosphorus and a major source of metabolic acid, protein restriction of varying degrees may be employed depending on the severity of uremic symptoms and acidosis. The more restricted protein diets used in severe uremia usually result in an inadequate protein intake. Therefore, a balance must be found between uremic symptoms and the patient's protein needs. The ambulatory patient is usually allowed 40 g of protein daily. In more severe cases the amount allowed is reduced to 10 or 20 g and in very severe cases may be temporarily restricted completely. Egg whites are particularly recommended. The remainder of the caloric requirements are provided by other low-protein foods high in carbohydrate (Appendix I). The salt intake must be regulated so that obligatory urinary loss of these electrolytes is corrected, but it should not be so high as to cause fluid retention and edema. Such dietary measures will reduce considerably the characteristic nausea and diarrhea of the chronically uremic patient. An increased fluid intake is desirable if the patient is putting out large volumes of dilute urine. Additional medical measures include calcium replacement, correction of acidosis, and medication to relieve nausea. Basic aluminum hydroxide gel is often given by mouth to bond phosphates and increase their excretion from the body via the gastrointestinal tract. This, in turn, will decrease the painful heterotopic calcifications seen frequently in chronic uremia. Antihypertensive medications, usually rauwolfia compounds or methyldopa, may be necessary. Diuretics in advanced uremia are usually ineffective.

Specific Nursing Considerations

The medical and nursing management in chronic renal failure is directed toward maintaining the patient for as long as possible in a state of reasonable physiologic balance. Under careful health supervision, many of these patients can live additional years of meaningful, productive life.

One aspect of medical management will be directed toward regulation of fluid intake and output. The volume of fluid intake will be determined by the patient's urinary output and blood levels of urea and electrolytes. In many patients, the volume of urine produced may seem adequate under ordinary circumstances. Actually, a larger urine output may be necessary to eliminate waste products because of the kidneys' loss of concentrating power. Consequently, some patients may need to take increased amounts of fluids. On the other hand, some patients will not be able to excrete a larger volume of urine with increased intake and may develop fluid retention. The doctor will determine fluid intake by carefully watching the patient's daily intake, output, and weight and balancing these against blood chemistry levels and the presence or absence of fluid retention and signs of congestive heart failure. The discovery of peripheral edema usually indicates that the vascular system is being overloaded and fluid intake should be curtailed. If the patient is in the hospital, it becomes apparent that the nurse must take adequate measures to ensure that *all* intake and output by whatever route be carefully measured and recorded! Each hospital nursing service tends to devise its own recording system. Most important is that all persons involved in patient care *know the system* for that hospital. Who is to empty and measure the water in the patient's carafe? What is the procedure for recording intake from the food tray? In some instances, it may be best to assign the responsibility for the accuracy of the intake and output to one nurse rather than depend on several individuals following the usual floor routine. What is ultimately important is that the patient's fluids be regulated and administered according to the planned medical regime. This is a nursing responsibility and is vitally important to the patient's care.

Diet becomes another matter of great importance in the medical management of these patients. The recommended fluid and salt intake will depend on the severity and stability of the patient's condition. Should the patient lose inordinate amounts of salt in the urine, his dietary intake will be increased proportionately. Many patients will require varying degrees of salt restriction. Salt restriction, initially, may be limited to the omission of the salt shaker and of salt in food preparation. Such highly salted foods as pretzels, potato chips, or crackers will also be prohibited. Should additional restriction become necessary, foods high in sodium content (cured ham, for example) may be eliminated and low-sodium foods will be ordered. Salt restriction will necessarily become more severe as the patient shows increasing signs of water retention as evidenced by peripheral or pulmonary edema, congestive heart failure, or decreased urinary output. On the other hand, as mentioned previously, the protein intake is restricted to some degree. The carbohydrate content is increased to provide calories and energy as well as to minimize protein breakdown. As renal failure progresses and blood nitrogen levels remain intractably high, the patient may be placed on a strict high-carbohydrate, moderate-fat diet, eliminating protein completely. This diet is a combination of a concentrated sugar, butter, and peanut oil. Since it is quite unpalatable, tube feedings may be necessary. Hard candy helps to cut the oily taste if the mixture must be taken by mouth. The potassium intake is often curtailed. If so, fruit juices, particularly citrus, as well as potassium-containing salt substitutes should be omitted. Ginger ale and other carbonated beverages help to relieve nausea and the monotony of stringent dietary restrictions.

Complicating the dietary management of these patients is the fact that most are anorectic, have little desire to eat, and are even repulsed at the thought or sight of food. Consequently, forethought and ingenious planning are necessary if the desired dietary regime is to be followed. The nurse is well advised to work closely with the dietitian, the patient, and his family. Wherever possible, the patient's food preferences should be considered. Often home-cooked food brought in by the family will be eaten when hospital food would be refused. The use of salt substitutes and various condiments such as dill, oregano, mint, cinnamon, and celery seeds can improve the flavor of otherwise bland, unappetizing meals. Food should be attractively served with attention to food colors; hot food should be served hot, cold served cold! Patients are often more receptive to food served in small quantities every three to four hours. Fluids, too, may need to be scheduled to meet the desires of the patient, particularly if they are limited. Following a very restricted diet is often one of the most upsetting and difficult tasks for the patient in renal failure. He needs much assistance, support, and understanding to help him manage successfully.

Another important principle in the management of these patients is the prevention of unnecessary complications. Because of chronic anemia, they tend to be more susceptible to infection. Consequently, the patient must be protected from those who have infections, particularly of an upper respiratory nature. It is also true that these patients tire easily and are often content to merely sit or lie quietly. Exercise should be planned at frequent intervals within the limits of the patient's tolerance. Whether this exercise consists of walking short distances or merely going through passive ranges of motion, turning and positioning in bed, it is essential to ward off hypostatic pneumonia, decubiti, thrombophlebitis, and diminution in mental alertness.

When electrolyte imbalance is severe, blood nitrogen levels markedly elevated, and urinary output drastically diminished, additional considerations beyond those mentioned are necessary in planning nursing care. First, careful, frequent observation of the patient becomes vital. Drastically elevated blood urea nitrogen levels may contribute to grand mal convulsive seizures; low calcium levels to tetany. Two simple physical signs to demonstrate hypocalcemia are Trousseau's and Chvostek's signs. Trousseau's sign is demonstrated by inflating a blood pressure cuff on the patient's arm to midway between systolic and diastolic pressure for several minutes. The sign is positive if the hand goes into palmar flexion. Chvostek's sign is positive if the facial muscles can be made to twitch by lightly tapping the facial nerve just below the temple in front of the ear. Tremors or muscular twitching may be the warning signs preceding either convulsions or tetany. Their appearance should be brought immediately to the doctor's attention. Under these circumstances, it is also advisable to pad siderails and have readily available a padded tongue blade, calcium gluconate, or calcium chloride for intravenous administration and an oral suction machine and airway.

The patient must also be watched for signs of increased intracranial pressure due to cerebral edema. Of particular importance is any change in level of consciousness or steady rise in blood pressure beyond that which is normal for the patient. Treatment of cerebral edema may be by intravenous administration of hypertonic glucose solution or intramuscular or rectal injection of magnesium sulfate solution.

Increased potassium levels may first become apparent to the nurse by an irregular pulse or tachycardia. Such hyperkalemia is usually treated with cationic exchange resins, which exchange sodium ion for potassium. These resins may be given either orally or rectally by enema. When administered rectally, a prescribed amount of resin is mixed with a specific volume of water and instilled by gravity, using a funnel and rectal tube. In order for the potassium exchange to take place, the patient must retain the fluid for several hours before it is expelled. If the material cannot be expelled, a low enema may be ordered to avoid impaction. Since the bowel may quickly absorb all instilled fluid, the volume to be used should be discussed with the doctor and, once expelled, the returns measured. The amount retained may be important in adjusting the patient's fluid intake.

Patients in uremia need meticulous mouth and skin care. The mucous membranes of the mouth are usually dry, cracked, and may be covered with small, white ulcerations. The tongue may be dry and swollen, making talking and eating difficult. This nose becomes easily obstructed with secretions, causing mouth breathing and additional dryness. The patient is often too weak to cough effectively, particularly since restricted fluids contribute to thick, tenacious secretions. The frequency of mouth care should be determined by the condition of the oral mucosa. It should be often enough—hourly, if necessary—to prevent drying and encrustations. Alkaline mouth wash, glycerine-lemon juice, one-half water and one-half hydrogen peroxide, are all appropriate mixtures for mouth care. A child-size, soft, bristled toothbrush is effective for brushing the teeth and tongue. If the gums bleed easily, a gauze-protected tongue blade, or hemostat may be preferable to the toothbrush. A mild cream or water-soluble jelly helps prevent peeling and cracking of the lips. If possible, the nasal passages should be kept open, to reduce the tendency toward mouth breathing. This may be accomplished by the use of cotton-tipped applicators. Nasopharyngeal and oral suctioning may be necessary to maintain open passages, remove secretions, and stimulate coughing. This is done only as needed and as gently as possible.

Patients in uremia tend to bleed and bruise easily. Frequently they complain of generalized aches and pains. Their skin becomes extremely dry and is easily abraded. Often pruritus is severe, possibly because of increased excretion of urates through the skin. In moving and turning these patients, care must be taken to avoid undue pressure when holding or lifting the patient. A drawsheet facilitates moving and can prevent sheet "burns" over bony prominences. If at all possible, skin adhesives are avoided. Should the patients become confused, wrist and ankle restraints must be well padded and fit snugly enough to prevent chafing. Often a Posey belt is sufficient restraint without resorting to securing the extremities. A liberal use of body lotion will help to minimize skin dryness. If itching is severe, vinegar (2 tablespoons to 1 pt water) added to the bath water helps to reduce itching by dissolving urate salts. Because hemorrhage from the gastrointestinal tract is always a possibility, any blood in the stool or gastric drainage should be reported to the doctor. In chronic renal failure mercurial diuretics are contraindicated since they may cause further kidney damage. Sedatives are used as needed, but judiciously, since small amounts may have exaggerated effects. Long-acting barbiturates are avoided.

If the patient in uremia can be stabilized by dietary means and medication, he will be followed on an outpatient basis by the doctor. The nurse must make certain that he and his family fully understand the specific regimen the doctor wishes him to follow. This would include directions for taking prescribed medications, thorough diet instructions, and emphasis on the importance of keeping scheduled doctor's appointments and reporting to him immediately any untoward signs or symptoms. It is also frequently helpful to these patients to be seen in their home by the visiting nurse in order to ensure that the patient makes appropriate adaptation of the medical regime to his home situation.

Acute Renal Failure

Acute renal failure is the sudden cessation of previously normal, or at least well-compensated, renal function. The known causes for acute renal failure are innumerable. They can be classified as *prerenal, renal, and postrenal,* although there is considerable overlap in these groups. Examples of prerenal causes are circulatory failure, severe dehydration, and salt depletion. Such renal failure can be corrected easily if the underlying disorder is treated promptly before any renal damage has occurred. Postrenal factors are primarily obstructions to the urinary passages, as with bilateral ureteral calculi, pelvic cancer, and the like; the main consideration is appropriate relief of the obstruction.

Statistically the "renal" type of acute failure is common. The causes are many. They include postoperative shock, transfusion reactions, serious crush injuries, intravascular hemolysis, overwhelming infections with septicemia, and an inexhaustible list of toxins. These poisons include many metals such as lead, mercury, gold, bismuth, uranium, and arsenic. Carbon tetrachloride, methyl and phenyl alcohol, various pesticides, drugs and other organic compounds such as glycols have been incriminated. Certain antibiotics used injudiciously have probably caused renal failure. These include polymyxin, colistin, neomycin, and kanamycin. Primary renal disorders may be accompanied by acute failure. Examples are corticorenal necrosis seen in pregnancy, acute glomerulonephritis with oliguria, and the terminal stages of chronic renal disease.

The microscopic changes in the kidney of acute renal failure are a massive epithelial necrosis and slough within the tubular lining. There will be areas of actual rupture of the basement membrane of the nephron with leakage of the contents into the medullary interstitial tissue. As healing occurs, new epithelial cells will regenerate. The areas of membrane rupture will be replaced with scar tissue.

The clinical course of acute renal failure may be divided into several stages. Initially, the underlying cause is most prominent, such as an episode of hemorrhagic shock and hypotension, nausea and vomiting following ingestion of a poison, and so forth. Within a period of several hours to one or two days, there will be a significant reduction in urinary output to 400 ml (and usually less) per 24 hours. Such oliguria or anuria (less than 100 ml per 24 hours) may last up to a month. Recovery will commence with an increasing urinary output followed by diuresis and eventual stabilization of renal function.

Treatment of Acute Renal Failure

The treatment of acute renal failure is extremely complicated. A successful outcome depends on highly competent medical attention and intensive nursing care. Trite as it may sound, an ounce of prevention is certainly worth a pound of cure. One can cite many examples. The number of mismatched transfusions can be kept to a minimum providing the data on the patient's chart and the slip from the blood bank are carefully cross-checked to avoid transfusion with the wrong sample. Intravascular hemolysis can be avoided if the labels on intravenous infusion bottles are read carefully and if irrigating solutions for transurethral operations are properly prepared. The two features in the treatment of acute renal failure are treatment of its cause and treatment of the renal failure itself. A complete discussion of the subject is beyond the scope of this text but several examples will clarify the principles involved.

There is good evidence that the use of an osmotic diuretic such as mannitol soon after an ischemic episode will prevent accumulations of proteinaceous debris in the tubules. For instance, there may be temporary renal ischemia during and immediately after surgery on the aorta. A known antidote for a specific poison may be indicated, such as British anti-Lewisite (BAL) for mercury poisoning. Dialysis, which will be discussed in the following chapter, may help remove excess amounts of poison from the body. Appropriate antibiotics may be necessary to arrest an infection responsible for septicemia, shock, and renal failure.

The treatment of the oliguria has improved over recent years with understanding of the physiology of renal failure. In the past, overzealous attempts at increased fluid intake to push the kidneys into producing urine resulted in fluid retention, cardiac failure, pulmonary edema, and death. At the outset, a small aliquot of intravenous fluid (up to 1500 ml) can be given fairly rapidly with observation of urinary output. A diuretic such as mannitol or ethacrynic acid can be administered simultaneously. If there is prompt acceleration of urinary output, additional fluid can be given. If there is no response, the pathologic changes of tubular epithelial necrosis and basement membrane rupture have probably begun, and additional overloading with fluid may be hazardous.

The period of watchful waiting begins. During the period of oliguria the water intake is limited to 400 ml daily as a baseline. Added increments are given to match urinary output, and appropriate increases for other sources of fluid loss; these include gastrointestinal loss by vomiting or diarrhea, fever, excessive perspiration, or an increased respiratory rate. Signs of congestive failure from overloading of fluids are watched for, such as pulmonary edema or dependent edema. The most accurate guide to fluid retention is the patient's weight. During the oliguric period he should not gain weight and ideally should lose 0.2 to 0.3 kg per day.

Caloric requirements are met by oral feedings if at all possible during this period. Since metabolism of body protein continues during this time, and since the excretion of the nitrogenous end products of this catabolism is sorely limited, no exogenous protein is given. Instead, a diet primarily carbohydrate is used, such as Karo syrup, ginger ale, and butter balls. An adequate supply of calories in this fashion further decelerates the body protein breakdown.

The level of serum electrolytes is monitored by frequent blood determination. Acidosis is corrected by infusion of sodium bicarbonate as necessary. However, unlimited amounts cannot be used, since there is a danger of overloading with sodium. Calcium is prescribed as the gluconate salt to ward off serious tetany from falling serum calcium levels. However, sodium bicarbonate and calcium gluconate cannot be administered in the same infusion, since there will be precipitation of insoluble calcium carbonate.

The most important ion in acute renal failure is potassium. A significant rise in the serum potassium may lead rapidly to death in cardiac standstill. A serious potassium rise can be recognized by characteristic electrocardiographic changes without waiting for actual blood levels. There are good methods to control the hyperkalemia. These include the use of the sodium form of cationic exchange resins to draw out excess potassium; they may be given orally or rectally by enema. An additional emergency method is to infuse hypertonic glucose (25 to 30 per cent) with added insulin (1 unit of insulin to 2 g of glucose). The insulin drives excess potassium into body cells, thereby lowering the serum level. The patient is maintained on this conservative regimen until diuresis occurs. This may be as soon as 48 hours after renal shutdown and up to as long as 31 days. If urinary output does not increase by this time, it is most probable that irreparable damage has occurred, and the kidneys will never function adequately on their own again. During the period of watchful waiting some form of dialysis may be necessary if the aforementioned measures are insufficient.

The beginning of recovery is the appearance of an increasing urinary output, the period of diuresis, which usually lasts three to ten days. The appearance of diuresis is not a time for relaxation of vigilance, since many patients have died in electrolyte imbalance during this phase of acute renal failure. During this time large volumes of urine, up to 12 liters daily, will be excreted. The tubules have yet to recover their ability to resorb significant amounts of sodium ion, so that the urine is essentially a plasma filtrate. Adequate replacement of water, sodium, and potassium during this period is important to keep up with the obligatory loss. As the diuresis abates, the blood urea levels gradually fall toward normal. The ultimate end result may be full recovery of renal function or only a slight permanent loss.

Special Nursing Considerations

Nursing considerations in the care of the patient in acute renal failure are similar to those in chronic renal failure as regards maintenance of the patient. An additional consideration, however, will be the active treatment of the underlying cause of failure. As indicated previously, such causes may have included hemorrhage with sustained low blood pressure, septicemia from massive infection, intoxication by chemical poisons, and mechanical obstruction of the urinary tract, to name but a few. What is important, then, is that the nurse understand the rationale for the treatment of the cause of the failure. The nurse may need, therefore, to monitor blood transfusions and take frequent blood pressure readings; or the patient may recently have undergone a surgical procedure and need all the care of the immediate postoperative patient. If renal failure is caused by a drug overdose, as with barbiturates, the patient may be unconscious.

Meticulous fluid and electrolyte balance is essential in acute renal failure, as in chronic failure. In acute failure, intake will be determined by the amount of urinary output plus the estimated insensible loss and loss from other sources. These other sources may include gastric drainage by nasogastric or gastrostomy tube, urinary drainage from nephrostomy, ureterostomy, cystostomy, or urethral catheters, and wound drainage from surgical incisions. Usually in acute renal failure, the urinary output is monitored by hourly measurement and specific gravity. In the diuretic phase, the hourly volume of intake intravenously is titrated to equal the hourly volume of urinary output, because diuresis can range anywhere from 200 ml to 1 liter of urine an hour. If such large volumes of fluid are not replaced promptly, the patient can quickly go into hypovolemic shock and severe electrolyte imbalance. When such large amounts of intravenous fluids are being administered, it is particularly important that intravenous bottles be properly labeled with date and time of administration to ensure accurate recording. As kidney function returns and the kidneys regain their ability to concentrate urine, this will be reflected in an increase in specific gravity above 1.010. This may take many months.

Because of the sudden onset of acute renal failure, these patients tend to be in a precarious crisis state for a period of hours or days until renal function returns or the patient dies. Because of the intensity of observations to be made and treatments to be instituted, these patients usually, if possible, need constant nursing care. Not the least of the nurse's responsibilities during this period is the emotional support and reassurance to a very frightened patient and a worried, distraught family. Convalescence following acute renal failure is usually a matter of several months, during which time the patient may benefit from counseling by a social worker with regard to financial assistance and planning for convalescent care.*

REVIEW QUESTIONS

1. Define the following terms: uremia, azotemia, cachexia, tetany.
2. Explain the effects of chronic renal failure on the following: blood urea nitrogen, serum potassium, calcium, sodium bicarbonate, red blood cell count, bleeding and clotting time.
3. What physical signs related to the abnormalities of the above might the nurse observe? Explain the implications for nursing care.
4. Describe Trousseau's and Chvostek's signs.
5. Discuss the rationale for dietary protein restriction in the care of uremic patients.

* References for Chapters 24–26 are listed at the end of Unit IV (pages 340–41).

6. Under the following headings indicate those factors to be considered in planning nursing care, including the rationale for all nursing activity: electrolyte balance, nutrition, oral hygiene and skin care, and complications to be prevented.

CHAPTER 25
Dialysis Therapy

SIGNIFICANT strides have been made in the care of selected patients in acute or chronic renal failure by the use of dialysis techniques. These methods, based on the following physicochemical principles, are used to remove excessive amounts of noxious substances from the patient when his own kidneys are incapable of performing this function adequately.

Diffusion is the process whereby a substance dissolved in one area of a body of liquid or gas will gradually spread until it is evenly distributed throughout. This is a consequence of the random *Brownian movement* as seen with visible particles but manifested at the molecular level. Therefore, any substance in greater concentration in one area will gradually diffuse until there is uniform dispersion. The rate of diffusion depends on many variables; these include the size of the molecules, temperature, magnitude of concentration differential between two points, and the nature of the medium wherein the diffusion is occurring. Larger molecules travel more slowly than smaller ones. Their velocity increases with temperature and difference in concentration. Finally, the more liquid the medium, the more readily diffusible it becomes.

Semipermeable Membranes

Should a membrane that is freely permeable to all compounds be interposed between two solutions of differing concentrations and composition, the components of these solutions will diffuse into each other until the concentration and composition of each compartment become identical. Such a membrane would be considered completely permeable. On the other hand, if the "pores" in the membrane are of a certain critical size, smaller particles will pass selectively but not larger ones. This then becomes a *semipermeable* membrane. However, permeability is not a simple matter of pore size alone. The electrical polarity of the membrane may determine whether or not a particle can traverse it. The fat solubility of a compound may determine its permeability, depending on the membrane involved. Furthermore, different diffusible substances will penetrate a membrane at different rates when all other variables are constant.

Solutions can be divided into two classes according to the size of the solute molecules. *Crystalloids* are smaller molecules that will permeate most semipermeable membranes. These are mostly inorganic salts, amino acids, sugars, and other organic compounds of lesser molecular size. Most proteins and polysaccharides will not permeate most natural membranes and are labeled *colloids*. A membrane that permits the passage of crystalloids but not colloids is known as a *dialyzing* membrane. The renal glomerulus is a semipermeable membrane through which an ultrafiltrate of plasma is transmitted into the urinary spaces. The pores of this membrane apparently allow all plasma constituents to filter through except for most of the protein molecules.

Osmosis and Osmotic Pressure

Osmosis is the diffusion of water or other solvents through a semipermeable membrane from an area of lower concentration to one of higher concentration. The impermeability of the membrane to certain solutes prevents them from diffusing through. Consequently the higher concentration of solute on one side of the membrane will draw water from the opposite side until the concentrations on either side will become as equal as possible. This "drawing power" of the more concentrated side is known as the *osmotic pressure*. The principles of diffusion, osmosis, and osmotic pressure in semipermeable membranes are constantly effective in the living organism. These principles are utilized in any artificial system or technique used to supplant inadequately functioning kidneys.

History and Development of Dialysis Therapy

For practical application, dialysis can be performed by one of two methods. The first is to dialyze against one of the patient's own membranes. The use of cationic exchange resins by enemas to replace potassium with sodium in effect uses the colon as a dialyzing membrane. One can theoretically use the lining of isolated loops of intestine as a dialyzer by continuous lavage. However, a large area of membrane is needed to achieve much transfer, and practically speaking, the peritoneal lining is best suited for this purpose. This method is known as *peritoneal dialysis*, *peritoneal lavage*, or *peritoneal irrigation*.

The second technique is to circulate a portion of the patient's blood through some type of semipermeable tubing which is immersed in a rinsing bath of predetermined composition to draw waste material and toxins from the patient's blood. The bath is known as the *dialysis bath* and, with the materials added during dialysis, is known as the *dialysate*. The technique utilizing circulation of the patient's blood outside the body is known as *extracorporeal hemodialysis* or simply *hemodialysis*. The machines used for this purpose are popularly known to the lay public as the artificial kidney. Figure 25-1 is a schematic illustration of dialysis principles.

Historically, there is a record of an artificial kidney used in animals over half a century ago. In this initial report, the animal's blood was circulated through a cylindrical collodion tubing immersed in a rinsing

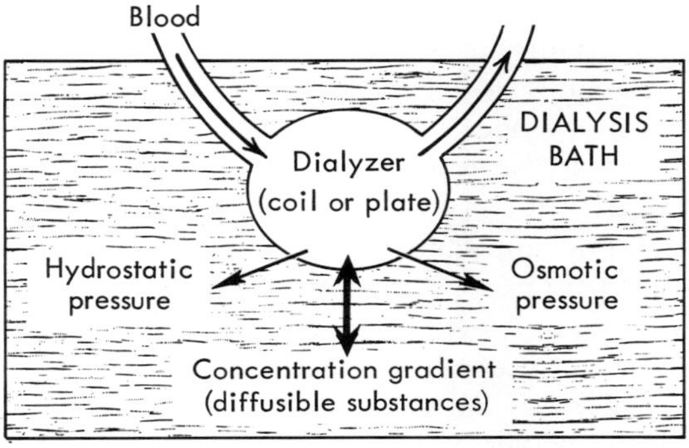

FIGURE 25-1. A schematic diagram of dialysis principles.

bath. Subsequently, various machines for human hemodialysis were designed which were dangerous, cumbersome, and inadequate. A major disadvantage of the older equipment was the need to add blood to the tubing, since a significant volume was necessary to fill the machine. In 1946 Kolff developed an artificial kidney requiring less blood and offering a larger area of dialyzing membrane. Other investigators have since fostered newer and more efficient designs. Probably the most commonly used presently are the Kolff disposable twin coil kidney and the Kiil dialyzer. With modern artificial kidneys, the volume of blood out of the patient is usually 500 ml or less. Unless the patient's blood volume is significantly diminished, there is no need to add blood to the system.

Indications and Goals of Dialysis

The aims of dialysis therapy are to remove the accumulated waste products of metabolism or dialyzable poisons from the bloodstream, to restore the electrolyte balance and pH of the circulating blood, and to withdraw excess body fluid from the patient. Among the drugs and poisons suitable for removal by this method are the barbiturates, bromides, salicylates, and thiocyanates.

The major uses of dialysis are in acute renal failure where there is a hope for eventual healing of the renal lesion and restoration of renal function and as a means to prolonging life in chronic failure. Any form of established acute tubular necrosis can be benefited, whether it be secondary to circulatory shock, "crush syndrome," transfusion reaction, or other cause. It must be reemphasized that dialysis is only supportive, and the initiating cause is treated simultaneously. Furthermore, the physician does not utilize dialysis therapy until conservative management is ineffective. However, as artificial kidney techniques improve, these methods are used earlier rather than later in the care of these patients.

Chronic or long-term dialysis has an important place in the management of certain patients in chronic renal failure. Selected patients who have no hope of recovery of renal function may be kept alive by dialysis several times weekly. Under suitable circumstances this can be performed on an outpatient basis at a chronic dialysis center or in the patient's home after a family number has been suitably instructed in the operation of the machine. The important usage of dialysis in this situation is in keeping alive the patient who is awaiting receipt of a kidney transplant from a suitable kidney donor. Dialysis may also be necessary to support the patient, if needed, during the posttransplantation period.

The chemical indications for dialysis are quite variable. Hyperkalemia often can be controlled adequately by cationic exchange resins, but if not (serum potassium greater than 7 mEq per liter), dialysis is indicated. A high blood urea nitrogen (150 mg per cent or higher) is usually an indication. More pertinent, however, is the clinical appearance of the patient. Signs of deterioration, such as decreased consciousness, coma or convulsions suggestive of increasing toxicity and acidosis, are most important.

The main contraindications to hemodialysis are a serious bleeding diathesis, particularly from the gastrointestinal tract, and circulatory instability such as severe hypotension or cardiac irregularities. Patients with septicemia often do poorly. The bleeding problem can be partially obviated by the technique of regional heparinization. Circulatory instability must be corrected by appropriate transfusions, cardiotonics, and so forth.

The chemical results of dialysis are predetermined by the composition of the dialysis bath. Urea, organic acids, and other retained products of metabolism diffuse from the blood into the bath by hydrostatic pressure. Thus such *ultrafiltration* will lower the serum levels of these substances. If the serum concentration of an electrolyte such as potassium is high, it can be decreased an intended amount by appropriately lowering its concentration in the bath. On the other hand, because of the usual acidosis, the concentration of sodium bicarbonate in the bath is raised to increase blood levels during dialysis. Concentrations of important blood constituents that are normal are kept constant by including a similar concentration in the bath. By increasing the total tonicity of the bath with dextrose to hypertonic levels, excessive edema fluid can be withdrawn from the patient.

Basic Preparations for Hemodialysis

To perform a hemodialysis, an arrangement must be made whereby arterial blood can be fed from the patient into tubing of the artificial kidney and a venous site is set up for the reentry of the dialyzed blood. This was accomplished in the past by insertion of large-bore needles or cutdowns into a vein and artery and is still suitable for a single dialysis. With the use of repeated dialysis, as in both acute and chronic renal failure, a need arose for a more practical method to connect patients to artificial kidneys.

One method is the surgical construction of a small *arteriovenous fistula* in the patient. This is accomplished by making a side-to-side anastomosis of the radial artery in the wrist to an adjacent vein under local anesthesia. Arterial blood will then travel through the fistula up the venous drainage of the arm. At dialysis, arterial blood is fed into the machine from a venipuncture proximal to the fistula. The dialyzed blood is returned to the patient through a higher venipuncture, as in the cephalic vein. After dialysis a pressure dressing is placed on the venipuncture sites for 24 hours, since these veins contain blood at arterial pressure. The advantage of the arteriovenous fistula is that it affords the patient greater mobility, as there are no indwelling tubes after the dialysis has been completed. The disadvantages include the repeated venipunctures, the possibility of infiltration during dialysis, bleeding from the puncture sites, and phlebitis.

The *arteriovenous shunt* is more commonly used. In this instance, selected Teflon tips are placed into the radial artery and an adjacent vein in the forearm. When the shunt is not being used, a short segment of Silastic tubing connects the arterial and venous cannulas (Fig. 25-2). If, after a period of time, the shunt becomes unusable, the opposite arm or a lower extremity can be utilized. The creation of an arteriovenous shunt did not become practical until relatively nonreactive materials

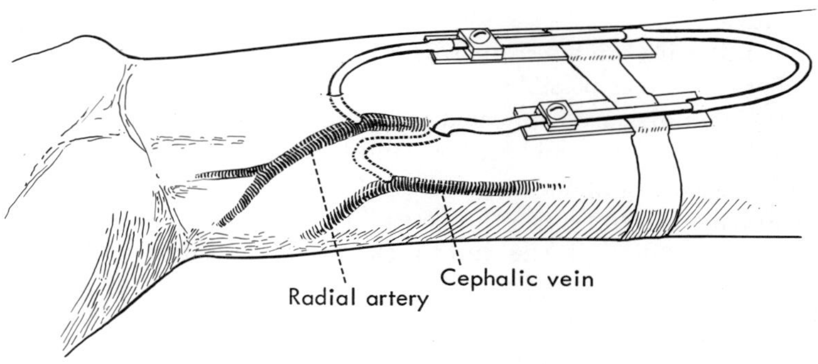

FIGURE 25-2. An arteriovenous shunt with Silastic bypass in place.

such as Teflon and Silastic became readily available. Even so, there is a significant danger of clotting in the bypasses, which would render it useless. Other inherent dangers include infection, blood leakage through exit sites, and serious hemorrhage on inadvertent separation of the external tubes or expulsion of the cannulae.

Consequently, the patient is carefully instructed in the ambulatory care of his shunt. The arm is kept clean and protected from moisture and injury at all times. When bathing, the arm should be held out of the bath. If need be, it can be wrapped in ordinary kitchen plastic wrap for further protection. This procedure is not recommended in that too tight a wrapping may induce clotting in the shunt. Heavy lifting or manual labor with this arm is avoided. The patient is instructed to examine the shunt at least every four hours for signs of infection, clotting, or bleeding. Because of the arteriovenous bypass, a prominent thrill is easily palpable in a functioning shunt. Its absence is readily noticeable and is a danger sign that blood is not circulating properly. Layering of the blood in the Silastic tubing is another sign of an impending clot, but since the tubing is translucent rather than transparent, this finding is less dependable than the absence of the thrill. Clamps should be readily available to the patient to obstruct both the arterial and venous sides of the shunt should it inadvertently come apart.

The general care of the shunt includes cleansing of each exit site and the intervening skin using a separate sterile sponge and applicator for each arm. Hexachlorophene soap is placed over each site and is wiped away in a direction away from the site. The patient must be impressed with the fact that wiping must never be toward the sites. The areas are wiped dry with sterile sponges. The exit sites are daubed with a suitable antibiotic ointment such as neomycin to reduce the likelihood of infection. Crusts can be removed with hydrogen peroxide. Gauze pads are placed above and beneath the tubing at the exit sites. Finally, an elastic bandage is wrapped around the arm, leaving the loop of the shunt visible above the dressing. The bandage is wrapped loosely, again to avoid clotting in the shunt.

When initiating and terminating dialysis, the cannulas are clamped for as short a time as possible, again with the intent of avoiding clotting. When the cannulas are connected to the dialyzing lines, the tubes must be properly aligned to avoid kinking and be so attached to the bedclothes as to afford some slack for movement of the arm or leg. All connectors are carefully taped to reduce the possibility of inadvertent separation. At the conclusion of dialysis, the shunt is cleaned as described in the previous paragraph. If, at any time, purulent exudate is noted at an exit site, a bacterial culture of this exudate is obtained. The shunt is always a potential source of serious systemic infection.

Several additional features of shunts are worth emphasizing. Initially on construction of a shunt there may be edema of the involved extremity until a collateral circulation has been established. This can be lessened by elevation of the extremity as much as possible. If a shunt has been placed in a lower extremity, weight-bearing on that leg is avoided for three weeks. Shunts are rarely placed above the level of the elbow or knee, since the volume of blood passing through the fistula may be large enough to embarrass the circulation and induce cardiac failure. Obviously, blood pressures are not taken in the cannulated arm. Venipunctures will not be necessary in most shunt patients for blood specimens, since the sample can be taken directly from the shunt itself.

Basic Details of the Artificial Kidney

The basic construction of the artificial kidney consists of a length of semipermeable tubing which is immersed in a dialyzing bath. The inflow end of the tubing is connected to the arterial side of the patient and the outflow to the venous system. Since the tubing is impermeable to bacteria, it is not mandatory that the bath be sterile. However, the solutions should be free of pyrogens and toxic substances.

The Kiil dialyzer consists of two grooved boards between which are two flat sheets of cellophane. As the boards are compressed together, the cellophane sheets form an envelope through which the patient's blood is circulated at an average rate of 150 ml per minute. The patient's own blood pressure is the propelling force in this dialyzer. Refrigerated rinsing bath is circulated around the cellophane sheets in a direction counter to the blood flow at a rate of 2 liters per minute and returned to a reservoir tank from which this solution is recirculated. The tank has a capacity of 400 liters so that the dialysate becomes considerably diluted. The blood returning to the patient is rewarmed to body temperature by immersing in warm water the tubing leading back to the patient. The Kiil dialyzer needs about 300 ml of blood to fill the cellophane tubing. Consequently, additional blood is not needed to prime the machine unless the patient is markedly hypovolemic. An external pump machine is unnecessary unless the patient is hypotensive. A disadvantage of the apparatus is that dialysis is slower than with the Kolff dialyzer. Usually a minimum of eight hours' exposure is required for an adequate dialysis.

The Kolff twin-coil dialyzer consists of two parallel lengths of cellulose tubing wound spirally as a coil within a semirigid plastic mesh support (Fig. 25-3). The coils are used once and discarded. The total length of coiled tubing is approximately 16 meters long and requires 350 to 500 ml of blood out of the patient at any one time. Smaller-capacity coils are available for use in children. An inflatable plastic cuff is used to control the blood volume in the coil. The cuff and coil sit in a metal canister through which dialyzing solution is circulated. An "inlet set" is inserted

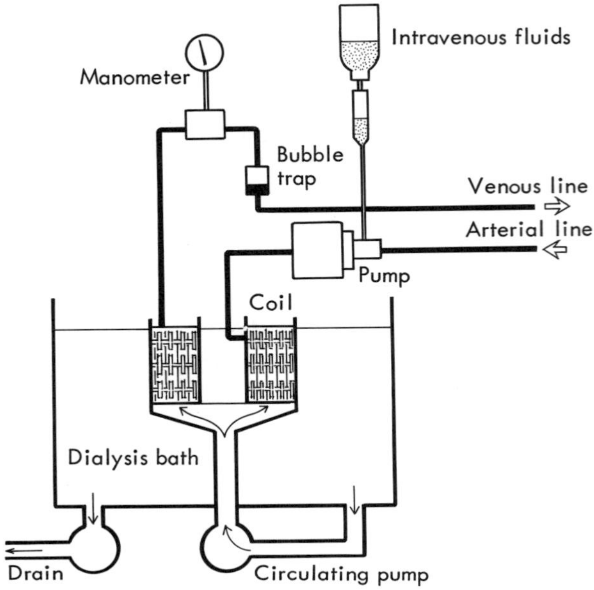

FIGURE 25-3. Schematic diagram of Kolff coil dialyzer.

between the patient's arterial cannula and the coil. The "inlet set" is threaded through a Sarns pump to give the blood a propelling force. The rate at which the blood travels through the tubing is controlled at this point. Usually the blood is propelled at 300 to 350 ml per minute. An "outlet set" is attached to the venous side where the returning blood can be observed for coagulation and where air bubbles are trapped to prevent embolization in the patient. The dialyzing bath is kept at body temperature.

To prevent clotting within the dialyzer, heparin is infused into the inlet set at the onset of dialysis and intermittently thereafter. During dialysis the patient becomes anticoagulated so that the normal Lee-White clotting time of 7 to 12 minutes is extended to as long as one hour. At the end of the procedure the patient's clotting time is allowed to return to normal spontaneously as the heparin is metabolized. In certain situations the technique of *regional heparinization* is employed. The indications for its use include postoperative patients, those with pericardial effusions, menstruating women, and patients with known or suspected bleeding, as from the gastrointestinal tract or intracranial lesions. Under these circumstances, the heparin added to the inlet tubes is neutralized with protamine sulfate at the outlet before the blood returns to the patient. The clotting times of blood from the patient and from the machine are monitored every 30 minutes. The patient's clotting time should be close to normal and that from the machine 15 to 20 minutes. The comparative features of the two commonly used dialyzers are listed in Table 25-1.

TABLE 25-1
COMPARISON OF TWO COMMONLY USED DIALYZERS

KOLFF COIL KIDNEY ("ULTRA-FLO")	KIIL DIALYZER
Urea clearance (dialysance)* = 150–210 ml/minute	Urea clearance (dialysance) = 75–100 ml/minute
4–6 hour dialysis	8–12 hour dialysis
Disposable coil	Not disposable
350–500 ml of blood for priming	No blood required for priming
Pump required	No pump required
Higher cost for each dialysis	Lower cost for each dialysis

* Dialysance defines the clearance capacity of the dialyzer.

Ultrafiltration

Excessive fluid is removed from the uremic patient during dialysis by the process of ultrafiltration, similar to what occurs in the normal glomerular membrane. This process can be accelerated by raising the pressure within the coil by tightening a screw clamp at the venous end. The rate of ultrafiltration will increase proportionately to the rise in coil resistance and pressure. This fluid withdrawal can be further enhanced by increasing the osmotic pressure in the dialysis bath. This is most commonly accomplished by adding appropriate amounts of dextrose to the bath. By simply increasing the coil pressure, as much as 10 lb of fluid can be withdrawn during a seven- to eight-hour dialysis. Therefore, weighing the patient before and after dialysis becomes quite important. Increasing the bath osmolality with dextrose seems to offset the side-effects of headache and vomiting from rapid fluid removal.

Studies During Dialysis

Blood studies are taken frequently from the patient who is being dialyzed for acute renal failure where there are rapid changes and deterioration of renal function. A hematocrit and clotting time are obtained before and after, as are blood determinations of the urea nitrogen and electrolytes. Additional studies may be ordered by the physician. Bank blood is made available by cross-matching should a transfusion be necessary during the procedure in these usually acutely ill patients.

For the stabilized patient in chronic renal failure, the following studies are obtained at weekly to monthly intervals, depending on the center: serum iron, phosphorus, calcium, alkaline phosphatase, fractionated bilirubin, transaminase, and electrolytes. An electrocardiogram is obtained monthly and a chest x-ray at less frequent intervals.

Specific Nursing Considerations

Although dialysis may be performed repeatedly in any one patient, a signed permit for the procedure should be obtained on each occasion. The first few dialyses may make the patient quite apprehensive. The patient who needs the procedure is seriously ill in the first place, and he may become frightened at the sight of the complicated-appearing apparatus in the second place. This apprehension is somewhat countered by widespread familiarity and confidence in dialysis techniques on the part of the general public by exposure from the press and television. It is not uncommon to watch chronic dialysis patients reading a magazine, watching television, or calmly taking a nap during their dialysis.

A discussion of the innumerable details pertinent to care and setting-up of equipment, management of the machinery, and so forth, is beyond the scope of this text. Detailed instruction manuals are written based on the experience of each dialysis center. However, certain salient points referable to the procedure will be discussed. The patient is weighed before and immediately after dialysis. The desired predialysis and postdialysis blood tubes and slips are prepared ahead of time. Bank blood is made ready if requested. The patient does not have to be fasting. After the dialysis has been completed, the arteriovenous shunt is reconnected, with the precautions outlined earlier in this chapter.

During the course of the dialysis vital signs are taken frequently, particularly at the start. Once these signs have stabilized, they are recorded at 30-minute intervals. The patient's fluid balance is maintained during dialysis as indicated by blood pressure levels and general condition. Blood specimens are obtained at specified intervals and heparin added as necessary to increase the clotting time. The patient is monitored to be certain that all lines flow freely and remain unkinked. Drugs, blood, and intravenous fluids are added as necessary. Clamps are readily available should any of the lines become disconnected. Pressures are adjusted in the coil as necessary. The dialysis bath is continuously observed for any signs of weakening of the wall with loss of blood into the surrounding bath. This may be a forewarning of an impending coil rupture with potentially a massive loss of blood in a short period of time. Using the Kolff kidney with a 300 to 350 ml per minute flow rate, a patient may hemorrhage significantly within a few minutes.

Problems Raised by Chronic Dialysis

The ambulatory problems of chronic dialysis patients are threefold—physical, psychologic, and socioeconomic. The physical problems are those related to a severe degree of chronic uremia; many of these patients have essentially no renal function because of the severity of their disease. Indeed, many are surgically anephric candidates for future renal transplantation. Prior to chronic dialysis therapy there were no such living patients.

Hypertension can be managed in many of these patients simply by restriction of sodium intake and removal of sodium and water during dialysis. Patients with no renal function at all are placed on a 400-mg sodium diet. Those with significant function are placed on a sodium intake commensurate with their ability to excrete sodium in the urine. At times small doses of antihypertensive medications, as described in Chapter 24, are necessary. The protein intake is kept at 40 g daily. The bone and joint problems related to calcium deposition are fairly well controlled with basic aluminum hydroxide gels. The peripheral neuropathies may be particularly troublesome; no effective treatment for this disabling complication is available. Sexual impotence is disturbingly common. The anemia of chronic uremia is seemingly well tolerated if the hematocrit is kept above 22 to 26 per cent by occasional transfusions of packed red blood cells as necessary.

The chronic dialysis patient has his share of psychologic problems. He realizes that he is living on "borrowed time." He has to depend on a machine to which he must be connected for six to eight hours at least twice weekly. He probably has an arteriovenous cannula in an extremity which requires constant care—a connection that may clot off at any time, separate with serious hemorrhage, or become infected. He is dependent on other people to help him. He may have financial worries.

There is presently enough experience in chronic hemodialysis patients to anticipate these problems and their management. Relatively well-motivated patients are chosen for these programs. The total cooperation of other members of the family, physicians, nurses, and social workers is vitally important.

The cost of dialysis is a major consideration. The average cost will be between $15,000 and $20,000 yearly for the chronic patient. With home dialysis the cost, after purchase of an artificial kidney, can be brought down to almost $5,000. Approximately 5,000 to 10,000 new patients will be available yearly who may be considered potential candidates for dialysis programs. Presently there are facilities for no more than 20 per cent of these candidates.

At this writing, the "state of the art" has advanced to the point that dialysis is primarily a nursing function of a highly specialized nature. In a well-organized dialysis unit, medical supervision becomes primarily of an advisory nature. The specially trained nurse will manage the routine dialysis by herself. The next logical step is becoming a reality. Under suitable circumstances dialysis can be performed in the home by a trained member of the family. The patient returns to the dialysis center once monthly for blood chemistries and general evaluation.

Peritoneal Dialysis

As discussed previously, the peritoneum can be utilized as an inert, semipermeable membrane for dialysis. It allows transfer of water and crystalloids, depending on their concentration on either side of the membrane, and is impermeable to proteins and larger molecules. Although the peritoneum is permeable to dextrose, this permeability is a relative matter. Therefore, solutions containing sufficient quantities of dextrose to make them hypertonic can be used for the removal of more rapidly traveling water and electrolyte molecules.

This method has the advantage that no complicated and expensive equipment is needed, and the procedure can be performed at the bedside rather than in a highly specialized dialysis unit staffed with highly specialized personnel. However, the technique has its drawbacks. The efficiency of dialysis per unit time is much less than with the artificial kidney machine, and a single dialysis may take 36 hours. However, since this is a slower process, biochemical problems from rapid changes in blood chemistry are much less common. On the other hand, there is a limit to the number of peritoneal dialyses that can be performed in any one patient—usually no more than 15 or 20 on an average, although there are some patients who have had as many as 50 or 60 dialyses. In general, this method is often not suited to the long-term, chronic dialysis patient. Finally, a recent intraabdominal operation and the presence of numerous intraperitoneal adhesions or peritonitis are relative contraindications to the use of this technique.

Technique of Peritoneal Dialysis

Peritoneal dialysis is performed by inserting dialyzing solution into the peritoneal cavity, allowing it to equilibrate with the patient's extracellular fluids, and removing the dialysate. Each cycle is known as an *exchange*, repeated enough times until dialysis is completed. The greatest equilibration across the peritoneal membrane occurs within the first hour and approaches the maximum amount by two hours. Therefore, a longer exposure during each exchange does not increase the efficiency of dialysis. Usually, 20 to 25 exchanges are necessary for a complete dialysis.

Initially, a midline paracentesis is performed under aseptic conditions. Written consent is required for the entire procedure. A plastic trochar is inserted through the abdominal wall into the peritoneal cavity, through which a plastic catheter is threaded and the trochar removed. The patient is either fasting or allowed only a small aliquot of water beforehand. The bladder must be emptied by either normal voiding or urethral catheterization. Although semipermanent cannulas have been devised from time to time for patients on chronic peritoneal dialysis, they have found little popularity. These catheters tend to become occluded by adhesions after a period of time and seem to offer little advantage over repeated paracenteses.

Once the catheter is secured in place, it is connected under sterile conditions by means of a Y tube to two suspended single liters of dialyzing solution prewarmed to body temperature. The solution is allowed to flow into the patient by gravity. This usually takes 10 to 15 minutes. After the two-hour exchange time has elapsed, the dialysate is drained by gravity to empty bottles on the floor (Fig. 25-4). New bottles of dialyzing solution are suspended and the cycle is repeated. Many clinicians add heparin to the solution, particularly at the outset of instillation to impede the precipitation of fibrinous deposits on the eyes of the catheter which may interfere with the free flow of fluid. Antibiotics are added to decrease the likelihood of peritonitis. Any antibiotic to which a patient gives a history of hypersensitivity is not used. Those agents, such as neomycin, that may be toxic if absorbed in significant quantities are avoided.

Solutions

The solutions used for peritoneal dialysis basically differ in their osmolality (determined by their dextrose concentrations) and the presence or absence of potassium salts. One and one-half per cent and 7 per cent dextrose solutions are commercially available. The former is used when the main aim of the dialysis is the removal and readjustment of solutes. The latter, more hypertonic solution is used when removal of excess accumulated body fluid is desired. All solutions for peritoneal dialysis are hypertonic to body fluids but vary only in degree. The concentration of electrolyte in these solutions is similar to normal body fluid except for the absence of potassium ion. If the patient is not hyperkalemic, potassium can be added. In most instances of renal failure there will be some need to lower the serum potassium levels, however. A small amount of bicarbonate or lactate is added to these solutions, since the patient is usually acidotic. The concentration of dextrose can be tailored as necessary by suitable mixtures of the commercially available solutions.

Specific Nursing Considerations

At the initiation of dialysis, the nurse suspends the prewarmed solution on an infusion stand, marks the fluid level in the inverted bottles with pencil or tape, fills the tubing, and attaches it to the Y tube and intra-

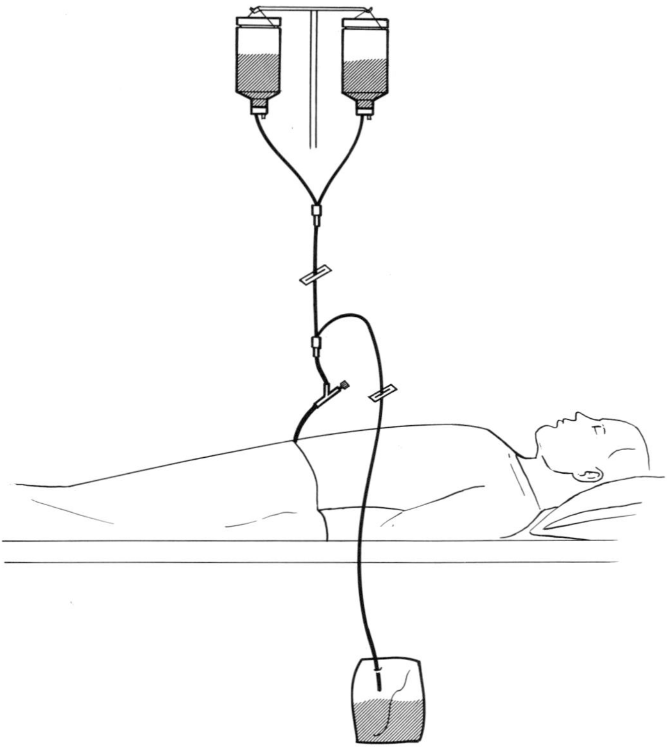

FIGURE 25-4. A typical setup for peritoneal dialysis.

peritoneal catheter. The solution is allowed to flow in while the patient is observed for any signs of abdominal pain or respiratory embarrassment. The blood pressure and pulse are recorded every 15 minutes until they stabilize, then every 30 minutes thereafter. If the markedly hypertonic solutions are used (7 per cent), the observations are taken every 15 minutes continuously because of the possibility of impending shock from too rapid fluid removal. After the fluid has run in, the tubing is clamped while there is fluid in it to preserve a siphon effect for later emptying and drainage of the intraabdominal dialysate. Usually the fluid will flow freely at the end of the exchange. If the flow is not free, drainage may be facilitated by turning the patient from side to side. At times, it will be necessary for the doctor to manipulate the intraperitoneal catheter to allow drainage.

During dialysis the patient remains supine in bed, although his head may be elevated to a 45-degree angle to relieve any discomfort or res-

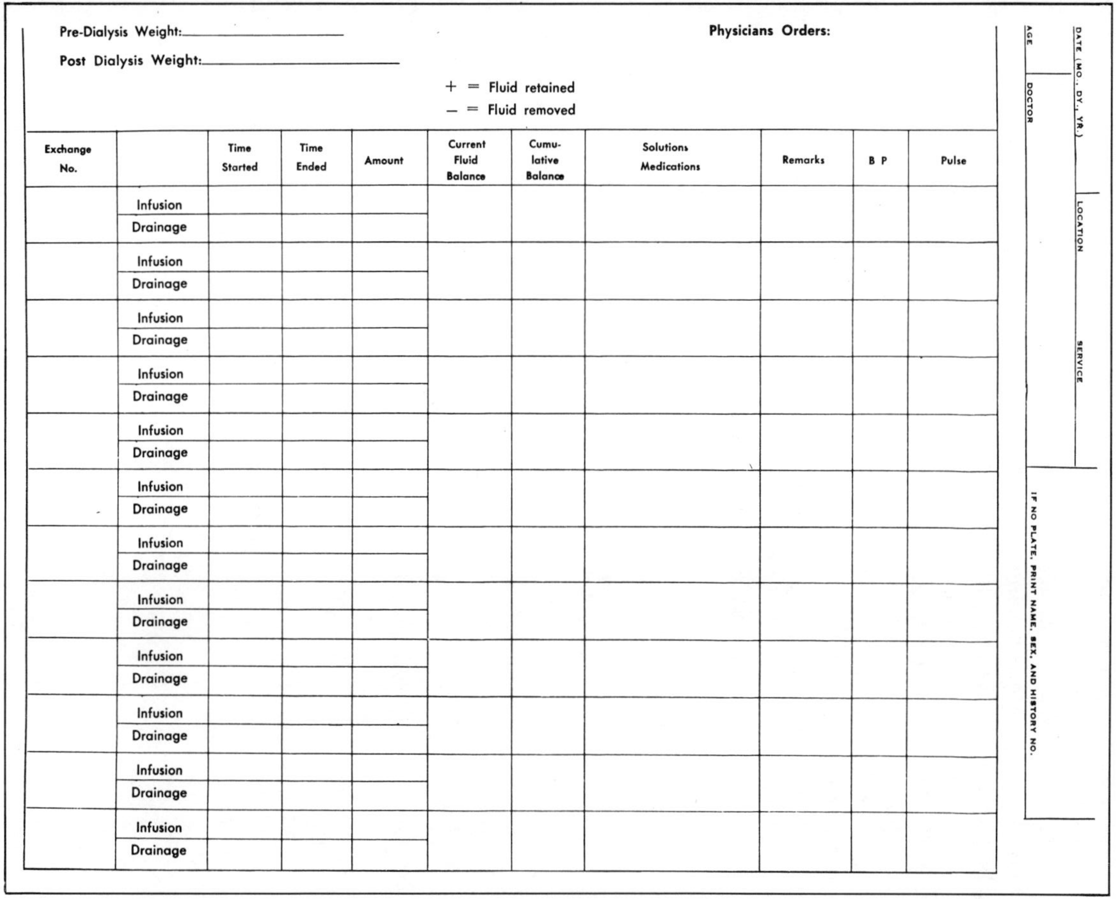

DATE (MO., DY., YR.) | LOCATION | SERVICE

AGE | DOCTOR

IF NO PLATE, PRINT NAME, SEX, AND HISTORY NO.

Pre-Dialysis Weight:______

Post Dialysis Weight:______

+ = Fluid retained

− = Fluid removed

Physicians Orders:

Exchange No.		Time Started	Time Ended	Amount	Current Fluid Balance	Cumu-lative Balance	Solutions Medications	Remarks	B P	Pulse
	Infusion									
	Drainage									
	Infusion									
	Drainage									
	Infusion									
	Drainage									
	Infusion									
	Drainage									
	Infusion									
	Drainage									
	Infusion									
	Drainage									
	Infusion									
	Drainage									
	Infusion									
	Drainage									
	Infusion									
	Drainage									
	Infusion									
	Drainage									
	Infusion									
	Drainage									
	Infusion									
	Drainage									

FIGURE 25-5. The standard peritoneal dialysis record sheet used at The New York Hospital–Cornell Medical Center.

piratory embarrassment from the pressure of the fluid. Careful attention is paid to all the patient's basic nursing needs—prescribed medications are given on time, blood specimens as necessary are obtained. The nurse must be most careful to note changes in vital signs or the level of consciousness, particularly when the more hypertonic dialyzing solutions are used. Most important is a careful record of volumes of fluid instilled and removed during the exchanges. A small error over a period of many exchanges may add up to quite a volume of fluid. Each hospital will have its own method of recording intake and output during peritoneal dialysis. Whatever the method might be, *know the system*! A copy of the standard peritoneal dialysis record used at The New York Hospital–Cornell Medical Center is shown in Figure 25-5.

At the conclusion of the dialysis the peritoneal catheter is withdrawn and a sterile dressing is applied over the puncture site. The wound is observed for any signs of bleeding. The abdomen is watched for signs of distention or peritonitis. Routinely, a culture is taken from the last exchange of the dialysate.

REVIEW QUESTIONS

1. Discuss the physicochemical principles on which dialysis therapy is based.
2. Describe the indications and goals of dialysis in acute renal failure; in chronic renal failure.
3. Differentiate hemodialysis and peritoneal dialysis.
4. Describe the arteriovenous shunt, its purpose, care, and possible complications.
5. What are the advantages and disadvantages of the Kolff versus the Kiil dialyzer?
6. What is meant by regional heparinization?
7. Describe the technique of peritoneal dialysis.

CHAPTER 26
Renal Transplantation

THE replacement of a worn-out, deteriorated organ by transplantation with a normally functioning one has been an age-old dream of mankind. At this writing, the spectacular implantation of a human heart, lung, or liver from one individual to another is highly experimental. On the other hand, kidney transplantation is meeting with enough success to approach practical reality for many patients with terminal renal disease.

Many factors are involved in successful renal transplantation. These include the suppression of rejection of the graft by the host, the availability of suitable donors, technical factors related to surgery, and the availability of a functioning dialysis unit and a capable team of surgeons, internists, and nursing specialists.

Technical Aspects

The transplanted kidney is nearly always inserted in a *heterotopic* position—i.e., one other than the normal renal location. The site used most often is the contralateral iliac fossa (Fig. 26-1), although it is technically possible to place the kidney on the same side. Among the reasons for not using the natural renal bed (*orthotopic* transplant) are problems concerning the blood supply to a long transplanted ureter, topographic arrangements regarding the vascular anastomoses, frequent disease in the renal site of the donor, and the necessity for simultaneous nephrectomy and implantation. The normal relationships of the kidney, front to back, are vein, artery, and pelvis. At implantation of a kidney, the organ is usually reversed 180 degrees, that is, turned over (left kidney to right iliac fossa, and vice versa), so that the pelvis is most anterior. The renal artery is anastomosed to a neighboring artery, usually the hypogastric, and the vein to the external iliac vein. By implanting as a mirror image, there is less likelihood of kinking and pressure on the ureter. The ureter is implanted into the bladder in such a fashion as to prevent reflux but to permit free downward flow of urine. The Paquin method previously described in this text, or modifications thereof, is commonly used. In the majority of situations the vascular anastomoses can be completed within 30 to 45 minutes after the donor kidney has been removed. If there is more than one renal artery, each artery must be anastomosed to the

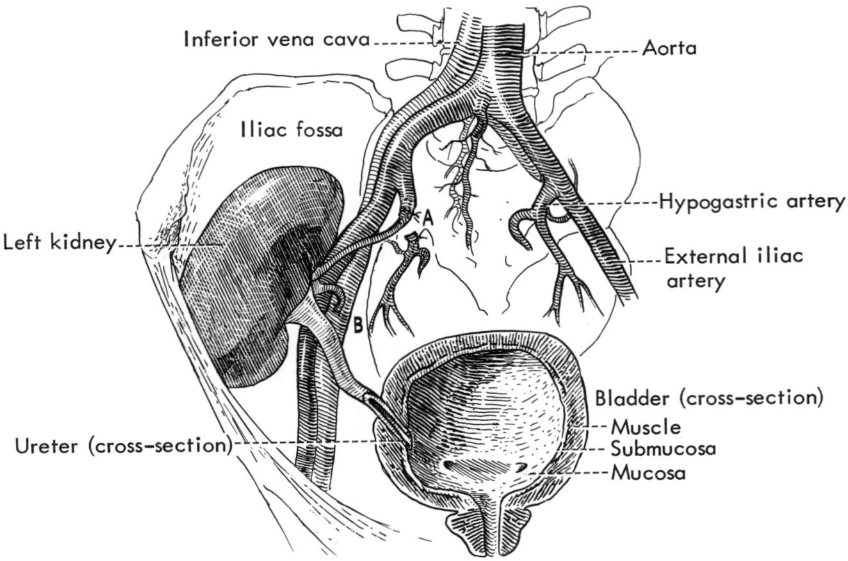

FIGURE 26-1. Relationships of a transplanted kidney. *A*, renal artery to hypogastric artery (end-to-end anastomosis); *B*, renal vein to external iliac vein (end-to-side anastomosis).

recipient's arteries, since the renal arterial supply is segmental. If one of the multiple renal arteries is ligated, the subtended renal parenchyma will become infarcted. However, the venous channels have multiple collaterals within the kidney. Consequently, when multiple renal veins are present, all but the largest ones can be ligated safely, and venous drainage of the entire kidney will be adequate.

The method by which urinary tract drainage is handled varies from center to center. For reasons to be discussed later, the transplant recipient is highly susceptible to infection. Consequently, many surgeons choose to keep foreign bodies in the urinary tract to the minimum by attempting watertight closure of the urinary tract, relying on an indwelling urethral catheter as the sole means of urinary drainage. On the other hand, some will employ cystostomy, ureterostomy, and nephrostomy tubes liberally, arguing that the risks of infection will be outweighed by the advantages of reliable unobstructed drainage.

The initial technical problems related to renal transplantation in man were settled during a series of transfers of kidneys between identical twins (isotransplants). These operations were performed in the relatively rare circumstances of a patient with end-stage renal disease who had an identical, healthy, and willing twin. It soon became evident that such transfers could be accomplished with almost uniform success and that the transplanted kidney would function normally. An interesting and unexpected result of isotransplant has been the occasional later development in the recipient of his original idiopathic disease, glomerulonephritis—and indeed even in the healthy donor! It is also technically feasible to move a patient's own kidney (autotransplant), to eliminate a gap in the ureter or to attach the kidney to better vessels, for example.

Graft Rejection

After most technically successful transplantations, the implanted kidney will begin to function promptly. There may be an immediate diuresis or the function may increase gradually. When the transfer has been made between identical twins, the donor kidney should function indefinitely without further specific treatment. However, if there is dissimilarity between the donor and recipient, the host's immune mechanisms will begin to react against the donor's foreign tissues. This usually occurs catastrophically in a matter of minutes if the donor and recipient are of different species (heterotransplant); but if they are of the same species (homotransplant), the reaction tends to be much slower, albeit variable. The kidney becomes infiltrated with chronic inflammatory cells, particularly lymphocytes. The renal tubular epithelium becomes necrotic, and thrombosis occurs in the smaller blood vessels of the kidney. This process is known as *rejection.* Clinically the rejection process is manifested by fever, a sharp decrease in urinary output, increasing proteinuria, and marked leukocytosis.

There is considerable evidence demonstrating the lymphoid cells of the host to be principal carriers of the immune mechanism. For this reason, some physicians have removed lymphoid masses such as spleen or thymus as part of the transplantation regimen, hoping such removals will alter the immune response of the host. For the same reason, attempts have been made to reduce the circulating lymphocytes by cannulation of the thoracic duct or by whole body radiation.

Selection of Donor Kidneys

There are many considerations in the selection of a suitable donor kidney. The most important is demonstration of enough antigenic similarity between donor and recipient to forecast a reasonable acceptance of the graft.

The first step in determining the relative compatibility of donor and recipient is identification of their blood types. Using the AB, A, B, O grouping system, donor and recipient must be of either the same or compatible blood groups. If this be the case, sera and cells of potential donor and recipient are cross-matched against each other. If there is agglutination between the two (positive cross-match) successful transplantation is most improbable in present experience.

If there is no reaction up to this point, donor and recipient are studied for various histocompatibility antigens present in the cells by means of *tissue typing*. A number of antigens (at least 11 are recognized) have to do with tissue rejection by formation of antibodies in the host.

If one of these antigens is present in the donor but not in the recipient, a major incompatibility exists, since the donor kidney will usually stimulate antibody production (and hence rejection) by the host. If more than one of these antigens is present in the donor and absent in the recipient, the severity of major incompatibility becomes greater. Conversely, a minor incompatibility is the presence of an antigen in the recipient that is absent in the donor. This is of relatively little importance since the donor does not reject the recipient. To study for the presence of these antigens, whole blood is processed through various steps until the lymphocytes are obtained as a separate aliquot. Groups of lymphocytes are incubated with the available antisera against the recognized antigens.

On the basis of such typing, donors and recipients can be matched against each other and a prognostic statement can be made regarding the likelihood of success. The results are classified as either *A*, *B*, *C*, or *D* matches. An *A* match represents antigenically identical twins who should not reject at all. A *B* match is one with no major incompatibility but any number of minor ones. A *C* match indicates only one major incompatibility; and *D*, two or more. At present, *D* and most *C* matches are usually absolute contraindications to a prospective transplantation.

A second important consideration is whether the kidney is obtained from a living donor or a fresh cadaver. The higher success rate, other factors being equal, follows the use of a kidney from a healthy living donor. However, the donor must undergo a painful operation which not only is unnecessary for his own well-being, but actually poses a threat to it. Fortunately, there have, thus far, been no immediate deaths in over 1000 living human donors. He must realize that he will have only one kidney to live on and that the transplantation has no guarantee of success to the recipient. The moral implications of such a sacrifice are complex; but it is generally agreed acceptable to give up a part to save the whole, and the mere fact of the extraordinary feature does not *ipso facto* indicate immorality.

Similarly, there is no need to overemphasize the problems peculiar to obtaining cadaver organs. For reasonable success, the kidney should be removed from the deceased as quickly as possible after death has occurred. The religious, legal, and medical considerations in defining the moment of death have assumed greater seriousness now that some of the dead person's tissue may be of value to living recipients. That "death" of all tissues does not occur simultaneously has raised significant problems. The cause of death in the donor is another factor. There have been instances of transplantation of cancer involving the donor kidney, for example. An ideal situation is when the deceased is a basically healthy individual who has died from an accidental injury such as a gunshot wound to the head.

Preoperative Considerations

A willing, potential donor who has been found to be antigenically suitable by typing methods undergoes a complete medical evaluation prior to operation. There should be no antecedent history of urinary tract disease. After demonstration of normal urinary tracts by pyelography, urinalysis, and total renal function studies, a renal arteriogram is made. The discovery of unrecognized arterial abnormalities, such as disease of the donor's renal arteries or multiple small arteries, may disqualify the donor. If the findings of these investigations are favorable and it is deemed the present and future risks of nephrectomy are no greater than that of the operation itself, the patient is accepted as a donor.

The preoperative preparation of the recipient includes an evaluation of his lower urinary tract. Obstructive uropathy, congenital or acquired, is best corrected prior to transplantation. The commonest congenital abnormality has been significant bladder outlet obstruction which has often been the direct cause for uremia. If there is obstructive prostatic enlargement, an appropriate corrective operation on the prostate is performed. Dialysis therapy, as needed, is employed during the preoperative and postoperative period. Bilateral nephrectomy may be done prior to, during, or after the transplantation operation. Pretransplantation nephrectomy is being done more commonly now, particularly since hypertension from the patient's underlying renal disease is easier to control afterward, and in some instances the patient's own kidneys may be a source of infection, especially during later immunosuppressive therapy. Many anephric patients have been kept alive by chronic (repeated) hemodialysis while awaiting a suitable donor, sometimes for months. During the day prior to operation, the planned immunosuppressive medications are begun and blood transfusions, if needed, are administered. If thoracic duct cannulation is to be used, the patient must be on reverse isolation, since, as his lymphocytes are removed, his resistance to infection is lowered.

Procedure During Operation

The operations are preferably performed in adjacent operating rooms. The operation on the recipient is begun first, during which time the vessels in the intended new home for the transplant are isolated and made ready for anastomosis. As this preparation progresses, the surgeon and anesthesiologist can judge how well the recipient, who is the poor risk and the weak link in the chain, will tolerate the procedure.

Accordingly, there is some leeway in canceling the elective operation on the donor should the recipient do poorly on the operating table. A selected person, either a physician or a nurse, is given the sole responsibility of communication between the two operating teams.

At the appropriate time, the recipient's surgeon will direct the donor team to begin the nephrectomy. The donor kidney is completely mobilized by delicate dissection to avoid unnecessary bruising. The renal artery and vein are dissected to their origins. The ureter is freed for an appropriate length with care to include as much periureteric fat as possible to preserve the ureteral blood supply. A few minutes before the recipient surgeon is ready for the donor kidney, he notifies the second team to complete the nephrectomy. The donor surgeon divides the ureter, after which the renal artery and vein are divided. In contrast to routine nephrectomy, clamps or ties are placed only on the donor's side of these vessels to retain maximum length for the recipient's surgeon to work with and to avoid damage to their delicate intima.

This kidney is next perfused with cold Ringer's lactate solution containing heparin and procaine. The perfusion into the artery continues (usually a minute or two) until the venous effluent is clear. This maneuver serves several purposes. By using a cold solution, the metabolism of the kidney is slowed, thus decreasing the effects of ischemia until the circulation is reestablished. By washing out the contained blood and instilling heparin, the degree of clotting within the vascular tree of the kidney will be diminished. The procaine acts to diminish vascular spasm.

The implantation of the kidney into the recipient is then accomplished by the technique described earlier in this chapter.

If the donor kidney is obtained from a cadaver, the organization necessarily varies depending on the circumstances. The kidneys are removed as soon as possible after death has occurred. The circulation and oxygenation of the kidneys are usually maintained by a heart-lung machine before and during the removal. In contrast to transplantation from a living donor, it is often difficult to have a suitably matched recipient ready at the time the cadaver kidney is available. A potential partial solution to this problem is the development of portable self-powered perfusion equipment which can be transported to the cadaver. The kidneys are inserted into sterile chambers and richly oxygenated, and cooled plasma is perfused through the kidneys with a pulsatile flow. Using this machinery, cadaver kidneys have been kept viable and usable for as long as 17 hours prior to implantation in the recipient.

Immunosuppressive Therapy

The key to long-term success of renal transplantation, other than in identical twins, is the control (or suppression) of the host's immune defense mechanisms. The donor kidney has a constant circulation of the recipient's blood, and the interface between the two is immense. Contrastingly, corneal grafts, which have a high success rate, have no blood circulation from the recipient, being supported by exchange of tissue fluids.

Any measures used to suppress the host's immune mechanisms interfere with his ability to fight infections (both a donor kidney and invading bacteria are foreign bodies). Total body irradiation to the reticuloendothelial system has been too drastic, so it is little used now. Splenectomy and thymectomy have not been proven useful. Thoracic duct cannulation for removal of lymphocytes is still used occasionally; but the duct cannula tends to malfunction, and the processing of the lymph and its reinfusion are cumbersome.

The most practical immunosuppressive agents now available are azathioprine (Imuran), steroids (cortisone and related compounds), and antilymphocyte serum (ALS), usually in some combination. Azathioprine interferes with nucleic acid synthesis, and therefore antibody formation, by the host. Presently it is being used indefinitely in the posttransplant patients for its immunosuppressive effects. The dosage is determined in part by its effect on the patient's white cell count, since an overdosage will depress the count to dangerously low levels. During a rejection episode the white count may rise to 40,000 or 50,000 per cubic millimeter, and an appropriately higher dosage is prescribed. The drug can be administered by mouth or intravenously.

The use of massive doses of steroids—in the form of prednisone, up to 400 mg daily, in conjunction with azathioprine—has diminished the severity of rejections more than either drug alone. The effect of steroids used as the sole immunosuppression is not great. With massive steroid therapy there is a significant risk of gastrointestinal bleeding from stress ulcers. This complication can be significantly prevented by the use of a strict ulcer regimen as for ordinary peptic ulcers.

Antilymphocyte serum (ALS) has been known to scientists since the turn of the century, but interest in it has been reawakened because of its immunosuppressive effect. ALS is an antiserum formed by one species to the lymphocytes of another. In this instance human lymphoid cells are injected into a horse, who in turn produces the antiserum. Up to the present, the supply of ALS has been limited, but preliminary experience with this material in transplantation patients has been encouraging. The antiserum produced is a complex one, since the initiating lymphocytes contain many antigens. ALS causes the destruction of circulating lymphocytes. The effect of a single treatment with ALS lasts about 50 days, the time the recipient needs to form a new supply of circulating lymphocytes. ALS is interesting in that it seems to be just as effective when there is a significant antigenic disparity between donor and host as when they are closely related. This is in contrast to azathioprine and steroids, which are much less effective when there are considerable antigenic differences. All of these immunosuppressives are in development stages and not fully assessed, especially concerning long maintenance therapy.

Results of Renal Transplantation

As of 1969, there had been 2347 kidney transplants reported to the Human Kidney Transplant Registry. This figure represents the majority of transplants performed worldwide up to that time. The following statistics refer to transplant survival rather than to patient survival, since if a transplantation is successful, the recipient can be kept alive afterward by chronic hemodialysis until another kidney is available.

Presently about one half of the donor kidneys have been obtained from living donors who are usually closely related to the recipient (such as a parent or a sibling). The other half are supplied by unrelated cadavers. The present estimated one-year transplant survival from an identical twin or sibling is 91 per cent, from a parent 83 per cent, other blood relative 67 per cent, and a cadaver 42 per cent. The overall one-year transplant survival from related living donors is 87 per cent. The two-year survival of related living donor kidneys is 77 per cent, and from the cadaver, 40 per cent. The longest surviving transplant from an identical twin is 12 years, and fraternal twin 10 years. Significant long-term data on closely related donors and cadaver implants are not available, since this type of transplantation has been performed in large numbers only during the past few years. The data on renal homotransplant survival are summarized in Table 26-1.

Table 26-1
Renal Homotransplant Survival

DONOR	1-YEAR SURVIVAL	2-YEAR SURVIVAL
Related, living	87%	77%
Cadaver	42%	40%

Specific Nursing Considerations

As emphasized previously, the patient who has reached a point in his kidney disease where repeated dialyses are necessary to sustain life is seriously ill. He relies constantly on the availability of an artificial kidney, personnel who can operate such machinery, and a functioning arteriovenous shunt, to name a few of the factors in his continuing existence. A successfully functioning transplanted kidney in such a patient offers the prospect of a future life accompanied by a greater sense of well-being and a relative independence as compared to the chronic dialysis patient.

There are innumerable stumbling blocks to success. These begin at the point when transplantation is first considered. A suitable donor kidney must be available. The best results are obtained when a kidney from a close relative is used. Consequently, the period during which related volunteers are screened by various typing methods for compatibility with the recipient is emotionally difficult for the entire family until the best prospect is selected. After this, the selected individual must prepare for additional examinations in the hospital, as described previously. Finally, the future donor must prepare himself to undergo a painful operation which is entirely voluntary. If a living donor is not available, the chronic dialysis patient lives a life of uncertainty, not knowing when a suitable cadaver kidney will appear, if ever.

A few of the areas of mishap during the transplantation operation, and its immediate postoperative complications, have been alluded to earlier in this chapter. Control of the rejection process not only is crucial to success during the hospital stay but is a factor in the continuing ambulatory care of these patients. Therefore, since these patients need medical care indefinitely, and since the procedures still fall in the realm of experimental medicine, the *team approach* to the care of these patients has been most worthwhile. In this instance, the team includes, along with the patient, a group of doctors and nurses who specialize in the management of dialysis and renal transplantation. Other members of the team will include the social worker, dietitian, and physical and occupational therapists. Dialysis is more often than not important, not only in the preoperative but also in the subsequent regulation of the patients with related electrolyte management problems in the posttransplantation period. During his time on repeated dialysis, the pretransplant patient will become well acquainted with the members of the team. He is encouraged to visit the transplant clinic where he can meet with other patients who have received kidneys. Often these relationships are a source of support and encouragement, for both the patient and his family. However, it becomes important for both nurses and doctors of the team to help the patient understand how his condition may differ from that of another, particularly to avoid mistaken comparisons in the face of another's setback.

Preoperative Preparations

The recipient and donor are admitted to the hospital several days prior to surgery. If the donor has undergone complete evaluation of his suitability at a previous admission, only routine studies will be needed preoperatively. Preparation of the recipient is more extensive. The blood volume is measured and appropriate lymphocyte-poor blood transfusions are given to reach optimum preoperative levels. A coagulation work-up is obtained to recognize possible bleeding tendencies. Baseline blood chemistries are obtained. Often a last preparatory dialysis is performed on the recipient 48 hours prior to operation. The blood and urine are cultured preoperatively and the stool tested for occult blood. Baseline x-rays of lamina dura of the teeth, distal clavicles, and hands are obtained for postoperative comparison to evaluate osteoporosis from prolonged steroid therapy.

Since transplantation surgery is experimental, accompanied by a risk, and no guarantee of success, the doctor will meet with the patient, the donor, and their families, either immediately before or after their admission to the hospital. The doctor explains the nature, risk, and related facets of the intended operations. In addition to the regular operative permit, a special permission form is signed by both donor and recipient, witnessed by the doctor and a notary public. The pertinent section of this form reads, "It is clearly understood by all parties to this instrument that no representations have been made to any of us regarding the success of attempted transplant, and we fully understand that said transplant is in the nature of an experiment and is being performed in the hope of saving the life of the recipient."

In addition to the usual preoperative instructions related to an extensive abdominal operation and urinary drainage systems, the patient is advised regarding the rationale and mechanism for reverse isolation techniques. Only members of the transplant team directly involved in his care will be allowed in the room. All will wear gown and masks. The patient is reassured to know that a nurse will be in constant attendance during the first few postoperative days. His family cannot visit directly, but he will be able to see them through the windows of his room.

Reverse Isolation

With the crippling of body defense mechanisms against bacteria by the use of immunosuppressive agents, the chronically ill patient who undergoes renal transplantation is particularly susceptible to infection. During the postoperative period, the patient is protected by being placed on a strict reverse isolation program. This period will vary from a minimum of five days to as long as two weeks. The walls and floor of the patient's single room are scrubbed down with a bactericidal solution prior to his return from the recovery room. The floor is mopped with the antiseptic every eight hours thereafter. The room is dusted with a damp cloth once daily. All personnel entering the room are gowned and masked after a surgical scrub. A bactericidal spraying of shoes is required. Those persons with any infection, particularly of the upper respiratory tract, must stay away from the patient. Materials brought into the room are appropriately sprayed whenever feasible. The door to the room is kept closed at all times.

The room should be well stocked with equipment and medications likely to be needed in the postoperative care. These include an adequate supply of intravenous solutions, syringes, dressings, containers for collecting and measuring urine, and other drainage and urine-testing equipment. Oxygen, suction, and an accurate bed scale should be there for use with the individual patient. Emergency medications should be immediately available in the unit. Particularly needed may be those used for control of hypotension, hypertension, convulsions, and electrolyte imbalance. Forethought in stocking the room not only serves to reduce the nurse's activity but will ensure fewer breaks in isolation technique, with greater safety for the patient.

Postoperative Care

Regulation of fluid and electrolyte balance assumes great importance in posttransplantation patients. During the first 24 to 48 hours, a massive diuresis of a liter or more per hour is not unusual. Such a diuresis is more common from kidneys from living related donors. This initial output is almost a pure glomerular filtrate. Dangerously large amounts of sodium and potassium can be excreted in a short time. Unless there is prompt replacement of the fluid volume and electrolytes lost in the urine, the patient may go rapidly into shock and die. On the other hand, the reverse situation may occur. It is not uncommon for cadaver kidneys to go into a period of acute renal failure lasting several weeks before there is significant function. In such situations, appropriate fluid restrictions, dialyses, and proper supportive therapy are required until the transplanted organ begins to function adequately.

As soon as feasible, a baseline weight of the patient is obtained. Daily weights are obtained using the technique described in the section on post-radical cystectomy care (see Chapter 20). During the first 72 hours (or longer, if massive diuresis continues) the urinary output is measured every 30 minutes, nasogastric drainage every 4 hours, and drainage on the dressings (by weight) every 8 hours. The volume of any irrigating solution used must be measured and deducted from the totals for the sake of accuracy. Periodically, an aliquot of urine is tested for specific gravity, albumin, sugar, acetone, and pH. Serum electrolyte values may be determined as frequently as every 4 hours during the diuresis. The total urine collection for each 24 hours is assayed quantitatively for electrolytes, urea, creatinine, and protein excretion.

The patency of urinary drainage systems is monitored continuously. A sudden cessation of urine output during the first few days most probably indicates catheter malfunction and should be reported to the doctor immediately. Necessary catheter irrigations should be performed by him rather than by the nurse. A slower decline in urine output more likely implies dehydration or renal failure.

Blood pressure, pulse, and respirations are recorded at least hourly during the first three days. A significant fall in blood pressure or a rise in the pulse rate may signify blood loss or dehydration. The diagnosis of either condition can be made by examination of the patient—determination of blood hematocrit and serum electrolytes. A rising blood pressure may indicate overhydration with possible resultant convulsive seizures. The body temperature is recorded every two hours. Should the patient develop a fever, cultures are taken from all possible areas, such as blood, wounds, urine, stool, and upper respiratory tract. A fever during the first three postoperative days is most likely the result of infection. Rejection crises can also be manifested by fever but are not likely to occur until later in the postoperative period.

During the subsequent postoperative period, the main concerns are adequate wound healing, control of rejection, and treatment of complications of immunosuppressive therapy. The blood urea nitrogen and creatinine clearance are followed daily. The patient is watched for signs and symptoms of uremia, as described earlier.

Preparations for Discharge

During the convalescent portion of his hospitalization, the transplant patient's maintenance schedule of immunosuppressive medications is established. He is thoroughly instructed by members of the transplantation team in all phases of home care. Particularly, the availability of a member of the team to the patient 24 hours a day is stressed, and appropriate telephone numbers are given to him.

The importance of accurate record-keeping at home and ingestion of prescribed immunosuppressive medications cannot be overemphasized to the patient. He is provided with a notebook to keep records of morning weights, morning and evening temperatures, and medications. He is instructed to bring the book with him on each clinic visit. He is taught how to test his urine daily for protein, using sulfosalicylic acid. He is provided with a set of standards from 0 to 4-plus proteinuria with which he can compare his own specimen. Instructions are given in the recognition of signs of homograft rejection. The patient is told to notify the transplant team immediately should there be a fever, a sudden decrease in urinary output, rapid weight gain, peripheral edema, or pain in the area of the transplanted kidney. Finally, he is advised against mingling in crowds or associating with people with any form of infection.

REVIEW QUESTIONS

1. Describe the basic surgical technique in renal transplantation.
2. Define the following terms:
   a. Isotransplant
   b. Homotransplant

c. Autotransplant
d. Heterotransplant
3. What is graft rejection? How is it manifested? How can it be controlled?
4. Discuss the considerations in selection of a donor kidney.
5. What is reverse isolation? Why and how is it implemented in the care of the posttransplantation patient?
6. Discuss the significant factors in the postoperative nursing care following transplantation.
7. Discuss the application and meaning of the team approach to care in transplantation.

REFERENCES—UNIT IV

Betson, Carol, and Linda Ude: "Central Venous Pressure," *Amer J Nurs*, **69**: 1466–68, 1969.

Bois, Marna S., Nancy B. Barfield, C. Elaine Taylor, and Christina Dyas Ross: "Nursing Care of Patients Having Kidney Transplants," *Amer J Nurs*, **68**: 1238–47, 1968.

Brescia, Michael J., Jame E. Cimino, Kenneth Appel, and Baruch J. Hurwich: "Chronic Hemodialysis Using Venipuncture and a Surgically Created Arteriovenous Fistula," *New Eng J Med*, **275**: 1089–92, 1966.

Brest, Albert N. and John H. Moyer, ed.: *Renal Failure.* A symposium sponsored by Hahneman Medical College, J. B. Lippincott Co., Philadelphia, 1967.

Burns, R. O., L. W. Henderson, E. B. Hager, and John P. Merrill: "Peritoneal Dialysis," *New Eng J Med*, **267**: 1060–66, 1962.

Calne, Roy Yorke: *Renal Transplantation*, 2nd ed. Edward Arnold, London, 1967.

Coil Dialysis Training Manual. Brooklyn–Cumberland Medical Center, Brooklyn, N. Y., July, 1968.

Downing, Shirley R.: "Nursing Support in Early Renal Failure," *Amer J Nurs*, **69**, 1212–16, 1969.

Felix, Kathleen S.: "Total Patient Care: The Team Approach in Transplantation," *Nurs Clin N Amer*, **4**: 451–60, 1969.

Ginsberg, Miriam K.: "A Study of Oral Hygiene Nursing Care," *Amer J Nurs*, **61**: 67–69, 1967.

Goldsmith, Edward I., John C. Whitesell, II, Kathleen Skelly, and Glenn D. Lubash: "Repeated Peritoneal Dialysis in Preparation for Renal Transplantation," *Surg Gynec Obstet*, **121**: 42–46, 1965.

Hampers, Constantine L., and John P. Merrill: "Hemodialysis in the Home—13 Months' Experience," *Ann Int Med*, **64**: 276–83, 1966.

Hampers, Constantine L., and Eugene Schupak: *Long-Term Hemodialysis: The Management of the Patient with Chronic Renal Failure.* Grune & Stratton, New York, 1967.

Juzwiak, Marijo: "Nursing the Kidney-Transplant Patient," *RN*, **31**, 34–41, 1968.

Kemph, John P.: "Psychotherapy with Patients Receiving Kidney Transplants," *Amer J Psychiat*, **124**: 623–29, 1967.

Kemph, John P.: "Renal Failure: Artificial Kidney and Kidney Transplant," *Amer J Psychiat*, **122**: 1270–74, 1966.

Leopold, Alice: "Psychological Problems in Hemodialysis, *RN*, **31**, 42–45, 1968.

Lieberman, Roger A., ed.: *Artificial Kidney Bibliography.* National Institute of Arthritis and Metabolic Disease, National Institutes of Health, Scientific Communications Office, Bethesda, Maryland.

MacLean, M. Moira, Helen Creighton, and Leonard B. Berman: "Hemodialysis and the Artificial Kidney," *Amer J Nurs*, **58**: 1672–75, 1958.

Maher, John F., and George E. Schreiner: "Hazards and Complications of Dialysis," *New Eng J Med*, **273**: 370–77, 1965.

Martin, Alfred J., Jr.: "Renal Transplantation: Surgical Technique and Complications," *Amer J Nurs*, **68**: 1240–41, 1968.

Meltzer, Lawrence E., Faye G. Abdellah, and J. Roderick Kitchell: *Concepts and Practices of Intensive Care for Nurse Specialists.* The Charles Press, Philadelphia, 1969.

Merrill, John P.: *The Treatment of Renal Failure: Therapeutic Principles in the Management of Acute and Chronic Uremia*, 2nd ed. Grune & Stratton, New York, 1965.

Pendras, Jerry P., and R. V. Erickson: "Hemodialysis: A Successful Therapy for Chronic Uremia," *Ann Int Med*, **64**, 293–311, 1966.

Rockwell, Janice Wood: "Nursing Care of the Patient with a Kidney Transplant," *Amer J Nurs*, **65**: 124–25, 1965.

Sand, Patricia, Goodhue Livingston, and Robert G. Wright: "Psychological Assessment of Candidates for a Hemodialysis Program," *Ann Int Med*, **64**: 603–21, 1966.

Schreiner, George E., and John F. Maher: "Hemodialysis for Chronic Renal Failure. III. Medical, Moral, Ethical and Socioeconomic Problems," *Ann Int Med*, **62**: 551–57, 1965.

Shea, Eileen, J., Donald F. Bogdan, Richard B. Freeman, and George E. Schreiner: "Hemodialysis for Chronic Renal Failure. IV. Psychological Considerations." *Ann Int Med*, **62**: 558–63, 1965.

Starzl, Thomas E.: *Experience in Renal Transplantation.* W. B. Saunders Co., Philadelphia, 1964.

Starzl, Thomas E.: "Reversal of Rejection in Human Homografts with Subsequent Development of Homograft Tolerance," *Surg Gynec Obstet*, **117**: 385–95, 1963.

Trusk, Carol W., "Hemodialysis for Acute Renal Failure," *Amer J Nurs*, **65**: 80–85, 1965.

Wright, Robert G., Patricia Sand, and Goodhue Livingston: "Psychological Stress During Hemodialysis for Chronic Renal Failure." *Ann Int Med*, **64**: 611–21, 1966.

Appendixes

I. Diets

Low-Purine Diet
Low-Calcium, Low-Phosphorus Test Diet
Moderately Low-Calcium, Moderately Low-Phosphorus Diet
Low-Oxalate Diet
Modified Giovannetti Diet

II. Positions and Draping for Examining Patients

III. Details of Catheterization Setup
Female Catheterization
Clean-Catch Urine for Culture
Urine Specimen for Culture—Male

IV. Bubble Suction

V. Guide to Instrument Setups for Some Commonly Performed Urologic Operations

VI. Teaching the Patient Home Catheter Care

VII. Questions Frequently Asked by Patients with an Ileal Conduit

VIII. List of Major Surgical Appliance Manufacturers

IX. Setup for Peritoneal Dialysis

APPENDIX I
Diets*

Low-Purine Diet

Foods containing over 150 mg of purine bodies in 100 g have been omitted from this diet. Foods containing moderate to large amounts of purine bodies (50–150 mg) have been omitted or restricted. Fried foods have been omitted from this diet, and the use of cream, butter, and other fats is restricted.

Approximate Food Value

Protein	80 g
Fat	80 g
CHO	200 g
Calories	1840

Vitamins and minerals *meet Nutritional Research Council Allowances, except possibly for iron.*

RECOMMENDED DAILY	FOODS TO INCLUDE	FOODS TO OMIT
	MILK	
1 pint or more	Whole milk, skim milk, buttermilk, milk beverages Cream limited to 2 oz daily	
	CHEESE	
	All kinds	
	EGGS	
1 or 2	As desired	
	MEAT, POULTRY, FISH	
Limited to 2 oz daily	2 oz of meat, poultry, or fish, except those listed under "Foods to Omit"	Glandular meats—sweetbreads, brain, kidney, liver, sausage, heart; anchovies, sardines. Meat extracts such as broth, gravies, and meat soups

(*Continued*)

* Reproduced by permission from "Manual of Diets," Department of Nutrition, The New York Hospital–Cornell Medical Center.

Low-Purine Diet (*Continued*)

RECOMMENDED DAILY	FOODS TO INCLUDE	FOODS TO OMIT
	BUTTER	
Limited to 1 tablespoon	Butter or margarine	
	BREAD	
2–4 servings bread or cereal as allowed	White bread, rolls and muffins, cornbread, white crackers	Whole-grain breads
	CEREALS	
	Refined such as Cream of Wheat, hominy grits, cornmeal, cornflakes, Rice Flakes, Rice Krispies, Puffed Rice, Corn Kix	Whole-grain cereals including oatmeal; wheat germ; bran
	CEREAL PRODUCTS	
	Spaghetti, noodles, macaroni, tapioca, rice	
	VEGETABLES	
3 or more servings including 1 green or yellow and 1 potato	All vegetables except those listed under "Foods to Omit"	Dried beans, peas, and lentils; asparagus, spinach, peas, mushrooms, cauliflower, Lima beans
	FRUITS	
2 servings including 1 citrus or tomato	All fruits and fruit juices	
	SOUPS	
	Milk soups made with any vegetable except those listed under "Foods to Omit"	Broths; soups made with a meat base, soups containing vegetables not allowed

RECOMMENDED DAILY	FOODS TO INCLUDE	FOODS TO OMIT
	DESSERTS	
	Fruit, pudding, ice cream, custard, junket, gelatin desserts, cake, and cookies Rich desserts and pastries in moderation only	Desserts containing mince meat or chocolate
	BEVERAGES	
	Milk beverages, carbonated beverages, fruit juice, Postum, and decaffeinated coffees Coffee, tea, or cocoa restricted to 1 cup daily	Alcoholic beverages Coffee, tea, or cocoa in excess of 1 cup daily
	MISCELLANEOUS	
	Sugar, syrups, honey, molasses, jelly, marshmallows, hard candy, gum drops, popcorn, peanut butter, salt, rich foods, and nuts in moderation only. Oils or mayonnaise limited to 2 teaspoons	Highly seasoned foods and condiments Fried foods; gravies Potato chips Chocolate

MEAL PLAN	SAMPLE MENU	SERVINGS G OR ML	SERVINGS HOSPITAL MEASURE
	BREAKFAST		
Fruit	Grapefruit	100	1/2 medium
Cereal	Cream of Wheat	130	1/2 cup
Egg	Soft-cooked egg	50	1
Bread	White toast	22	1 slice
Butter	Butter	5	1 pat
Milk	Milk	240	1 glass
Beverage	Coffee	150	1 cup
Milk for coffee or cereal	Milk for coffee or cereal	60	2 ounces
Sugar	Sugar	14	2 packets

(*Continued*)

Low-Purine Diet (*Concluded*)

MEAL PLAN	SAMPLE MENU	SERVINGS G OR ML	SERVINGS HOSPITAL MEASURE
	LUNCHEON		
Soup	Cream of tomato soup	150	1 soup cup
Egg or cheese	Macaroni and cheese	100	1/2 cup
Vegetable	Green beans	75	1/2 cup
Salad	Coleslaw	50	1/2 cup
Dressing	Mayonnaise	5	1 tsp
Dessert	Pears	100	1/2 cup
Bread	White bread	22	1 slice
Butter	Butter	5	1 pat
Milk	Milk	240	1 glass
	DINNER		
Meat	Pot roast	60	2 oz
Potato	Baked potato	100	1 medium
Vegetable	Carrots	75	1/2 cup
Dessert	Fruited gelatin	150	1/2 cup
Bread	White bread	22	1 slice
Butter	Butter	5	1 pat
Milk	Milk	240	1 glass

Low-Calcium, Low-Phosphorus Test Diet

This diet contains 150 mg of calcium and 600 mg of phosphorus and is planned as a two-week test diet to be used on a research unit. Other services will not have the facilities necessary for serving this type of constant diet. The patient is given a choice of meat, fruits, and vegetables as indicated under "Foods to Include" at the start of the diet. These foods must then be used consecutively for the entire test period.

Approximate Food Value

Protein	40 g
Fat	35 g
CHO	205 g
Calories	1295

Vitamins and minerals *do not meet NRC Allowances*

AMOUNT TO BE SERVED AND EATEN	FOODS TO INCLUDE	FOODS TO OMIT
	MILK	
None	None	All milk, cream and milk beverages

AMOUNT TO BE SERVED AND EATEN	FOODS TO INCLUDE	FOODS TO OMIT
	CHEESE	
None	None	All cheese
	EGGS	
1 only (2 oz of meat may be substituted for 1 egg daily)	Raw, poached, soft or hard cooked	Scrambled eggs or fried eggs unless fat used for frying is subtracted from daily allowance
	MEAT	
$2\frac{1}{2}$ oz only. (2 oz of meat may be substituted for 1 egg daily)	Beef, lamb, veal, pork or poultry	All glandular meats, including brain, heart, liver, kidney, sweetbreads; game (pheasant, rabbit, venison, grouse); sardines and fish roe
	BUTTER	
15 g	Butter or margarine	Butter or margarine in excess of allowance
	BREAD, CEREAL AND CEREAL PRODUCTS	
As indicated under "Foods to Include"	1 slice white bread 2 slices whole-wheat bread 5 saltines	All cereals and cereal products Bread and saltines in excess of allowance Bread made from self-rising flour
	VEGETABLES	
1 serving of 100 g	Potato, corn, or Lima beans Rice may be substituted for one of the vegetables	All vegetables not listed under "Foods to Include" including beet greens, celery, chard, parsely, spinach, dried peas, beans, and lentils Creamed vegetables

(*Continued*)

Low-Calcium, Low-Phosphorus Diet (*Continued*)

AMOUNT TO BE SERVED AND EATEN	FOODS TO INCLUDE	FOODS TO OMIT
	VEGETABLES (*Continued*)	
1 serving of 50 g	Beets, green beans, cabbage, carrots, cauliflower, eggplant, onions, peas, pumpkin, winter squash or turnips	Creamed vegetables
2 servings of 50 g each	Asparagus, cucumber, lettuce, mushrooms, radishes, summer squash, or tomatoes	
	FRUITS	
3 servings of 100 g each including 1 serving of citrus fruit or tomato	Apples, apricots, bananas, berries, cherries, cranberries, grapes, grapefruit, melons, oranges, peaches, pears, pineapple, plums, tangerine or tomato juice, and orange juice	All dried fruits Rhubarb and other fruit not specified under "Foods to Include"
	SOUPS	
	None	All
	DESSERT	
	Fruit only, as allowed	All prepared desserts, including pies, cakes, cookies, puddings, ice cream
	BEVERAGES	
	Coffee, tea, ginger ale	
	MISCELLANEOUS	
	Sugar, salt, pepper, cinnamon, as desired Jelly limited to 20 g, if desired	Chocolate, candy, honey, condiments having a calcium or phosphate base Nuts Fried foods, salad dressing, mayonnaise and gravy

MEAL PLAN	SAMPLE MENUS	SERVINGS G OR ML	SERVINGS HOSPITAL MEASURE
	BREAKFAST		
Fruit	Orange juice	100	weighed
Egg	Poached	50	1
Bread	White toast	22	weighed
Butter	Butter	5	weighed
Jelly	Jelly	10	weighed
Beverage	Black coffee	as desired	1 pot
Sugar	Sugar	as desired	1 packet
	LUNCHEON		
Vegetables	Lettuce	50	weighed
	Tomato	50	weighed
Bread	Whole wheat	44	weighed
Butter	Butter	5	weighed
Fruit	Banana	100	weighed
Beverage	Tea	as desired	1 pot
Sugar	Sugar	as desired	1 packet
	MIDAFTERNOON NOURISHMENT		
Beverage	Ginger ale	as desired	210
Saltines	Saltines	8	weighed
Jelly	Jelly	5	weighed
	DINNER		
Meat	Broiled chicken	75	weighed
Vegetables	Baked potato	100	weighed
	Green beans	50	weighed
Butter	Butter	5	weighed
Fruit	Honeydew melon	100	weighed
Beverage	Tea	as desired	1 pot
Sugar	Sugar	as desired	1 packet
	EVENING NOURISHMENT		
Beverage	Tea	as desired	1 pot
Saltines	Saltines	12	weighed
Jelly	Jelly	5	weighed
Sugar	Sugar	as desired	1 packet

Moderately Low-Calcium, Moderately Low-Phosphorus Diet

This diet contains 500–700 mg calcium and 1000–1200 mg phosphorus.

Approximate Food Value

Protein	70 g
Fat	75 g
CHO	220 g
Calories	1835

Vitamins and minerals *meet NRC Allowance, except for calcium and possibly iron.*

RECOMMENDED DAILY	FOODS TO INCLUDE	FOODS TO OMIT
	MILK	
Limited to ½ pt	Limit to 1 cup (½ pint) whole milk, skim milk or buttermilk Sweet or sour cream may be substituted for part of the milk	Milk or cream in excess of 1 cup daily
	CHEESE	
Limited to 2 oz	Pot cheese, cottage cheese, or cream cheese limited to 2 oz daily	All other cheeses
	EGGS	
Limited to 1	Limited to 1 whole egg daily Egg whites as desired	
	MEAT, POULTRY, FISH	
Limited to 4 oz	Limited to 4 oz of beef, lamb, pork, veal, chicken, turkey, fish, frankfurters, and cold cuts One egg may be substituted for for 2 oz of meat	Brain, heart, liver, kidney, sweetbreads, game (pheasant, rabbit, venison, grouse), sardines, fish roe, herring
	BUTTER	
2 tablespoons	Butter or margarine	

RECOMMENDED DAILY	FOODS TO INCLUDE	FOODS TO OMIT
	BREAD AND CEREALS	
2–4 servings bread or cereal as allowed	White bread, rolls and crackers except those made from self-rising flour Farina, cornmeal, hominy grits, white rice, cornflakes, Rice Krispies and Puffed Rice	Whole-grain breads, cereals and crackers; rye breads; all breads made with self-rising flour; oatmeal, bran, branflakes, wheat germ and all dry cereals except those allowed
	CEREAL PRODUCTS	
	Macaroni, spaghetti, noodles, white rice	Brown and wild rice
	VEGETABLES	
3 or more servings including 1 green or yellow and 1 potato	All vegetables except those listed under "Foods to Omit"	Broccoli, beet greens, chards, collards, mustard greens, spinach, turnip greens, dried beans, peas, lentils, and soybeans
	FRUITS	
2 servings including 1 citrus or tomato	All fruits except rhubarb	Rhubarb
	SOUPS	
	All soups including cream soup made from daily milk allowance, except those listed under "Foods to Omit"	Soup containing spinach or dried peas, beans, or lentils
	DESSERTS	
	Fruit pies and cobblers (except those containing rhubarb), fruit ices, gelatin	All desserts except those listed under "Foods to Include"

(*Continued*)

Moderately Low-Calcium, Low-Phosphorus (*Continued*)

RECOMMENDED DAILY	FOODS TO INCLUDE	FOODS TO OMIT
	DESSERTS (*Continued*)	
	Puddings made with daily milk and egg allowance Angel food cake and meringues Do not use package mixes	
	BEVERAGES	
	Coffee, Sanka, tea, and carbonated beverages	Chocolate, cocoa, Postum, beer, and ale
	MISCELLANEOUS	
	Sugar, jellies, jams, honey, salt, pepper, spices, fruit flavored hard candies Vegetable and animal fats, gravy, mayonnaise and salad dressings	Nuts, peanut butter, chocolate, condiments having a calcium or phosphate base
	Pickles, olives, catsup, prepared mustard Pretzels, potato chips, popcorn One serving of cake or a candy bar may be included once a week	Tums and artificial sweetners containing calcium or phosphate base

MEAL PLAN	SAMPLE MENUS	SERVINGS G OR ML	SERVINGS HOSPITAL MEASURE
	BREAKFAST		
Fruit	Orange juice	120	1 juice glass
Cereal	Farina	130	1/2 cup
Egg	Soft cooked	50	1
Bread	White toast	22	1 slice
Butter	Butter	10	2 pats
Jelly	Currant jelly	25	souffle cup
Milk	Milk	120	1 juice glass
Beverage	Coffee	200	1 pot
Sugar	Sugar	14	2 packets

MEAL PLAN	SAMPLE MENUS	SERVINGS G OR ML	SERVINGS HOSPITAL MEASURE
	LUNCHEON		
Juice	Tomato juice	120	1 juice glass
Meat or substitute	Sliced turkey	60	2 oz
Vegetable	Green beans	75	1/2 cup
Salad	Head lettuce	50	1/2 cup
Dressing	French dressing	10	2 tsp
Dessert	Canned pears	100	1/2 cup
Bread	White bread	22	1 slice
Butter	Butter	10	2 pats
Milk	Milk	120	1 juice glass
	DINNER		
Meat	Roast lamb with gravy	60	2 oz
Potato	Steamed potato	100	1 medium
Vegetable	Carrots	75	1/2 cup
Dessert	Apple pie	120	1/8 pie
Bread	White bread	22	1 slice
Butter	Butter	10	2 pats
Beverage	Tea	200	1 pot
Lemon	Lemon		1 wedge
Sugar	Sugar	7	1 packet

Low-Oxalate Diet

Foods Omitted Because of High Oxalic Acid Content

Spinach
Potatoes, sweet
Beans
Endive
Beets
Swiss chard

Tomatoes
Dried figs
Plums
Strawberries

Cocoa
Chocolate
Tea

Data adapted from:

McLester, James S., and William J. Darby: *Nutrition and Diet in Health and Disease*, 6th ed. W. B. Saunders Co., Philadelphia, 1952.

Mattice, Marjorie R.: *Bridges' Food and Beverage Analyses*, 3rd ed. Lea & Febiger, Philadelphia, 1950.

Modified Giovannetti Diet

This diet contains 20 g protein.

RECOMMENDED DAILY	FOODS TO INCLUDE	FOODS TO OMIT
	MILK	
Limited to 1/2 cup (4 oz)	Limited to 1/2 cup of whole milk only	Milk, or cream in excess of 1/2 cup daily
	EGG	
Limited to one	Limited to 1 whole egg daily, poached, scrambled, hard cooked, or used in cooking	Eggs in excess of one a day
	BUTTER AND FATS	
As desired	Butter or margarine as desired. Oil	Salad dressings, mayonnaise, gravy
	BREAD	
2 slices	Limited to 2 slices of white bread. If additional bread is desired it must be the special homemade bread. This bread can be eaten as desired and is best when toasted with jam and butter	Whole wheat, rye, rolls, commercial biscuits or muffins
	CEREAL	
1 serving 1/2 cup	Cooked cereal made with water or cold cereal	
	CEREAL PRODUCTS	
1 serving 1/2 cup cooked	Rice, macaroni, spaghetti, noodles	Brown and wild rice
	VEGETABLES—Fresh or Frozen	
3 servings 1 serving = 1/2 cup cooked	Corn, green beans, carrots, broccoli, cauliflower, potato, tomato, wax beans, lettuce, cabbage, eggplant,	All vegetables except those listed under "Foods to Include." Canned vegetables

RECOMMENDED DAILY	FOODS TO INCLUDE	FOODS TO OMIT
	VEGETABLES (*Continued*)	
	asparagus, mustard greens, turnip greens, mushrooms, green pepper, cucumbers, radishes, onions, dandelion greens *Peas, beets, and spinach are high-protein vegetables and should be eaten only twice a week*	
	SOUPS	
1 serving	Homemade vegetable soup or potato soup (special recipe)	Cream soups, soups made with meat base, commercial canned or frozen soups
	FRUITS	
5 servings	All sweetened fruits, fresh or canned, and fruit juices	
	CONDIMENTS	
As desired	Pepper, onion powder, garlic powder, herbs	Salt, onion salt, garlic salt, Accent, allspice, catsup, mustard
	MISCELLANEOUS	
As desired	Sugar, honey, syrup, hard candies, marshmallows, jelly, jams, jelly candies. Desserts made from special recipe. Fruit ices (Italian ices). Carbonated beverages	Chocolate, nuts, pretzels, potato chips, commercial cakes, pies, cookies, ice cream, peanut butter, pickles, olives, sherbet, Jello

NOTE

It is extremely important that the patient eat just those food items that are listed under "Foods to Include" in the amounts stated. The calorie requirement must be maintained in order for the diet to be of value to the patient. Extra calories can be gotten by eating the special desserts, the special bread and muffins, and by adding sugar or syrup to fruits and juices.

(*Continued*)

Modified Giovannetti Diet (*Continued*)

RECOMMENDED DAILY	FOODS TO INCLUDE	FOODS TO OMIT

Meat and cheese are not allowed on the diet unless used as a substitution as listed below. No fish is permitted on the diet.

SUBSTITUTIONS

1. 2 level tablespoons of cream cheese for 1/4 cup of milk,
2. 1 oz meat for 1 egg (only 2 times a week).
3. 1/2 cup ice cream for 1/2 cup milk (only 1 time a week).

MEAL PLANS

BREAKFAST	NOON MEAL SPECIAL VEGETABLE PLATE	EVENING MEAL SPECIAL FRUIT PLATE
Pear nectar Cornflakes with brown sugar 1 toast, butter, jam 1/4 cup milk Tea, honey, sugar	Hard-cooked egg Buttered corn Buttered wax beans Baked potato 1 bread, butter, jelly Ginger ale	Peach halves Bing cherries Small apple Special bread, butter, jelly Fruit ice 1/4 cup milk Tea, sugar
	3 P.M. Small glass juice (4 oz) with sugar Special muffin, butter, jelly	8 P.M. 1 glass (8 oz) lemonade with Karo syrup
Peach nectar Puffed rice Brown sugar 1 toast, butter, jam 1/4 cup milk Tea, sugar	Scrambled egg Carrots, buttered Green beans, buttered Boiled potato 1 toast, butter, jelly, Coca-Cola	Pear halves Canned plums Applesauce Special muffin Special dessert Ginger ale 1/4 cup milk Tea, sugar
	3 P.M. Special bread toasted, jam, butter 4 oz orange juice with 1 tsp sugar	8 P.M. 1 glass lemonade with honey

RECOMMENDED DAILY	FOODS TO INCLUDE	FOODS TO OMIT
Cranberry juice cocktail Rice Krispies Special bread, butter, jam 1/4 cup milk Tea, sugar	Sandwich hard-cooked egg on white toast with lettuce and tomato Baked apple (see recipe) Ginger ale	Baked potato Buttered corn Special bread, butter, jam Tapioca pudding (see recipe) 1/4 cup milk Tea, sugar
Apple juice with sugar Cream of rice (made with 1/4 cup milk) Maple syrup Special muffin, butter, jam Tea, sugar	French toast (2 slices regular bread and 1 egg and 1/4 cup milk) Pancake syrup Pineapple slices Ginger ale	Sweet potato Fried greens Special bread, butter, jam Fruit ice, Ginger ale
	3 P.M. Fruit ice and ginger ale mixed	8 P.M. Orangeade

PINEAPPLE TAPIOCA PUDDING

INGREDIENTS

1 1/2 cups water
1/4 cup quick-cooking tapioca
1/2 cup sugar
1 1/2 cups crushed pineapple
1 tablespoon lemon juice

PROCEDURE

1. Combine water, tapioca, and sugar and cook, stirring constantly for 3 minutes.
2. Remove from heat and stir in fruit.
3. Cool, stirring occasionally.
4. Divide into four dessert dishes.

POTATO SOUP

INGREDIENTS

1 potato, cubed
1 tablespoon butter
2 tablespoons dry mix
1 cup water

PROCEDURE

1. Cube potato and boil in 1 cup water.
2. Melt butter in frying pan and add flour, slowly mixing constantly.
3. When flour and butter are well blended, add to potato mixture.
4. Let soup simmer slowly and add salt and pepper to taste.

POTATO PANCAKE

INGREDIENTS

1 medium potato
5 tablespoons oil
3 tablespoons dry mix
1/2 teaspoon grated onion

PROCEDURE

1. Grate potato, add flour, grated onion and pepper.
2. Fry in oil. Makes five pancakes.

APPENDIX **II**

Positions and Draping for Examining Patients*

Dorsal

1. Patient lies supine in bed with legs together, arms at side.
2. One pillow is permitted under head.
3. No specific type of draping needed.

Dorsal Recumbent

1. Patient lies flat on back, knees separated, and legs flexed so that soles of feet rest flat on bed.
2. One pillow only under head.
3. Draping
   a. Cover patient with bath blanket fanfolding bedclothes to foot of bed.
   b. Place bath blanket diagonally over patient: corners 1 and 3 over far and near leg respectively, corner 2 over chest, and corner 4 on bed between legs.
   c. Cover entire far leg and foot with corner 1 of blanket: fold end under foot to hold it in place. Repeat with near leg using corner 3. Be sure inner aspect of thigh is covered.
   d. When doctor is ready to examine patient, corner 2 may be raised which will expose only part to be examined.

Sims' Position or Left Lateral Prone

1. Patient lies on left side obliquely across bed or table, buttocks brought to edge of mattress.
2. Direct patient to place her left arm behind back, incline body forward so that she lies partly on chest.
3. The thighs are flexed: the right one more than the left.
4. The knees are flexed: the right one more than the left, so that it crosses the left and rests on the bed.
5. Draping: Place bath blanket or sheet over patient; cover feet well, leave loose near hips.

* Reproduced by permission from "Nursing Procedure Manual," Nursing Service, The New York Hospital–Cornell Medical Center.

Knee-Chest Position

1. Cover patient with bath blanket or sheet.
2. Patient rests on chest and knees, knees slightly separated, thighs perpendicular, face turned to side, arms free on both sides. (No pillows should be used, but one small pillow may be used for under head until patient becomes accustomed to position.)
3. Place bath blanket across patient diagonally and drape as for dorsal recumbent position.

Lithotomy Position

1. Patient should be on an examining table.
2. Cover patient with bath blanket or sheet. Remove bath robe, pajama bottoms, and slippers.
3. Place disposable paper pad at foot of table and tuck under table pad to protect sheet. If pillow is used, cover with disposable paper also.
4. Flex thighs on abdomen and place feet in stirrups. Thighs are outside of rod. Have patient move down on table on her back until the buttocks are slightly beyond the edge of table.
5. Drape as in dorsal recumbent position.

APPENDIX **III**

Details of Catheterization Setup*

Female Catheterization

Note: Either of the following two methods may be used.

EQUIPMENT

1. Catheterization set from sterile supply room containing
   a. 8 cotton balls
   b. Disposable cup
   c. Kelly forceps
   d. 2 Robinson catheters #14
   e. Emesis basin
2. Tray
3. Disposable pad or covered treatment rubber
4. Flashlight
5. Paper bag
6. Lubicating jelly
7. Antiseptic solution as specified by department
8. Containers for specimens as needed.

PREPARATION OF PATIENT

1. Fanfold top bedding and cover patient with bath blanket.
2. Place disposable pad or covered treatment rubber under buttocks.
3. Assist patient to lithotomy position and drape with bath blanket.
4. Adjust flashlight and paper bag.

PREPARATION OF EQUIPMENT

1. Wash hands.
2. Place catheterization set on bed between patient's legs.
3. Open set, keeping inside of wrapper sterile.
4. Using Kelly forceps, remove cup from basin.
5. Using Kelly forceps, remove two cotton balls from cup and place beside emesis basin.
6. Pour antiseptic solution over remaining cotton balls in cup.
7. Expel small amount of lubricating jelly into paper bag then into emesis basin.

* Reproduced by permission from "Nursing Procedure Manual," Nursing Service, The New York Hospital–Cornell Medical Center.

PROCEDURE	KEY POINTS
1. Wash hands thoroughly.	
2. Using dry cotton balls over fingers, separate labia.	
3. Cleanse area with moistened cotton balls, using one at a time in a downward stroke on a. Side of meatus farthest from self b. Side of meatus nearest self c. Directly over meatus	
4. Pick up one catheter with Kelly forceps, place it on sterile field at far side of basin.	This catheter may be used if first catheter is contaminated.
5. Pick up other catheter with Kelly forceps 2 inches below tip, rotate in lubricant, and introduce into urethra until urine drains.	End of catheter rests in emesis basin.
6. Hold catheter in place with Kelly forceps or fingers while collecting specimens.	
7. Permit rest of urine to drain into emesis basin.	Do not remove more than 1000 ml of urine at one time without consulting physician.

Alternate Procedure

ADDITIONAL EQUIPMENT

1. 1 pair of sterile rubber gloves

PREPARATION OF PATIENT

Same as above.

PREPARATION OF EQUIPMENT

1. Wash hands.
2. Place catheterization set on bed between patient's legs.
3. Open set keeping inside of wrapper sterile.
4. Pour antiseptic solution over cotton balls in disposable cup.
5. Expel small amount of lubricating jelly into paper bag then into emesis basin.

PROCEDURE	KEY POINTS
1. Put on sterile gloves.	
2. Remove disposable cup from emesis basin and place in convenient place.	

3. Separate labia with one hand.	This hand is no longer sterile.
4. Using Kelly forceps cleanse area with moistened cotton balls, using one at a time in a downward stroke on: a. Side of meatus farthest from self b. Side of meatus nearest self c. Directly over meatus	Have cotton ball cover tip of forceps as much as possible to prevent injury to patient.
5. Place Kelly forceps at edge of sterile field.	
6. Pick up one catheter with hand and place it on sterile field at far side of basin.	This catheter may be used if first catheter is contaminated.
7. Pick up other catheter with hand about 2 inches below tip, rotate in lubricant, and introduce into urethra until urine drains.	
8. Hold catheter in place while collecting required specimens.	
9. Permit rest of urine to drain into emesis basin.	Do not remove more than 1000 ml of urine at one time without consulting physician.

COLLECTION OF SPECIMENS FOR CULTURE

1. Permit a few drops of urine to flow into basin before pinching off catheter.	
2. Place end of catheter over edge of basin so that culture tube can be held underneath it.	
3. Using the third and fourth fingers of the hand to hold catheter, remove cotton plug of culture tube with a twisting motion.	
4. Collect approximately 10 ml (one-half tube) of urine, holding tube on slant to minimize air contamination.	Never fill culture tube more than one-half full or allow cotton plug to become wet.
5. Replace cotton plug carefully with a twisting motion away from you.	
6. Complete information on label of tube.	

MICROSCOPIC EXAMINATION

Collect 100 ml of urine in a clean specimen bottle.

Clean-Catch Urine for Culture

Note: This procedure may be carried out in the bathroom or at the bedside and may be done by either patient or nursing personnel.

EQUIPMENT

1. Sterile packet containing
   one 250-ml graduate
   two cotton balls
2. Paper cup
3. pHisoHex solution
4. Paper bag
5. Sterile culture tube
6. Emesis basin or bedpan

PREPARATION OF EQUIPMENT AND PATIENT

1. Open packet.
2. Pour a few drops of pHisoHex solution and a small amount of warm tap water into the paper cup.
3. Arrange clothing to enable you to obtain urine specimen.
4. Wash hands well with soap and water.
5. Place cotton balls in pHisoHex solution in paper cup.

PROCEDURE FOR FEMALE PATIENTS

1. Spread labia with fingers of one hand.
2. Wash inside labia and meatus, front to back with pHisoHex cotton balls. Discard cotton balls in paper bag.
3. Keeping labia separated, have patient void small amount in toilet or bedpan, then void small amount of urine into sterile graduate for specimen collection.

PROCEDURE FOR MALE PATIENTS

1. Instruct patient to retract foreskin.
2. Wash head of penis with pHisoHex cotton balls by starting at the meatus and washing toward the foreskin. Discard cotton balls in paper bag.
3. Have patient void small amount in toilet or emesis basin, then void small amount of urine into sterile graduate for specimen collection.

SPECIMEN (nursing personnel will do the following):

1. Use sterile technique to open and close culture tube.
2. Hold culture tube on a slant and with free hand pour approximately 10 ml urine into it. (Never fill more than half the tube.)
3. Place tube in upright position.
4. Label and *refrigerate specimen immediately*.

Urine Specimen for Culture—Male

EQUIPMENT

1. Male urine culture set containing
   a. Graduate, 250 ml
   b. Cotton balls
2. Emesis basin
3. Antiseptic solution as specified by department
4. Culture tube (properly labeled with patient's name, history number, floor, and date)

Note: This procedure to be carried out in the bathroom whenever possible.

PROCEDURE	KEY POINTS
1. Instruct patient to retract foreskin until specimen is obtained.	
2. Cleanse meatus with antiseptic solution.	
3. Instruct patient to void a small amount into emesis basin.	
4. Have patient void into graduate.	Patient to avoid contact with interior of graduate.
5. Remove cotton plug from culture tube with back surface of fingers of one hand.	Hold plug between fingers while picking up culture tube in that hand. Avoid touching end of plug that goes back into tube.
6. With free hand pour 10 ml of urine from graduate into culture tube, holding tube on a slant. (Do not fill tube more than one-half full.)	Take care not to spill urine on outside of tube.
7. Replace plug in tube.	
8. Keep tube in an upright position at all times.	
9. Before discarding remaining urine check to see if the patient is on measured output.	
10. Rinse, wash, and dry graduate.	

APPENDIX IV
Bubble Suction*

EQUIPMENT

1. 50-inch length of sterile rubber tubing
2. 40-inch length of sterile rubber tubing
3. 2 lengths of rubber tubing 8 inches long
4. 6-inch length of rubber tubing
5. Sterile Y tube
6. Drainage bottle with screw cap (empty)
7. Drainage bottle with screw cap partially filled with water
8. 2 rubber washers to fit inside of screw caps
9. Bottle holders for both drainage bottles
10. Large spring clip
11. Wall suction or suction machine

PROCEDURE	KEY POINTS
1. Attach 6-inch length of tubing to long prong of screw top and place in bottle partially filled with water so that tubing is 2 inches below level of water.	Distance of tubing under water controls the amount of suction to the catheter.
2. Attach both drainage bottles in bottle holders on upper section of bed frame.	
3. To each arm of Y tube, attach one 8-inch rubber tubing and connect other ends of rubber tubing to the short prongs of screw tops on both drainage bottles.	
4. To the remaining end of the Y tube add 50-inch length of rubber tubing and attach to wall suction or suction machine.	
5. Attach 40-inch length of rubber tubing to the apparatus on the patient or catheter as ordered and connect to the long prong of the screw top on the empty drainage bottle.	

* Reproduced by permission from "Nursing Procedure Manual," Nursing Service, The New York Hospital–Cornell Medical Center.

6. Coil rubber tubing on bed, and clip to draw sheet with large spring slip. — Allows patient free movement in bed without pull on catheter or allowing tubing level to drop.

BUBBLE SUCTION

If not working, check:
Suction turned on? Washer in screw caps? Chip in neck of bottle? Crack in bottle? Is the tubing latex?
If water is bubbling up into short tube, increase the length of air inlet so as to be able to lower water level.

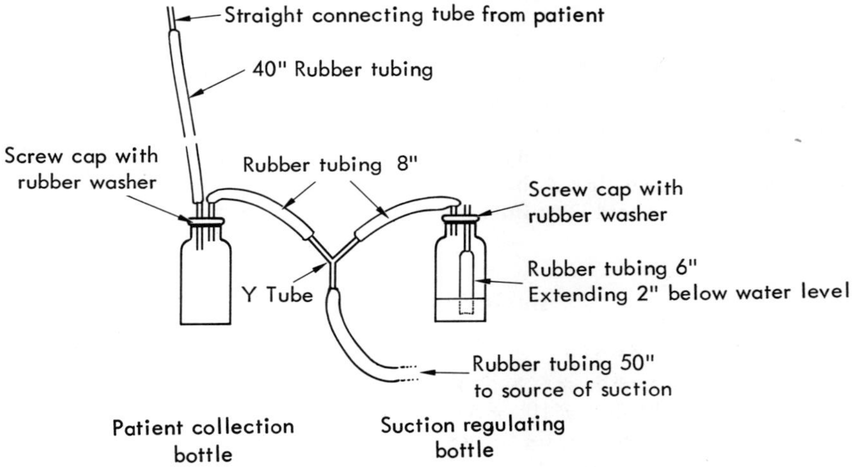

APPENDIX V
Guide to Instrument Setups for Some Commonly Performed Urologic Operations

The following lists are offered as guides to setting up instruments for urologic operations (Chapter 16). Additional instruments, catheters, and the like should be readily available in the operating suite if the situation calls for them. The type and size of suture material may vary from surgeon to surgeon for the same operative procedure. A basic major and minor instrument tray will be outlined with additional instruments for the selected operation.

Basic Major Tray

CUTTING INSTRUMENTS

3 scalpel handles, #3, #4, and #7
2 each of knife blades, #10, #20, and #15
1 Mayo scissors, straight, 6¼ inches
1 Mayo scissors, curved, 6¼ inches
1 Metzenbaum dissecting scissors, curved, 7 inches
1 suture scissors
1 "old" suture scissors (for cutting catheters, drains, etc.)

CLAMPS

12 Halstead hemostats, straight, 5½ inches
12 Halstead hemostats, curved, 5½ inches
12 Crile hemostats, curved, 6¼ inches

FORCEPS

2 dressing forceps, serrated, no teeth, 5½ inches
2 tissue forceps, 1 and 2 teeth, 5½ inches
2 dressing forceps, serrated, no teeth, 10 inches
6 sponge forceps, serrated or smooth jaws, 10 inches
6 Backhaus towel clamps, 3½ or 5 inches
4 Judd-Allis tissue forceps, 4 and 5 teeth, 6 inches

RETRACTORS

2 each of small, medium, and large Richardson retractors
2 Kelly retractors, medium blade

2 McBurney appendix retractors
2 Cushing vein retractors
1 malleable copper retractor, 1¼ by 13 inches
2 Volkman rake retractors, 4-pronged, blunt, 8½ inches

SEWING INSTRUMENTS

1 set of assorted needles
3 Crile-Wood fine needle holders, 6¼ inches
3 Mayo-Hegar medium needle holders, 6 inches

ACCESSORY INSTRUMENTS

1 grooved director, 5 inches
1 silver probe, 5 inches
Assorted suction tips and tubing

Basic Minor Tray

CUTTING INSTRUMENTS

2 scalpel handles, #3 and #4
2 blades, #10 and #20
1 Mayo scissors, straight, 6¼ inches
1 Metzenbaum dissecting scissors, 7 inches
1 suture scissors

CLAMPS

6 Halstead hemostats, straight, 5½ inches
6 Halsted hemostats, curved, 5½ inches
6 Crile hemostats, curved, 6½ inches

FORCEPS

1 dressing forceps, serrated, no teeth, 5½ inches
1 tissue forceps, 1 and 2 teeth, 5½ inches
3 sponge forceps, serrated or smooth jaws
4 Backhaus towel clamps 3½ inches
2 Judd-Allis tissue forceps, 4 and 5 teeth

RETRACTORS

2 Cushing vein retractors
2 Volkman rake retractors, 2- or 3-pronged, blunt, 8½ inches
2 Meyerding or Lang retractors, right angle, small

SEWING INSTRUMENTS

2 Crile-Wood needle holders, fine, 6¼ inches
2 skin hooks
Small assortment of straight and curved needles

ACCESSORY INSTRUMENTS

1 grooved director, 5 inches
1 silver probe, 5 inches
1 small suction tip
1 medicine glass, 60 ml (for local anesthetic)
Appropriate syringes and hypodermic needles for anesthetic infiltration

Instruments for Operations on the Kidney

Nephrectomy: Major Tray

RETRACTORS

1 Harrington splanchnic
1 large Deaver
1 small Deaver
2 medium Kelly abdominal
2 large Kelly abdominal
1 narrow blade Doyen
1 wide blade Doyen

LONG INSTRUMENTS

6 Mixter gall duct forceps, $6\frac{1}{4}$ inches
6 Mixter gall duct forceps, $7\frac{3}{4}$ inches
6 Wylie hemostats
3 Mayo-Hegar needle holders, 10 inches
1 Guyon-Pean pedicle clamp
1 long Metzenbaum dissecting scissors
1 long Mayo scissors straight
1 Herrick pedicle clamp
1 Young pedicle clamp

SUTURES

6 plain catgut 00 reels
4 plain catgut 00 (cut $\frac{1}{3}$ lengths)
1 chromic catgut 0 (cut $\frac{1}{3}$ lengths)
1 silk 000
1 silk 0
8–12 chromic 0 (cut $\frac{1}{4}$ lengths)
4 packages 000 silk on milliner's needles

Often a rib will be resected by the surgeon to facilitate his exposure in operations on the kidney. The following rib instruments should be available:

1 Alexander periosteotome
1 Langenbeck periosteal elevator
2 Doyen rib raspatories (right- and left-handed)

1 Stille-Giertz rib shears
1 Sauerbruch rib rongeur
1 Finochietto rib spreader
1 Bailey rib contractor

Pyelolithotomy

In addition to the instruments for nephrectomy, the following are useful:

STONE FORCEPS

4–6 Randall stone forceps of assorted curvature
1 straight Blake gallstone forceps
1 curved Blake gallstone forceps

SUTURES

4 chromic atraumatic 0000 catgut (for closure of renal pelvis)

CATHETERS

Red rubber, 8–14 French } to pass down ureter for determination
Ureteral, 5–6 French } of patency
Malecot, 18–24 French, should nephrostomy be required

Complete Nephrolithotomy and Partial Nephrectomy

As for pyelolithotomy, with addition of selected vascular instruments for control of the renal artery:

2 Blalock pulmonic stenosis clamps
2 Satinsky vena cava clamps
4 Johns Hopkins bulldog clamps of assorted sizes

SUTURES

Many 0000 chromic catgut ureteral sutures will be needed to ligate blood vessels on the cut kidney surface

Pyeloplasty

For reparative procedures on the renal pelvis, the following delicate instruments should be available in addition to the pyelolithotomy setup:

1 Stevens tenotomy scissors, straight
1 Stevens tenotomy scissors, curved
2 Adson-Brown forceps, fine, 5 inches
2 Potts fixation forceps, $5\frac{1}{2}$ inches
12 Halstead mosquito forceps, straight, 5 inches
12 Halstead mosquito forceps, curved, 5 inches
Assorted size latex catheters to splint the ureter

Instruments for Surgery of the Ureter

The instruments used for ureterolithotomy and reconstruction of the ureter are essentially the same as for similar operations on the kidney.

Ileal Conduit (Bricker Procedure) Major Tray for Laparotomy

Instruments for intestinal and ureteral anastomosis

- 4 Allen intestinal anastomosis clamps, 1 and 2 fine teeth
- 4 Barnes-Redo intestinal forceps
- 6 Halstead mosquito forceps, straight, 5 inches
- 18 Halstead mosquito forceps, curved, 5 inches
- 6 Babcock intestinal forceps
- 1 small Metzenbaum dissecting scissors
- 1 small Mayo scissors, straight
- 1 Stevens tenotomy scissors, curved
- 1 Stevens tenotomy scissors, straight
- 2 Adson-Brown forceps, fine, 5 inches
- 2 Potts fixation forceps, 5½ inches

LONG INSTRUMENTS

- 6 Mixter gall duct forceps, 6¼ inches
- 4 Mixter gall duct forceps, 7¾ inches
- 6 Wylie clamps
- 6 Judd-Allis intestinal forceps, 7½ inches
- 3 Mayo-Hegar needle holders, 10 inches
- 1 Metzenbaum dissecting scissors, 9 inches
- 1 Mayo straight scissors, 10 inches
- 2 tissue forceps, serrated, 10 inches

RETRACTORS

Same as listed for nephrectomy

SUTURES

- 4 plain catgut 00 reels
- 4 plain catgut 00 (cut ⅓ lengths)
- 1 chromic 0 (cut ⅓ lengths)
- 2 silk 000 (for intestinal anastomosis)
- 4 chromic catgut 0000 atraumatic ureteral (for ureterointestinal anastomosis)
- 2 chromic catgut 00 atraumatic
- 1 chromic catgut 0 atraumatic
- 8–12 chromic catgut 0 (cut ¼ lengths)
- 4 packages 000 silk on milliner's needles
- 15–20 large silver wire stays (used for cancer patients)

Ureterosigmoidostomy

Same instruments as for ileal conduit

Operations on the Bladder and Prostate

Suprapubic Cystotomy: Basic Major Tray

ADDITIONAL INSTRUMENTS

1 catheter stylet (mandarin)
6 Judd-Allis intestinal forceps
6 Mixter gall duct forceps
6 Wylie hemostats
2 Jackson retractors
1 Balfour self-retaining retractor
Malecot catheters, 24–30 French
Foley catheters available of assorted sizes

Segmental Resection of Bladder

Suprapubic cystotomy setup plus the following instruments:

4 Mixter gall duct forceps, $7\frac{3}{4}$ inches
6 Judd-Allis intestinal forceps, $7\frac{1}{2}$ inches
6 Babcock intestinal forceps
1 Deaver retractor, small
1 Deaver retractor, large
1 Kelly retractor, medium
1 Kelly retractor, large
1 Doyen retractor, medium
1 Doyen retractor, large
1 Balfour self-retaining retractor
2 Jackson retractors
1 long, curved scissors
1 long, straight scissors
2 tissue forceps, serrated, 10 inches

CATHETERS

As for cystotomy, ureteral catheters 5 and 6 French should be available

Radical Cystectomy (Anterior Pelvic Exenteration)

Basically the same setup as for ileal conduit. Silver wire stay sutures may be used for through-and-through closure. A perineal prostatectomy setup (see below) may be needed if the surgeon plans to perform the combined abdomino-perineal approach in the male patient.

Ureteroneocystostomy and Plastic Revision of the Bladder Neck

Same instrument tray as for segmental resection of the bladder with the addition of:

1 Stevens tenotomy scissors, straight
1 Stevens tenotomy scissors, curved
2 Adson-Brown forceps, fine, 5 inches
2 Potts fixation forceps, $5\frac{1}{2}$ inches
6 Halstead mosquito forceps, straight, 5 inches
6 Halstead mosquito forceps, curved, 5 inches

Suprapubic Prostatectomy

Same as for segmental resection of the bladder with the addition of

Lowsley prostatic lobe-holding forceps
O'Connor perineal drape

Retropubic Prostatectomy

As for suprapubic prostatectomy. In either operation, various models of self-retaining retractors may be requested by the surgeon.

Perineal Prostatectomy (Simple and Radical)

As for suprapubic prostatectomy with the deletion of self-retaining retractors and the addition of the following instruments:

1 Young prostatic tractor, 8 inches
1 Lowsley seminal vesicle tractor, curved, 9 inches
1 Young prostatic enucleator
2 Young lateral retractors
1 Young bulb retractor
1 Young anterior retractor
1 Young bifid retractor

Transurethral Resection

(see Chapter 22)

Operations on the Penis and Scrotum—Vasectomy, Hydrocelectomy

Orchiectomy, Meatotomy

Minor instrument tray

Circumcision

Minor instrument tray

Chordee Repair

Minor instrument tray with the addition of

2 Stevens tenotomy scissors, straight and curved
2 Adson-Brown forceps, fine, 5 inches
2 Potts fixation forceps, $5\frac{1}{2}$ inches
6 Halstead mosquito forceps, straight, 5 inches
6 Halstead mosquito forceps, curved, 5 inches
Urethral sounds, 12, 14, 16, 18 French
Red rubber catheters, 8, 10, 12, 14, 16 French

Hypospadias Repair

Same as for chordee repair with addition of:
Retention sutures of wire, nylon, or silkworm gut
Catheter stylet
Setup for cystostomy diversion
Malecot catheters, 16, 18, 20, 22 French for temporary urinary diversion

APPENDIX VI
Teaching the Patient Home Catheter Care

While the patient is still in the hospital, it is best that the nurse assemble for him as many of the needed supplies as possible. Although the equipment can be purchased subsequently, the nurse cannot be certain when he will, or that he will, purchase the correct equipment. Certainly, his hospital instruction will be far more effective if he actually learns the various care procedures using the same equipment he will be using at home.

The following list includes those supplies needed for irrigating the catheter, for bedside drainage, and for changing catheter tapes. Although a majority of these items must be purchased, several are items that the patient may already have at home.

1. Irrigating solution ordered by the doctor if it is commercially prepared. If normal saline is to be used, the nurse must teach the patient how to make a sterile solution at home.
2. Asepto bulb and syringe. One bulb and syringe should be included for each catheter to be irrigated. A 2-oz bulb and a medium syringe are appropriate for urethral or cystostomy catheters. A ½-oz bulb and a small syringe are best for ureteral or nephrostomy catheters. The nurse should mark the syringe(s) with the volume of solution to be used with an ampul file.
3. Small glass bottle. This bottle is used to hold the irrigating solution. In the hospital a glass laboratory specimen bottle can be used for purposes of demonstration. At home the patient can use a small jelly or salad dressing jar. A separate jar is needed for each catheter to be irrigated. If two catheters are to be irrigated, the patient may elect to sterilize the bulb, syringe, and jar between irrigations rather than doubling his equipment.
4. Container for irrigation returns. In the hospital an emesis basin can be used for purposes of demonstration. At home the patient can use a coffee can or such other washable container.
5. One roll of ½-inch tape. Adhesive is needed to secure catheters and to replace soiled tapes.
6. Compound tincture of benzoin. This is used to protect the skin, as well as to improve adhesion of the tape.
7. Gauze pads, 2 by 2 inches.
8. 70 per cent alcohol. The gauze and alcohol are used to clean the end of the catheter and the glass connector.
9. Medium-sized plastic or glass connectors. Connectors are necessary to connect catheters to drainage tubing. Two connectors should be provided

for each catheter. Connectors are changed when the catheter is irrigated and as necessary if encrustations begin to form on the inner lumen.

10. Rubber drainage tubing with $\frac{3}{16}$-inch or $\frac{1}{4}$-inch lumen. Five feet of rubber tubing are needed for bedside drainage. If two catheters are to be drained by a Y-tube connection, an extra foot of tubing is necessary to make the connection. If two catheters are to drain separately, two 5-foot sections of tubing are needed for bedside drainage.
11. Leg bag. Plastic or rubber leg bags may be worn. Two leg bags should be provided for each catheter to be drained unless, of course, a Y tube is used.
12. Adhesive remover. Commercial preparations are best for removing tape because they cause less skin irritation and, usually, are less flammable. Ether, benzene, or acetone may be used, but the patient must be warned of their flammability. Under no circumstances should they be used while smoking or near a flame (the pilot light on a stove, for example). They should be stored in a cool, well-ventilated cupboard.
13. Small bottle brush. This is used to clean syringes, leg bags, and connectors.
14. Ten-inch saucepan with cover. Such a pan should be available on the nursing unit for teaching purposes. The patient will probably have such a pan at home. He should be instructed to use it only for sterilization of his catheter equipment. The pan must be deep enough to permit complete immersion of the equipment being sterilized.
15. String or wire basket. Ten-inch pieces of string tied to the bulb, the syringe, and the solution bottle, and then loosely wrapped around the handle of the pan, make it possible to lift the equipment from the water without contamination. A wire basket, like those used to fry with deep fat, can be used for the same purpose. The articles are placed in the basket, sterilized, the water poured off, and the articles lifted out as soon as cooled.
16. Two-quart container for bedside drainage. Two containers are needed if two catheters are to be drained separately. The container(s) may be of plastic or glass. Household bleach, wax, and cleaning solutions often come in containers appropriate for such use.
17. Vinegar. This is used when cleaning equipment (see page 237) and will probably be among the patient's household supplies.

If the patient is to change his ureterostomy catheters at home, he will need the following additional supplies:

1. Two catheters for each ureter of the type and size specified by the doctor. These should be obtained by the nurse and sent home with the patient.
2. A hemostat or Kelly clamp with which to handle the sterile catheter. This, too, should be obtained by the nurse and sent home with the patient.
3. A tube of sterile, water-soluble, lubricating jelly. This should be obtained by the nurse and sent home with the patient.
4. A saucer in which to put the lubricating jelly.

Irrigation Instructions for the Patient

To prepare for your irrigation, collect the following equipment:

1. Irrigating solution ordered by the doctor
2. Rubber bulb and Asepto syringe

3. Glass syringe
4. Solution bottle
5. Three 10-inch lengths of string
6. Several gauze pads saturated with 70 per cent alcohol
7. Saucepan and lid
8. Container for irrigation returns

Sterilizing Equipment

In order to prevent infection, the rubber bulb, glass syringe, and solution bottle must be sterilized before each irrigation. Sterilize them in the following way:

1. Tie a 10-inch length of string around the bulb, the neck of the glass syringe and the neck of the solution bottle.
2. Place these articles in the saucepan, wrap the strings snugly around the pan's handle, and fill the pan with enough water to completely cover the articles.
3. Place the saucepan on a lighted burner, cover with the lid, and allow the water to come to a boil. When the water is bubbling vigorously, begin timing, allowing the water to boil 10 minutes.
4. After 10 minutes, turn off the heat. Leave pan covered and allow the water to cool. If time is limited, pour off the hot water, being careful not to touch the articles. Proceed when articles are cool enough to handle.
5. Unwind the strings from the saucepan handle. Lift the solution bottle from the pan. Empty any water collected in the bottle into the sink, *not* back into the pan. Do not touch the inside of the bottle. Next, remove the glass portion of the syringe, and place it in the solution bottle. Do not touch the sides or the tip of the syringe. Lift the bulb from the pan, squeeze the bulb to remove any water, and insert it into the glass syringe. Be sure to push the bulb firmly into the syringe. If desired, you may cut off the strings with scissors so as not to interfere with the rest of the procedure.
6. Fill the solution bottle one-half full with irrigating solution. Squeeze the bulb of the syringe, and fill it with the desired amount of solution. You are now ready to irrigate your catheter.
   Note: If two catheters are to be irrigated, sterilize two sets of equipment or use one set and sterilize between irrigations.

Making a Sterile Solution of Normal Saline

1. In a saucepan sterilize a glass quart jar and its lid, as previously described.
2. In another saucepan place 1 tsp of table salt in 1 qt of tap water. Cover the pan and boil the solution for 10 minutes.
3. When 10 minutes have elapsed, turn off the heat. Leaving the lids in, allow both saucepans to cool to room temperature.
4. Carefully pour the water from the pan containing the jar and its lid; do not touch the insides of the jar or the lid.
5. Pour the salt solution into the jar, and screw the lid on tightly.

6. This solution should be made up and kept on hand at all times. If the jar is tightly sealed and the inside not touched, the solution will remain sterile for a week.

Irrigating the Catheter

1. Situate yourself so that you can easily reach both the catheter and the irrigating equipment. It is best to sit in a straight chair in front of a table.
2. Disconnect the catheter from the drainage tubing and place both the catheter and the tubing ends in the waste container.
3. Wipe the end of the cather with 70 per cent alcohol. Insert the syringe tip into the catheter. Instill the solution by pressing the bulb gently and evenly until all the fluid has been instilled.
4. When the fluid is in the catheter, pinch off the catheter with the fingers and disconnect the syringe from the catheter. Allow the solution to drain into the waste container. Repeat steps 3 and 4 three times.
5. When the irrigation is completed, wipe the end of the glass connecting tip with 70 per cent alcohol and reinsert the tip into the catheter.
   Note: Discontinue the irrigation procedure (1) if the irrigating solution does not drain back, (2) if excessive pressure is needed to force the solution into the catheter, or (3) if sudden pain occurs. Call your doctor.

When you have finished irrigating your catheter, discard the waste material and the excess irrigating solution in the toilet. Wash the waste container, the solution bottle, and the bulb and syringe with soap and water. Allow the equipment to dry. Keep all your irrigating equipment in a covered box until ready for the next irrigation.

Care of the Leg Bag and Bedside Drainage

At least twice a week wash the glass connectors, all the rubber tubing, the leg bag, and the night drainage bottle with soap and water. Use the bottle brush to clean the glass connectors and openings at both the top and the bottom of the leg bag. After washing, soak for 15 minutes in a solution of vinegar and water, adding $\frac{1}{4}$ cup of vinegar to each quart of water. After soaking, rinse the equipment with cold water and allow to dry. Hang the leg bag so that it drains completely. Wash the equipment more frequently if an odor develops or if the glass connectors become cloudy.

Changing the Ureteral Catheter(s)

1. Set up for catheter irrigation(s), as previously described.
2. Set up for changing catheter tapes, as previously described.
3. In addition, sterilize one clamp, a saucer, and one catheter of correct size for each ureterostomy. Tie a 10-inch string on the hemostat handle and wrap the string around the saucepan handle.
4. Sterile surgical lubricating jelly.

While you are still hospitalized, the doctor and nurse will determine when your ureteral catheters are draining most efficiently. When this is done, they will mark the distal end of each catheter just as it exits from the stoma, using indelible ink or red nail polish. After marking, the catheter will be withdrawn and a ruler used to measure the distance in inches from the tip of the catheter to the mark. This will be done for each catheter, and the measurements will then be used to mark each subsequent catheter. With each ureterostomy, the catheter size will vary, as well as the length of insertion. It may, therefore, be necessary to mark the catheters "R" (right) and "L" (left). These markings serve as a guide for placement; but with alterations in the placement of the catheter tip, as the result of position changes (sitting, standing, lying), it may be necessary to occasionally move the catheter in or out by one-quarter inch to ensure optimal drainage. If there is leakage around the catheter, it should be repositioned. The same is true when the cathether does not irrigate normally.

Inserting the Ureteral Catheter(s)

1. All equipment for irrigating, taping, and handling the sterile catheters should be readily available and conveniently placed.
2. Unwind the string and lift the clamp from the saucepan. Using the clamp to hold the saucer and the catheter(s) in the pan, drain off the water. Do not touch the end of the clamp, the inside of the saucer, or the cathether(s) with your fingers or any other unsterilized object.
3. Using the clamp, lift the saucer from the pan and place it on the table. Leave the catheter(s) in the saucepan.
4. Heat the sterile end of the clamp on the sterile saucer.
5. Discard a small amount of lubricating jelly in the waste container. Then place an amount about the size of a 25-cent piece on the sterile saucer.
6. Remove the tapes and the used catheter from one ureterostomy.
7. Sitting straight in your chair, pick up the appropriate catheter with the clamp. Grasp the catheter first with the clamp about 2 inches from the tip; the extreme outer end may be held with the fingers of your free hand.
8. Breathing deeply to relax abdominal muscles, use the clamp to gently feed the catheter into the ureter and the renal pelvis to the mark indicated on the catheter. If you encounter resistance, stop momentarily. Such resistance is normally caused by peristalsis or ureteral spasm, which usually subsides quickly, allowing the catheter to be advanced.
9. Hold the catheter in position with your free hand. Place the clamp on the sterile saucer. Irrigate the catheter. If the catheter irrigates easily, tape the catheter. If irrigation returns are sluggish or if unusual pressure is needed to instill solution, reposition the catheter $\frac{1}{4}$ inch in or out until the irrigation is normal.

   Note: Compare the renal pelvis to an upright funnel. The catheter is inserted through the spout into the basin of the funnel. If it is inserted too high, above the level of accumulated fluid, it will not drain properly. If the catheter is not inserted far enough and is still in the spout, it also will not drain properly. Optimum drainage will occur when the catheter tip is just above the spout in the basin of the funnel.

10. Tape the catheter in position as described, and attach it to the leg bag.
11. Repeat the entire procedure if a second ureterostomy catheter is to be changed.

Changing Catheter Tapes

Tapes should be changed whenever they become soiled and always when the catheter(s) is changed. Before attempting to change tapes:

1. Soak the edges with adhesive solvent in order to remove them more easily.
2. Cut two 4-inch strips of tape, and round the corners to prevent curling. Set the strips aside within easy reach—e.g., on the table edge.
3. Hold the catheter firmly and, without pulling, remove first the upper and then the lower tapes.
4. Clean the skin, first with solvent to remove adhesive residue, and then with soap and warm water. Dry the skin gently but thoroughly.
5. Let the catheter fall naturally from the opening (in a dependent position). Apply tincture of benzoin to the skin where tape is to be applied.
6. When the tincture of benzoin is tacky, place one strip of tape on the skin.
7. Place the second piece of tape over both the catheter and the bottom tape. Usually the tape is placed approximately 1 inch below the skin opening.
8. For greater comfort, shave the skin around the stoma to remove hair in the area where the adhesive is to be applied.

General Information

1. Drink lots of fluids, at least $2\frac{1}{2}$ qt per day.
2. Notify your doctor if
   a. You have pain in your kidney or bladder
   b. You develop a fever or
   c. Your catheter does not drain or if there is blood in your urine

APPENDIX **VII**

Questions Frequently Asked by Patients with an Ileal Conduit

The following questions are those frequently asked by patients and can serve to guide the nurse in planning the scope and content of the teaching program.

When Should I Change My Appliance?

Most people change every four to seven days. Some go as long as ten days. Changing is best determined by what you feel is best for you. Factors that will influence the frequency include the condition of the skin and stoma, odor, comfort, the fit of the appliance, and the character of the drainage. The longer the appliance is worn, however, the more difficult it is to keep the bag clean and odor-free.

To determine the optimal wearing time for you, gradually increase the time between changes—that is, two days increased to three days increased to four days, and so on, until you reach your maximum. This may be when leakage occurs, when you feel itching or discomfort under the faceplate, or when an odor becomes detectible. With experience most people develop a sixth sense that tells them when to change. Once you have determined your maximum, reduce it by one day and establish this interval as your routine. A regular schedule of changing will ensure your comfort and safety.

How Do I Remove the Appliance?

Always use a solvent to remove the appliance. Never just rip it off. First, empty the pouch. Then, using a medicine dropper or gauze, drop solvent on the adhesive and gently work the faceplate away from the skin. Peel the adhesive residue from your skin with your fingers to use a solvent. Never rub the skin vigorously. If every last particle is not removed, don't worry about it. After using solvent, always wash the skin with mild soap and water.

Apply adhesive to the faceplate before applying it to the skin. To ensure that the faceplate is completely dry and dust-free, wipe it lightly with solvent. If you are using cement, apply it according to the manufacturer's instructions. The usual procedure calls for application of two, thin, evenly spread layers of cement, allowing two to three minutes' drying time between layers. After applying the second layer, set the appliance aside, faceplate up, and proceed to prepare the skin.

To absorb drainage, cover the stoma with a "wick" made of absorbent material (gauze, cotton, facial tissue). Dry the skin thoroughly. Following the same procedure as before, apply cement to the skin. Should urine run over the skin or cement, dry the area thoroughly and reapply the cement. After application of the cement, with the "wick" still in place, line up the faceplate opening over the stoma. Touch the lower rim to the abdomen, remove the "wick," and quickly press the plate over the stoma. Hold the appliance firmly in place for several minutes. Adjust the belt to give firm but comfortable support.

If you prefer to use double-faced adhesive discs, first make certain the faceplate is clean and dry. Remove the protective backing from only one side of the disc. Carefully center the disc opening over the faceplate opening. Press the adhesive surface of the disc firmly to the faceplate. Use your index finger to smooth the disc in place, removing any creases. Remove the protective backing from the opposite side of the disc and set the appliance aside, faceplate up. With the "wick" in place, dry the skin thoroughly. Center the faceplate opening over the stoma and complete the procedure as above. Many patients carry convenient, double-faced discs in their pocket or purse in case of an accident.

How Do I Take Care of My Appliance?

You should have at least two appliances, including belts. Worn alternately, they will last longer and will more easily be kept clean and odor-free.

To clean them, first remove the valve outlet and rinse the pouch with tap water to remove any residual urine. In a basin, used only for this purpose, wash the appliance in soap and warm water. If preferred, detergent may be used. Using a bottle brush, scrub the inside of the pouch, paying particular attention to the outlet and valve. Again, rinse the appliance. To help control odor, the bag should be soaked in a cleaning solution for several hours after washing. Such a solution can be made with household bleach (1 tsp bleach to 1 qt water) or with vinegar (1/4 cup vinegar to 1 qt water). The vinegar solution not only helps to control odor, but also seems to reduce the formation of sediment on the inner pouch surfaces. Commercial cleaning solutions can also be purchased from most appliance manufacturers and should be used according to instructions. Most commercial solutions, as well as bleach, will damage the rubber if used in too concentrated a form.

Cement can be peeled from the faceplate with the fingers or removed with solvent. Because solvents are composed of hydrocarbons, however, they cause rubber to deteriorate gradually and, thus, should be used sparingly in direct contact with rubber. If you choose to use a solvent, be sure to wash the rubber with soap and water immediately thereafter. Although many people remove the cement from the appliance each time it is cleaned, others allow several layers to build up. This, they believe, actually improves adhesion.

After cleaning, hang the appliance in air and dry thoroughly. This is best accomplished by hanging the pouch with sides separated and valve outlet open. A drying rack, specifically designed for this purpose, can be purchased from the manufacturer. Less expensive, however, is one fashioned from a coat hanger. When the appliance is dry, dust it inside and out with cornstarch or talcum. Either will keep the rubber soft and pliable and will prevent the pouch sides from sticking together. Many patients use a scented talcum because it leaves a clean, pleasant odor. Be sure to store your ostomy equipment in a cool, dry place. Leg bags and night drainage equipment should be cleaned daily following the same procedure.

How Often Should I Buy a New Appliance?

This is a highly individualized matter. The major determinants are the appearance of your used appliance and whether or not you can continue to keep it clean and odor-free. These factors are very much influenced by how long and how often you wear each appliance. If you own only one appliance, you may have to replace it within several months. Owning at least two appliances and alternating their use, however, increases the length of time each will be serviceable. How you clean and care for the appliance are also important. The injudicious use of harsh cleaning solutions will certainly damage the rubber or plastic. With reasonable care, an appliance that is alternated with another should last six months or longer.

Semidisposable rubber or plastic pouches, with proper care and rotation of use, will also last weeks and even months. The faceplates of the two-piece appliances are frequently serviceable for a year or more.

When you reorder your appliance, be sure to remeasure your stoma size to determine whether or not a new size is necessary. The opening should be approximately 1/8 inch greater than the diameter of the stoma. Measuring is particularly important in the first six months following surgery. After that, the size of the stoma will not change appreciably.

How Should I Care for My Skin?

It is recommended that on the days when you change your appliance you plan to take a long, leisurely tub bath. The water should be warm, not hot, and of a depth that the stoma is immersed. Because the stoma contracts naturally upon contact and also because of peristalsis, water will not enter the conduit or ureters. The warm water cleanses the skin and improves circulation. Take this opportunity to examine the skin and stoma carefully for any signs of irritation.

The immediate treatment of any local irritation depends upon its severity. A cardinal rule, however: no matter how minor the problem, don't ignore it.

METHOD I

For skin that is slightly to moderately inflamed, itching, or burning:

1. Change your appliance and treat your skin every two or three days until the irritation subsides. Change your appliance more frequently if the skin does

not respond to treatment or if there is noticeable itching or discomfort under the faceplate between changings.
2. Take a warm bath each time you change your appliance.
3. Expose the skin area to a heat lamp for 20 to 30 minutes, using a goose-necked lamp with a 60-watt bulb, $1\frac{1}{2}$ to 2 ft above the abdomen. During exposure, use toilet tissue to cover the stoma and absorb drainage. Discard the tissues in a paper bag. *Never* expose the stoma to a sun lamp or to direct sunlight.
4. Prepare the appliance in the usual manner.
5. Holding the "wick" over the stoma, pat the skin dry with a soft towel. With a piece of gauze dipped in water, moisten the skin surface around the stoma, particularly the areas of irritation. With a dry piece of gauze dipped in karaya powder, dust the powder on the moistened surface. Coat the skin with a thin, even layer. Allow the karaya to dry and dust off the excess.
6. Apply cement on top of the karaya and proceed to apply the appliance as usual.

METHOD II

For skin that is moderately to severely inflamed, accompanied by raw or broken skin areas, follow the steps in Method I with the following additions:
1. On the broken areas apply an extra-thick coating of karaya. Or, if you prefer, use zinc oxide or aluminum hydroxide ointment on the open areas.
2. Place a gauze or tissue patch over the broken area. This is particularly important if ointment is used, since its oily base interferes with adhesion.
3. Apply cement over the patch and proceed as usual.
4. If your skin does not show improvement after several days of treatment, change to Method III.

METHOD III

For skin that is severely inflamed, blistered, or weeping, switch from permanent to temporary bags and follow steps outlined in Method II at least twice a day until the skin surface has healed and the inflammation subsided.

Many patients prefer to treat moderate or severe skin irritations with karaya discs, either the plain disc used as a gasket on a permanent appliance or the disc that is mounted on the faceplate of a temporary appliance. The plain disc is used as a seal between the skin and the faceplate of the permanent appliance. No adhesive is used; the belt holds the appliance firmly in place. Many severe irritations have healed quickly with the karaya disc. When using karaya discs, however, make certain urinary drainage is adequate. Karaya tends to become quite sticky and gummy when exposed to body heat and moisture. Occasionally, the surface of the bag can become stuck tight over the stoma, obstructing the outflow of urine.

If the skin under the pouch becomes reddened, it may denote a sensitivity to the rubber or plastic or a heat rash caused by perspiration. Usually a pouch cover made of white flannel or cotton will eliminate this irritation.

Stomal swelling is usually caused by a faceplate opening that is two small or one that has not been properly centered, causing pressure. Direct injury may also cause swelling. This is sometimes the case with children, although surprisingly not so often as one might expect.

Sediment that collects inside the pouch and produces a sandpaperlike surface may cause stoma irritation sufficient to induce bleeding. You should review your cleaning procedure as well as the frequency of changing the appliance.

Sometimes, in the immediate area of the stoma, the skin becomes tough, thick, irregular, inflamed. If this tissue follows a clearly defined, circumscribed area, matching the faceplate opening, the opening is too large. Until a faceplate of the correct size can be obtained, foam pads are quite useful. These pads are available from most appliance manufacturers. The opening is cut to fit the stoma, leaving no skin exposed. It is cemented to the skin, and the appliance is then cemented to the pad. When the skin condition around the stoma has improved, the stoma is measured so that a new appliance can be ordered.

Stoma and skin problems are most frequently caused by improper use of cement or solvent. Other causes may include an improperly fitted faceplate, improper application or removal procedures, skin sensitivity to rubber, cement, or solvent, or poor nutrition. As important as treating the irritation immediately is discovering the cause of the irritation. Knowing why it occurred will oftentimes dictate the treatment and, most certainly, will help to determine its prevention.

Do I Have to Use Night Drainage?

The two major reasons for using bedside drainage at night are to ensure free flow of urine from the stoma and to prevent accidental leakage. If night drainage were not used and the pouch became too full, pressure against the stoma could interfere with the outflow of urine and possibly cause a kidney infection. It is a certainty, too, that turning over onto a pouch of urine in one's sleep is likely to cause enough pressure to break the watertight seal between the skin and the faceplate or, in the case of a two-piece appliance, the seal between the pouch and the flange.

For night drainage you will need 5 ft of rubber tubing ($\frac{3}{16}$ or $\frac{1}{4}$ inch in diameter), a 2-qt collection container, and a valve adapter so that the tubing can be connected to the pouch outlet. Some manufacturers sell the complete bedside drainage set. Adapters, however, can be purchased as a single unit if you choose to make your own drainage set. Rubber tubing can be procured at either a drugstore or a surgical supply house. Empty 2-qt glass or plastic bottles, such as one might find among one's household supplies, make adequate collection containers. If a cap is used on the container, make two openings—one for the tubing, the other to act as an air vent. If no cap is used, the tubing can be taped to the edge of the mouth of the bottle. It is important that the end of the tubing be positioned so that it is never in contact with the urine collecting in the bottle. The bottle may be placed at the side or at the foot of the bed, whichever is more comfortable. Pin the tubing to the mattress (be sure the pin is large enough not to obstruct the lumen of the tubing) so that the tubing hangs straight from the mattress to the container; gather the remaining long coil on the bed to allow free movement. If the container is placed at the end of the bed, the tubing must be an additional 2 to 3 ft long. To keep the pouch from twisting and kinking, many patients find it helpful to wear a pair of lightweight underpants. This is particularly helpful with children.

Although bedside night drainage is preferred, some people are extremely unhappy at the prospect. A compromise that seems to have worked satisfactorily is the wearing of a leg bag. A short piece of tubing connects the pouch outlet with the leg bag inlet. The leg bag should be constructed in such a way that the inlet valve prevents backflow of urine into the appliance. Still other people prefer, rather than night drainage or even a leg bag, to wake themselves several times a night so that they may empty the pouch into the toilet. Those who use this technique have not found that it interferes with their rest or sleep.

I Like to Play Tennis! Will I Still Be Allowed?

Certainly! Once you have recovered from surgery and unless specifically contraindicated, your doctor will probably encourage you to return to all the activities you enjoyed before surgery. About the only caution one need consider is contact sports, such as football. Most doctors prefer that such sports be avoided. Your doctor, however, may feel differently, so check with him.

Many patients prefer to wear their appliances while swimming. If it is worn, the belt should be changed afterward. Others, however, prefer to wear only a cloth pad over the stoma. Whether or not you wear your appliance is a matter of personal choice, determined by where you swim and the amount of time you spend in and out of the water.

Do I Have to Change My Diet?

No, unless, of course, your doctor feels there is a specific reason to do so. The mere fact of diversion, however, does not impose dietary restrictions. It *is* important that you maintain an adequate fluid intake—at least $2\frac{1}{2}$ qt of liquid a day. Again, fluids are restricted only if there is a specific reason indicated by your doctor. A high fluid intake serves as a natural internal irrigation to keep the kidneys functioning properly. Also, if the urine is more dilute, there are fewer problems with urine odor or sediment formations from urine salts.

Certain foods impart distinct odors to the urine. Asparagus causes a musty smell. Some patients believe fish imparts a "fishy" odor. What may be troublesome for one person may not be for you. Follow your usual diet. In good time you will discover those foods you should avoid.

Urine color may also be changed by certain foods and medications. Ingestion of a large quantity of beets, for example, gives the urine a reddish cast. Cathartics containing phenolphthalein may also cause a red coloration.

If there is a persistent change in the amount, odor, or color of your urine, check with your doctor.

What Happens if My Appliance Leaks so Often I Have to Change It Every Day?

Barring an unusual stomal or dermal condition, if you have to change your appliance more than once every 48 hours, you are not getting adequate results. People are often quick to attribute leakage problems to faulty construction or design of the appliance. While these factors are occasionally the culprits, careful investigation demonstrates that the problem usually is not inherent in the appliance, but rather in how it fits and how it is used. The answers to certain questions may give the clue.

When does leakage occur and is it related to any particular activity? If leakage occurs consistently at night, for example, it means your night drainage routine is not effective. If you use bedside drainage, the tubing may be kinking, allowing the pouch to become too full. Experiment with placement of the tubing and the collection container until you find a way to prevent this. You may need to modify your sleeping habits. Rather than sleeping on your abdomen, learn to sleep on your side. Another example is that of the shoe salesman who had just returned to work following construction of an ileal conduit. He was distraught that his appliance seemed to leak only when he was at work. His job, of course, required much getting up and down, stooping and bending. He soon discovered that by placing his pouch at a specific angle, leakage no longer occurred.

Where does the faceplate leak and does it tend always to be in the same spot? Appliances have been changed unnecessarily when it has been falsely assumed that the leak is between the faceplate and the skin. The real problem is often a valve outlet that has not been closed tightly or, perhaps, needs a new washer. Children frequently have trouble tightening the valves. In the two-piece appliance, the pouch may not be securely attached to the faceplate flange. Verifying the location of the leak will save a lot of time and energy.

If leakage occurs consistently between the faceplate and the skin, the problem, most likely, is related to one of two things. First, meticulously review each step of your application procedure. Skin cement that is put on in thick, uneven coats may create a problem. Failing to observe the proper drying time and the presence of moisture on the skin are other factors to consider. If you use double-faced discs, are you applying them in such a way that there are no creases or wrinkles? If you are satisfied that your application procedure is correct, check the fit of your faceplate. Is the curvature of the plate appropriate for you? The convexity of the plate is too great if the outer rim pulls away from the skin soon after application. On the other hand, if the faceplate is flat and the skin area around the stoma, retracted, the convexity is not great enough. It may be that having the manufacturer buff an edge that protrudes on a bony prominence is all that is needed. Are there any defects in the skin surface, such as surgical scars? When such irregularities exist, a foam pad cemented between the faceplate and the skin may solve the problem.

Careful investigation of when and where leakage occurs, a review of your application procedure, and a check of the fit of the faceplate will usually indicate why the appliance leaks. Once the "why" is known, the problem is easily solved.

What Do I Do About Urine Odor?

Odor may have a single cause or may be a combination of several factors. A solution to odor control, therefore, is the identification of the cause(s). The first and obvious question is how long you wait between pouch changes. If you are changing it every seven to ten days, reduce the time to four to five days. Are you wearing one appliance continuously? If so, buy another so that you can alternate them. Always change to a clean, odor-free appliance. How are you cleaning the appliance? Do you always flush the pouch daily with tepid water? This is done by removing the valve outlet, draining the bag and, with a syringe, instilling tap water. A meat baster serves this purpose very nicely. Rather than water, some people prefer a deodorizing solution. It must be one, however, that will not cause stoma irritation. What has been your average daily fluid intake? If it has been low, the urine may be more concentrated and, thus, have a stronger odor. Occasionally, urinary tract infections cause unpleasant odors.

If all attempts to control odor fail and you have been using a single-piece pouch appliance, it may be advisable to switch to a two-piece appliance with disposable pouches. These pouches can be changed and cleaned daily and then discarded when necessary.

How Often Should I See My Doctor?

During the first year following surgery, the doctor will probably want to see you every three months, just to make certain everything is going properly. Thereafter, he will probably want to see you yearly for a routine examination. It is important that you keep these scheduled appointments. Very often minor problems can be solved if treatment is prompt.

Between your regularly scheduled visits, however, do not hesitate to contact him if you (1) have pain or tenderness in the region of the kidney, associated with an elevated temperature; (2) notice a persistent change in the color, odor, or volume of urine for which you can find no explanation; (3) have persistent or recurring skin or stoma irritations or problems with your appliance.

What Do I Do When I Want to Travel?

There are three major areas of consideration when planning a trip. These include (1) preparation to meet a medical emergency; (2) the type of equipment you should take; and (3) how and where you can obtain additional supplies if needed.

Place with your identification papers a statement indicating that you have a urinary ostomy and its specific type. Your doctor's name, address, and telephone number should also be included. If you are going to travel outside the United States, it is advisable to carry a letter from your doctor documenting your medical history and treatment. Included should be your own written instructions regarding care of the ostomy. This information would prove invaluable to anyone giving you care who is not familiar with your condition.

Most people carry their ostomy equipment in a bag used only for that purpose. An airline bag or makeup kit does nicely. Your supplies should include an extra appliance and belt, cement, and solvent. You should also carry materials necessary to treat skin irritation, such as karaya powder, foam pads, and temporary bags. Don't forget your night drainage and cleaning materials—e.g., soap, brush, drying rack, cleaning solution, and talcum. Double-faced discs are handy to have in case of an emergency. Hospital-type, disposable plastic drainage bags and tubing are easily cleaned and compact to carry. These can be purchased from a surgical supply house.

Obtaining additional ostomy equipment when traveling in the United States present no major problem. The local telephone directory will list surgical supply houses. If this is not available, call the local hospital and speak to the surgical nursing supervisor. If there is an ileostomy club, they most certainly can tell you where to purchase supplies. If worse comes to worse, wire your home supplier. If the supplies are sent air mail, special delivery, you should receive them anywhere within the United States in 48 hours.

If you intend to travel abroad, probably the best source of information will be the ileostomy club nearest you. Among its membership you will undoubtedly find several people who have traveled outside this country. They will be able to give you many helpful tips.

With thought and careful planning, there is no reason why you cannot indulge your wanderlust, from a camping trip in the northwoods to climbing the Matterhorn!

Should I Dilate the Ileal Stoma?

Ask your doctor. Many doctors feel it is unnecessary, and it can be injurious if done improperly. Others feel dilating prevents the stoma from becoming too constricted and, possibly, interfering with drainage. It is a cardinal rule never to introduce an object into the stoma unless specifically instructed to do so by your doctor. If he feels dilation is necessary, he will show you how.

APPENDIX **VIII**

List of Major Surgical Appliance Manufacturers

Atlantic Surgical Co., Inc.
2287 Babylon Turnpike
Merrick, L.I., N.Y. 11566

C. R. Bard, Inc.
Murray Hill, N.J. 07971

Con-Seal, Inc.
Box 310, Lenox Hill Station
New York, N.Y. 10021

Davol Rubber Co.
Providence, R.I. 02901

The Dierker Co.
6529 Santa Monica Blvd.
Los Angeles, California 90038

Thomas Fazio Laboratories, Inc.
P.O. Box 35
Assonet, Mass. 02702

Gricks, Inc.
202-11 Jamaica Ave.
Hollis, N.Y. 11423

Lapides Urinary Ileostomy Device
American Cystoscope Makers, Inc.
8 Pelham Parkway
Pelham Manor, N.Y.

Marlen Manufacturing and Development Co.
5156 Richmond Road
Bedford, Ohio 44146

The Marsan Manufacturing Co., Inc.
5924 South Pulaski Road
Chicago, Illinois 60629

The Perma-Type Co., Inc.
1559 New Britain Avenue
West Hartford, Conn. 06110

Perry Products
3803 East Lake Street
Minneapolis, Minn. 55406

The Torbat Company
1185 Jefferson Boulevard
Warwick, R.I. 02886

United Surgical Supplies, Inc.
Largo, Flordia 33540

Suggested Instruction Booklets

Manual for Ileostomy Patients
Published by QT Inc., Boston
c/o The Medical Foundation
227 Commonwealth
Boston, Mass. 02116

Count Your Blessings,
by Maj. and Mrs. John R. Jeter, Jr. Published by the authors for a nominal fee
311-1 Third Street
For Leavenworth, Kansas 66027
(Booklet is a teaching manual for parents of children with ileal conduit)

APPENDIX IX
Setup for Peritoneal Dialysis*

Equipment

Adult Service

Peritoneal dialysis set—adapter with 3-inch rubber tubing is now in set Trocaths, 2 Drainage bag	Obtain from sterile supply room
Inpersol solution, 1.5%, 1000 ml, 48 bottles Inpersol solution, 7.0%, 1000 ml, 12 bottles	Obtain from pharmacy *prior to* procedure
Inpersol administration sets, 2	

Heparin, 1000 units/ml		1 vial
Potassium chloride		12 vials
Normal saline, 30 ml vial		1 vial
Procaine, 2.0%		1 vial
Betadine, for skin prep.		
Sterile 4″ × 3″ gauze		2 boxes
Sterile combine pads		8
Sterile gloves		
Sterile scissors		
Syringes	50 ml	2
	10 ml	24
	2 ml	24
Needles, 18-gauge		30, for mixing and adding medications

Container for discarded needles and syringes
Alcohol sponges
Adhesive tape, ½″ and 1½″
Montgomery straps
Disposable pads
Rubber-tipped hemostats—3
IV pole
Calibrated cylinder or pitcher for measuring drainage
Bed scale to weigh patient before, during, and after dialysis
Retraints
Masks

* Reproduced by permission from "Nursing Procedure Manual," Nursing Service, The New York Hospital–Cornell Medical Center.

Peritoneal dialysis record sheets
Vacutainers and culture tubes as ordered by physician

Optional Equipment

Catheterization set
Skin prep. tray with disposable razor, pHisoHex
Salt-poor albumin for IV use

Pediatric Service

Peritoneal dialysis set—will need additional sterile medicine glass Trocaths, Pediatric, 2 Drainage bag	Obtain from sterile supply room

Catheterization set

Inpersol solution, 1.5%, 1000 ml—6–20 bottles Inpersol solution, 7.0%, 1000 ml—6–20 bottles Inpersol administration sets — 2 Abbott Inpersol catheters — 2 #16 for small children #18 for older children	Obtain from pharmacy *prior to* procedure

Postdialysis suture set
Anticoagulant
Antibiotic as ordered

Potassium chloride		12 vials
Sterile gloves		
Syringes	10 ml	10
	2 ml	10
Needles, 20 gauge		10, for mixing and adding medications
Container for discarded needles and syringes		
Screw clamps		3
Urine specimen bottles		8, for specimen from each dialysis

Skin preparation set
Disposable pads
IV pole
Calibrated cylinder or pitcher for measuring drainage
Bed scale to weigh patient before, during, and after dialysis
Restraints
Masks
Peritoneal dialysis record sheets
Vacutainers and culture tubes as ordered by physician

Preparation of Patient	*Key Points*
1. Obtain signed permission for treatment with specific procedure indicated.	Explain as needed and sign as witness.

2. Encourage patient to void. Catheterize all children unless indwelling catheter is in place.	This helps to avoid accidental puncture of the bladder.
3. Weigh patient and record weight.	
4. Place patient in supine position.	
5. Cover patient with bath blanket, and fanfold top bedding to bottom of bed.	
6. Expose abdomen and shave to pubis p.r.n. (not in pediatrics).	
7. Record blood pressure, pulse, and respirations.	Include temperature in pediatrics.
8. Apply restraints as necessary.	

NOTE: 1. *If ordered by doctor* during dialysis, *weigh patient* after *completion of drainage and* before *starting another exchange.*
2. *Check per cent of solution carefully.*

Procedure	*Key Points*
1. Warm bottles of solution to room temperature in a basin of water.	This may help to prevent abdominal cramps and a drop in body temperature when solution is instilled.
2. Place tray in convenient working area and uncover.	
3. Assist physician with skin preparation and the drawing of bloods, p.r.n.	
*4. Add medications as ordered by physician to one bottle. Attach administration set, expel air, clamp tubing, and hang bottles on IV pole.	Adding medications to only one bottle lessens the chance of contamination.
*5. After catheter is in place and administration set has been connected, clamp outflow tube leading to large drainage bottle.	
*6. Unclamp inflow tubes leading from suspended dialysis solution bottles and note time.	It should take no longer than 10 to 15 minutes for inflow of solution. Utilize gravity by lowering height of bed and raising level of bottles.
7. Take bood pressure, pulse, and respirations throughout procedure as ordered by physician.	In pediatrics, observations are made every 15 to 20 minutes, and temperature is taken 10 to 15 minutes after fluid has entered abdomen, and every hour thereafter.

* Done by physician in Pediatrics Department.

*8. Clamp inflow tube after solution is instilled and note time.	Care should be taken to prevent entrance of air.
*9. Record on dialysis record and medication record the *amount*, *times*, and *type of solution used*, and *the medication(s) added to it*.	*In pediatrics*, nurse records medication on medication record.
*10. Leave solution in abdomen as ordered by physician.	Length of time varies (30–60 minutes). In pediatrics: 60 minutes.
*11. Unclamp outflow tubing.	Gravity drainage should occur rapidly in a steady, forceful stream and can be facilitated by raising height of bed or changing position of patient. It should take no longer than 10 minutes for adults and 20 minutes for a child.
12. Measure drainage and record on dialysis record.	
*13. Compare amount of fluid instilled with fluid removed, and record difference.	Plus sign (+) in front of figure signifies fluid retained by patient. Minus sign (—) signifies fluid removed from patient in excess of amount instilled. Notify physician of an excessive fluid (200–500 ml) retained or removed from patient.
*14. Repeat steps 4–13 as ordered by physician.	Number of exchanges varies.
15. At termination of dialysis, obtain culture of final drainage and tip of peritoneal catheter. Send to bacteriology laboratory *immediately*.	
16. Apply dry sterile dressing at termination of dialysis.	In pediatrics, incision is sutured.
17. Weigh patient and record weight.	It is important to use the same scale for both predialysis and postdialysis weighing. More frequent weights may be indicated, depending upon nature of dialysis.

Index